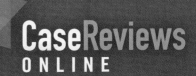
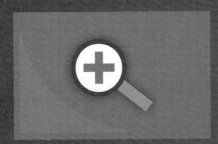
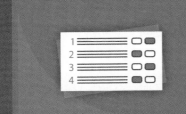

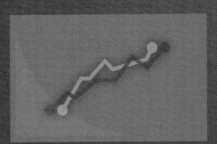
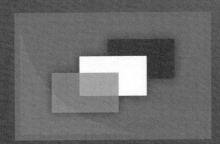
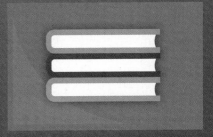

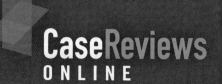
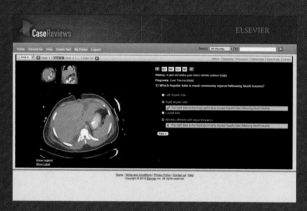
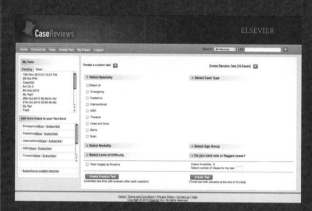
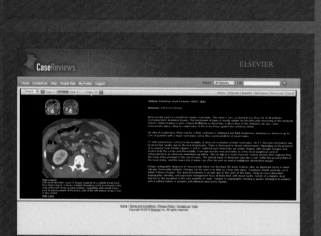
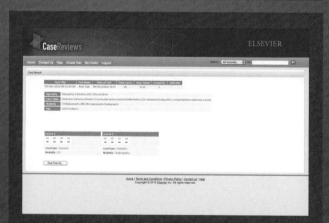

CASE REVIEW
Duke Review of MRI Principles

Series Editor
David M. Yousem, MD, MBA
Professor of Radiology
Director of Neuroradiology
Russell H. Morgan Department of Radiology and Radiological Science
The Johns Hopkins Medical Institutions
Baltimore, Maryland

Other Volumes in the CASE REVIEW Series
Brain Imaging, Second Edition
Breast Imaging
Cardiac Imaging
Emergency Radiology
Gastrointestinal Imaging, Second Edition
General and Vascular Ultrasound, Second Edition
Genitourinary Imaging, Second Edition
Musculoskeletal Imaging, Second Edition
Nuclear Medicine, Second Edition
Obstetric and Gynecologic Ultrasound, Second Edition
Pediatric Imaging, Second Edition
Spine Imaging, Second Edition
Thoracic Imaging, Second Edition
Vascular and Interventional Imaging

ELSEVIER
MOSBY

Wells I. Mangrum, MD
Practicing Radiologist
Sacred Heart Hospital
Eau Claire, Wisconsin

Kimball L. Christianson, MD
Fellow, Division of Abdominal Imaging
Department of Radiology
Duke University Medical Center
Durham, North Carolina

Scott M. Duncan, MD
Diagnostic and Interventional Radiologist
Radiology Associates Inc.
Jeffersonville, Indiana

Quoc Bao "Phil" B. Hoang, MD
Assistant Chief of Radiology
Southeast Louisiana Veterans Healthcare System
New Orleans, Louisiana

Allen W. Song, PhD
Professor of Radiology, Psychiatry, Neurobiology, and
    Biomedical Engineering
Director, Brain Imaging and Analysis Center
Duke University School of Medicine
Durham, North Carolina

Elmar M. Merkle, MD
Chairman, Department of Radiology and Nuclear
    Medicine
University Hospitals Basel
Basel, Switzerland

CASE REVIEW

Duke Review of MRI Principles

CASE REVIEW SERIES

ELSEVIER
MOSBY

1600 John F. Kennedy Blvd.
Ste 1800
Philadelphia, PA 19103-2899

DUKE REVIEW OF MRI PRINCIPLES: CASE REVIEW SERIES   ISBN: 978-1-4557-0084-4

Copyright © 2012 by Mosby, an imprint of Elsevier Inc.

Library of Congress Cataloging-in-Publication Data
Duke review of MRI principles / Wells Mangrum ... [et al.].
      p. ; cm.—(Case review series)
      Review of MRI principles
      Includes bibliographical references and index.
      ISBN 978-1-4557-0084-4 (pbk. : alk. paper)
      I. Mangrum, Wells.   II. Title: Review of MRI principles.   III. Series: Case review series.
      [DNLM: 1. Magnetic Resonance Imaging–Case Reports.   2. Magnetic Resonance Imaging–Problems and Exercises. WN 18.2]
      616.07′548–dc23
                                                                                                  2011051754

Senior Content Strategist: Don Scholz
Content Development Specialist: Rachel Miller
Publishing Services Manager: Pat Joiner-Myers
Designer: Steven Stave
Marketing Manager: Carla Holloway

Working together to grow
libraries in developing countries

www.elsevier.com | www.bookaid.org | www.sabre.org

ELSEVIER   BOOK AID International   Sabre Foundation

Printed in the United States of America

Last digit is the print number: 9   8   7   6   5   4   3   2   1

We would like to collectively acknowledge and thank the faculty and residents of Duke Radiology, in particular Elmar M. Merkle and Daniel Boll for their influential roles in the early stages of the book. To our residency program director, Charles Maxfield, and our fellowship directors, Jay Baker, James Eastwood, Clyde Helms, Tracy Jaffe, and Paul Suhocki, we say thank you for being supportive of the project. We also extend our heartfelt thanks to our former chairman, Carl Ravin, who created the framework at Duke Radiology within which we were able to write this book during residency and fellowship training.

For my lovely wife Tami, thanks for always being supportive and believing in me. I feel fortunate to have you as my wife. Somewhere in my youth or childhood, I must have done something good. Thanks also to my parents for their advice that they gave along the way. "Our doubts are traitors and make us lose the good we oft may attain by fearing to attempt." To my two boys, you bring me endless joy as your father. I love you both very much.

—Wells

To Olivia, Leifur, Magnus and Paia for all their love and support.

—Kimball

First, I would like to thank Wells for his persistence and his foresight; this project never would have gotten off the ground, much less gotten published, without him. I also want to thank the other coauthors of the book. The struggles of this process brought us together, and our accountability to each other pushed us through.

Special appreciation goes to Tim Amrhein, who really came through in a pinch. His insight was crucial in the editing and revision process. I owe you one, Tim.

Finally, to my wife Kristen, and my boys Carter, Tyler, and Chase: thanks for supporting me through the peaks and valleys of this process. I couldn't have done it without you. You all mean the world to me.

—Scott

I want to thank my best friend and wife, Kim, for your love, patience, and understanding during the writing of this book. I am truly blessed to have you in my life. To my big brothers (Duc, Tuan, and Khan) and big sisters (Diana, Lan-Phuong, Nikki, Tina, and Linda), thank you for all of your encouragement and support throughout my life. To my parents, Ngo and Hoa, thank you for your countless sacrifices on my behalf. I wish you were both still here to share in all of your children's success, and I hope you are proud of me.

Finally, to Linda Gray and Carl Ravin, thank you for granting me an opportunity of a lifetime here at Duke. It has truly been an honor and a privilege to be amongst such an extraordinary collection of people.

—Phil

To my family, especially my wife Jan-Ru, for her patience and loving support.

—Allen

To my wife Christina, the true source of my academic time, and my beloved daughters Paula and Anna.

—Elmar

Timothy J. Amrhein, MD
Division of Neuroradiology, Department of Radiology,
Duke University Medical Center, Durham,
North Carolina
*T2 Contrast; Chemical Shift Type 2 Artifact;
Flow-Related Contrast; Time-of-Flight Imaging;
Phase Contrast*

Mustafa R. Bashir, MD
Assistant Professor, Department of Radiology, Duke
University Medical Center, Durham, North Carolina
Perfusion Magnetic Resonance Imaging

Erica Berg, MD
Women's Imaging Fellow, Duke University Hospital,
Durham, North Carolina
Inversion Recovery

Kimball L. Christianson, MD
Fellow, Division of Abdominal Imaging, Department
of Radiology, Duke University Medical Center,
Durham, North Carolina
*Proton Density; Gadolinium-Based Contrast Agents;
Motion, Pulsation, and Other Artifacts; Time-Resolved
Contrast-Enhanced Magnetic Resonance
Angiography; Diffusion MRI*

Manjiri M. Didolkar, MD, MS
Instructor of Radiology, Harvard Medical School;
Attending in Radiology, Musculoskeletal Radiology,
Beth Israel Deaconess Medical Center,
Boston, Massachusetts
T1 Contrast

Scott M. Duncan, MD
Diagnostic and Interventional Radiologist,
Radiology Associates Inc., Jeffersonville, Indiana
*T2 Contrast; Chemical Shift Type 2 Artifact; Flow-
Related Contrast; Time-of-Flight Imaging; Phase
Contrast*

Quoc Bao "Phil" B. Hoang, MD
Assistant Chief of Radiology, Southeast Louisiana
Veterans HealthCare System, New Orleans, Louisiana
*T1 Contrast; Preparatory Pulses; Inversion Recovery;
Motion, Pulsation, and Other Artifacts*

Steve Huang, MD
Assistant Professor, The University of Texas MD
Anderson Cancer Center, Houston, Texas
Motion, Pulsation, and Other Artifacts

Ramsey K. Kilani, MD
Adjunct Associate in Radiology, Duke University and
Duke University Medical Center, Durham,
North Carolina
Diffusion MRI

Charles Y. Kim, MD
Assistant Professor, Department of Radiology, Duke
University; Attending Physician, Vascular &
Interventional Radiology, Duke University Medical
Center, Durham, North Carolina
*Time-Resolved Contrast-Enhanced Magnetic Resonance
Angiography*

Christopher D. Lascola, MD, PhD
Assistant Professor, Department of Radiology,
Assistant Professor of Neurobiology, and Director,
Molecular Neuroimaging Laboratory, Department of
Radiology, Duke University Medical Center, Durham,
North Carolina
Proton Density

Mark L. Lessne, MD
Assistant Professor, Department of Radiology,
Interventional Radiology Center, The Johns Hopkins
University School of Medicine, Baltimore, Maryland
Motion, Pulsation, and Other Artifacts

Matthew P. Lungren, MD
Resident (PGY 5), Duke University Medical Center,
Durham, North Carolina
Preparatory Pulses

Wells I. Mangrum, MD
Practicing Radiologist, Sacred Heart Hospital,
Eau Claire, Wisconsin
*Susceptibility Artifact; Perfusion Magnetic Resonance
Imaging; Magnetic Resonance Spectroscopy;
Functional Magnetic Resonance Imaging*

Elmar M. Merkle, MD
Chairman, Department of Radiology and Nuclear
Medicine, University Hospitals Basel, Basel,
Switzerland
*T1 Contrast; Gadolinium-Based Contrast Agents;
Preparatory Pulses; Inversion Recovery; Susceptibility
Artifact; Motion, Pulsation, and Other Artifacts;
Time-Resolved Contrast-Enhanced Magnetic
Resonance Angiography; Diffusion MRI; Perfusion
Magnetic Resonance Imaging*

Michael J. Paldino, MD
Instructor in Radiology, Harvard Medical School;
Staff Neuroradiologist, Children's Hospital Boston,
Boston, Massachusetts
Perfusion Magnetic Resonance Imaging

Jeffrey R. Petrella, MD
Associate Professor, Department of Radiology, Duke University School of Medicine; Director, Alzheimer Imaging Research Laboratory, Department of Radiology, Duke University Health System, Durham, North Carolina
Magnetic Resonance Spectroscopy; Functional Magnetic Resonance Imaging

Christopher J. Roth, MD
Assistant Professor, Department of Radiology, Duke University Medical Center, Durham, North Carolina
Functional Magnetic Resonance Imaging

Allen W. Song, PhD
Professor of Radiology, Psychiatry, Neurobiology, and Biomedical Engineering, and Director, Brain Imaging and Analysis Center, Duke University School of Medicine, Durham, North Carolina
T1 Contrast; Proton Density; Gadolinium-Based Contrast Agents; Preparatory Pulses; Inversion Recovery; Susceptibility Artifact; Motion, Pulsation, and Other Artifacts; Time-Resolved Contrast-Enhanced Magnetic Resonance Angiography; Diffusion MRI; Perfusion Magnetic Resonance Imaging; Magnetic Resonance Spectroscopy; Functional Magnetic Resonance Imaging

James T. Voyvodic, PhD
Associate Professor, Department of Radiology, Duke University Medical Center, Durham, North Carolina
Functional Magnetic Resonance Imaging

Rodney D. Welling, MD
Resident in Radiology, Department of Radiology, Duke University Medical Center, Durham, North Carolina
Proton Density

I have been gratified by the popularity and positive feedback that the authors of the Case Review Series have received upon the publication of the first and second edition of their volumes. Reviews in journals and word-of-mouth comments have been uniformly favorable. The authors have done an outstanding job in filling the niche of an affordable, easy-reading, case-based learning tool that supplements the material in The Requisites series. I have been told by residents, fellows, and practicing radiologists that the Case Review Series books are the ideal means for studying for oral Boards and subspecialty certification tests.

It was recognized that while some students learn best in a noninteractive study-book mode, others need the anxiety or excitement of being quizzed or put on the "hot seat." The selected format for the Case Review Series (which consists of showing a limited number of images needed to construct a differential diagnosis and then asking a few clinical and imaging questions) was designed to simulate the Boards experience. The only difference is that the Case Review books provide the correct answer and immediate feedback. The limit and range of the reader's knowledge is tested through scaled cases; ranging from relatively easy to very hard. The Case Review series also offers a brief authors' commentary, a link back to The Requisites volume, and an up-to-date reference in the provided literature.

Because of the popularity of the series, we have been rolling out the second and third editions of the Case Review Series volumes. The expectation is that the these editions will bring the content up to the current knowledge limits of the field, introduce new modalities and new techniques, and provide new and even more graphic examples of pathology. To adjust to the upcoming change from an oral boards examination to a computer-based one, the Case Review Series is also changing. Our intention is to move to an even more engaging live platform through the use of the internet. Thus the questions are being reframed into multiple choice format, the links will be dynamic to on line references and The Requisites volumes, and feedback will be interactive with correct and incorrect answers. Please go to the website www.casereviewsonline.com to see how the Case Review Series evolves to best prepare trainees for the boards and practitioners for reading specialty cases. Personally, I am very excited about the future. Join us.

David M. Yousem, MD, MBA

In 2001 we decided to reorganize our four-year residency training program by combining it with a subsequent year of subspecialty fellowship training, resulting in a 5-year combined residency/fellowship training program. We further reorganized the time into 3 years of general radiology followed by 2 years of subspecialty (fellowship) radiology, and this design came to be known as the 3/2 program. Imbedded within the two years of subspecialty training experience was a protected 6 months of time designed to allow for "intellectual exploration." It was anticipated that most residents would use this time to pursue classic research investigations, but allowance was made for other creative experiences that reflected the fundamental premise of "intellectual exploration." One of the most innovative experiences that arose out of this opportunity was the development, by a group of residents, of this textbook integrating the fundamental principles of MR physics with clinical applicability across a broad range of MR imaging procedures. As a program we are absolutely delighted with the initiative undertaken by this special group of residents and the dedication and focus they demonstrated in bringing this project to a successful conclusion. This has been a project that arose from, and has been driven by, residents, assisted by faculty radiologists and medical physicists. We believe this project underscores the kinds of contributions that can be made by radiology trainees when given the appropriate opportunity, encouragement, and support to pursue the intellectual challenges that present themselves during resident/fellowship training. The 3/2 program allows trainees to make tangible contributions to the betterment of the field of diagnostic imaging and, thus, ultimately benefits not only the trainees but also practitioners in the field and, most important, the patients they serve.

Carl E. Ravin, MD
Professor and Former Chair, Department of Radiology, President,
Private Diagnostic Clinic, PLLC, Duke University Medical Center, Durham, North Carolina

We can recall the intimidation that we felt when we opened our first MRI and looked at the long list of MRI sequences performed for the scan. Eventually, we all overcame that initial fear and began to approach each MRI sequence individually. We can remember asking what is the purpose of this type of sequence? What clinical information should I derive from this sequence? What are the limitations of this sequence?

Through the course of residency we acquired answers to these questions from multiple different sources. We probably learned the most from our mentors whom taught us the pearls of clinical MRI interpretation as we worked beside them at Duke Hospital. We also learned from books on MRI by PhDs that explained the physics behind MRI. But often times we found it difficult to see the clinical relevance in the principles that we were taught by the physicists. Finally, we learned from books written by MDs that discussed clinical MRI applications. There are some excellent books out there, but these too have some limitations. First, the clinical MRI books written by MDs frequently focus on only one organ system and do not attempt to show how the same MRI principles are used across the different organ systems (i.e., neuroradiology, musculoskeletal radiology, cardiac MRI, body MRI). Second, the clinical MRI books are frequently organized by disease and not by MRI principle. Third, these books are not case based.

It was surprising and sometimes frustrating to us that we could not find a case-based review of MRI principles and their relevance to clinical practice. We have found the case review format to be an excellent way to teach and learn our ways in radiology. The success of the Case Review series and hot-seat board review courses reveals that many other residents feel the same way.

Four of us were Duke radiology residents when we decided that we could attempt to solve this disconnect in the medical literature by writing a book ourselves. Using the research time allotted to us from the 3/2 training program at Duke Radiology, we began writing late in our second year of residency and completed our work early in our fellowship year at Duke. We recruited two of our attendings, Allen W. Song and Elmar M. Merkle, to serve as our advisors. Their role was to review our material to give us some additional pointers and to help verify the contents. Tim Amrhein, a current fourth year radiology resident at Duke and future neuroradiologist, stepped in late in the process, co-authoring several chapters and also providing substantial feedback on the remaining chapters. Together we have put together this case review of MRI principles. We hope this book will help to dispel the common initial fear of MRI and replace that fear with a fascination of the amazing utility of MRI.

Wells I. Mangrum, MD
Kimball L. Christianson, MD
Scott M. Duncan, MD
Phil B. Hoang, MD
Allen W. Song, PhD
Elmar M. Merkle, MD

Chapter 1

T1 Contrast

Phil B. Hoang, Manjiri M. Didolkar, Allen W. Song, and Elmar M. Merkle

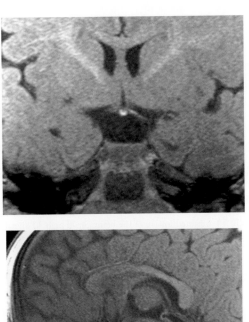
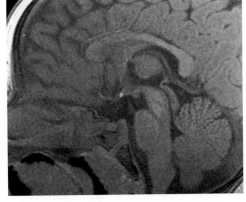

1. What weighting are these images?

2. Which parameter gives the most T1 weighting on a spin echo sequence, a long or short TR?

3. Do tissues that produce high signal on T1-weighted images have a long or short T1 relaxation time?

4. Where do you normally expect to find the neurohypophysis?

5. The patient presented with short stature; what is the diagnosis?

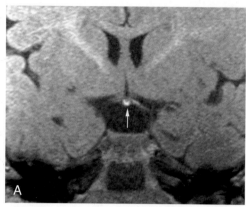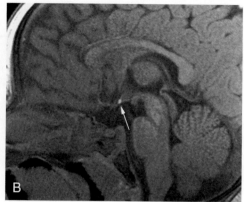

FIGURES 1A AND 1B. Coronal (A) and sagittal (B) T1-weighted images of the brain. Small high T1 signal focus at the superior aspect of the infundibulum *(arrows)* is demonstrated. Lack of the expected "bright spot" of the neurohypophysis within the posterior sella is observed on the sagittal image (B).

1. These are T1-weighted images.

2. A short time to repetition (TR) (400 to 800 msec) on a spin echo pulse sequence gives you T1 weighting.

3. Tissues that produce high signal on a T1-weighted image (such as fat) exhibit a short T1 relaxation time.

4. The neurohypophysis is normally located in the posterior sella.

5. Ectopic neurohypophysis.

Discussion

The normal T1 "bright spot" of the neurohypophysis is due to the proteins bound to vasopressin. Absence of the bright spot in its expected position or location within the posterior sella is consistent with ectopic neurohypophysis, a cause of short stature in children. The diagnosis is made by recognizing the abnormal position of the neurohypophysis on a T1-weighted (T1W) image, which in this case was in the superior aspect of the infundibulum.

Part I: Basic Spin Principles and T1 Relaxation

Because of its abundance in the human body, hydrogen is the most frequently imaged nucleus in clinical magnetic resonance imaging (MRI). Hydrogen has a considerable angular magnetic moment, with its single, positively-charged proton acting as a tiny, spinning bar magnet. Protons normally spin in random directions in the absence of an external magnetic field; because of this random movement, the magnetic vector sum of these protons is typically zero.

When placed in a strong external magnetic field (B_0), these protons align either parallel (low energy) or antiparallel (high energy) with respect to B_0; more protons tend to align parallel to B_0 since less energy is required to do so. Because they possess both magnetic *and* angular momentum, the protons precess, or wobble, around the axis of B_0 instead of spinning in a tight circle; this precession motion confers both longitudinal (M_z) and transverse (M_{xy}) components in the magnetic moments of the protons. Protons tend to precess at a certain frequency while under the influence of B_0, which is called the Larmor frequency. The Larmor frequency defines the frequency at which the radiofrequency (RF) pulse is broadcast to induce proton resonance, or excitation. The Larmor frequency is proportional to the strength of the main magnetic field; at 1.5 Tesla, the Larmor frequency of hydrogen protons is 63.8 MHz, and it is approximately 127 MHz at 3 Tesla.

The **vector sum** of the magnetic moments of the precessing protons (M_z and M_{xy}) results in a net equilibrium magnetization (M_0). This magnetization vector is primarily in the longitudinal direction (M_z) since more protons align in parallel with B_0. The transverse component (M_{xy}) does not contribute significantly to M_0, as the protons do not spin in phase with each other and effectively cancel each other out. As the energy of B_0 increases, so does the energy differential between protons in the low (parallel) and high (antiparallel) states, with increasing numbers of protons aligning parallel to B_0. This results in a significant directional (vector) component of the net magnetization. However, the receiver coil, which is the component of the MRI machine that detects signals, is sensitive only to variations of the magnetization vector; the original main magnetization along the z direction, even though it is precessing, is viewed as a "stationary" vector from the receiver coil perspective. Given this, something must be done to perturb the system and generate detectable signal changes that can be picked up by the receiver coils; this comes in the form of an RF excitation pulse.

Application of the RF pulse (a short burst of electromagnetic energy) results in energy absorption by protons. In order for this energy transfer to occur, the RF pulse and precessing protons must have the same frequency. This results in a change in the energy level of the protons, which go from the low-energy (parallel) state into the high-energy (antiparallel) state. Simultaneously, there is a gain in the protons' phase coherence, as the protons receive their initial phase that is synchronized. This produces a net *loss* of longitudinal magnetization and a net *gain* in transverse magnetization, respectively. Conceptually speaking, this is better known as the "tipping" of net magnetization vector from the longitudinal axis (B_z) into the transverse plane (B_{xy}), such that the precession motion can be visible and signal changes detectable by the receiver coils. The degree of transverse magnetization generated depends on both the amplitude of the RF pulse and length of time it is administered; **complete rotation of protons into the transverse plane is the result of a 90° RF pulse**.

After cessation of the excitation pulse, the resonating protons "relax" back into their equilibrium state, which occurs by two mechanisms: transverse (T2) and longitudinal (T1) relaxation. While these two mechanisms occur concurrently, they do so at different rates. Briefly, transverse relaxation refers to loss of phase coherence due to interactions between spinning protons (spin-spin). This leads to a net decrease in transverse magnetization, and is also referred to as T2 decay. This concept is discussed in greater detail in Chapter 2.

In T1 relaxation, the resonating proton returns to its thermal equilibrium state by transferring energy to the other nuclei in its surrounding, or lattice. This mechanism is commonly referred to as spin-lattice relaxation, and results in a net increase in longitudinal magnetization. T1 relaxation occurs at an exponential rate; at time T1, longitudinal magnetization has returned to 63% of its final value, and at time 3*T1, longitudinal magnetization has returned to 95% of its final value. The differences in tissue T1 relaxation are responsible for the contrast on a T1W image and depend on the efficiency of energy transfer from proton to lattice. Tissues with short T1 relaxation times (fat) generate high signal, while tissues with long T1 relaxation times (water) generate low signal.

Differences in T1 relaxation are primarily attributed to the natural movement unique to a molecule. In short, the more similar the molecule's natural motional frequency is to that of the Larmor frequency, the more efficiently energy transfer to its lattice occurs. This results in a short T1 relaxation time. Small molecules, such as those found in free water (cerebrospinal fluid), move rapidly; on the other side of the spectrum, macromolecules such as protein move at a slower pace. While the motional frequencies of these molecules differ immensely, both exhibit long T1 relaxation times because both move at a frequency much different than the Larmor frequency. Intermediate-sized molecules, such as fat, move at frequencies very similar to the Larmor frequency and thus exhibit short T1 relaxation times.

The term *T1 shortening* refers to a decrease in the T1 relaxation time of a tissue, leading to greater signal intensity on a T1W pulse sequence than is expected. This change is usually under the influence of agents that induce T1 relaxivity of nearby free water protons. The mechanisms exhibited by these agents include paramagnetic (gadolinium, manganese, methemoglobin) or hydration layer (proteins, ionic calcium) effects. The most commonly known paramagnetic agents are the gadolinium chelates used in contrast-enhanced sequences; these agents, as well as the mechanisms of T1 relaxivity exhibited by these agents, are discussed in greater detail in Chapter 4.

Part II: T1 Contrast and Pulse Sequence Considerations

An important point to consider when interpreting any magnetic resonance (MR) image is that image contrast is not exclusively due to differences in T1, T2, or proton density; these contrasts all make some contribution. However, by manipulating certain operator-dependent parameters, we can have *more* of one contrast and *less* of the others. This is why we use the terms *T1, T2,* and *proton density* weighting when describing the contrast in an image.

Spin Echo

In a conventional spin echo (SE) sequence, the 90° RF pulse is followed by a 180° refocusing pulse, which is administered at the halfway point of the echo time and is used to bring the protons back into an in-phase (i.e., synchronized) state. The parameter with the greatest effect on T1 contrast on a conventional SE sequence is the time to repetition (TR), which is the time interval between successive excitation pulses. A moderate TR can be determined to optimize the T1 contrast. The TRs for T1W SE sequences are typically in the range of 400 to 800 msec. As the TR lengthens, most tissues recover their longitudinal magnetization and produce signal; while this will increase overall signal-to-noise ratio in the image, it will diminish T1 contrast (Fig. 1).

While modifying TR can optimize T1 contrast, adjusting the length of the second parameter, the time to echo (TE), governs T2 contrast. The TE is the time interval between the excitation pulse and signal collection; this parameter has the greatest effect on decreasing the contribution from T2 contrast (Fig. 2). To minimize the T2 contrast (so that T1 contrast is dominant), the TE should be kept as short as possible (15 to 25 msec). A moderate TE would generate significant T2 contrast (see Fig. 2).

Gradient-Recalled Echo (GRE)

This class of pulse sequences uses an excitation pulse with a variable "flip" angle (< 90°) and rephases protons with gradients of equal magnitude and duration but *opposite* polarities.

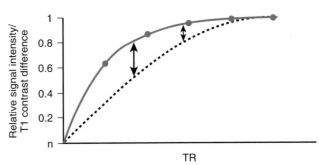

FIGURE 1. Following the excitation pulse, tissues regain longitudinal magnetization (M_z) at rates determined by their specific T1 relaxation time. A short TR maximizes differences in T1 contrast (*large arrow*). A longer TR minimizes T1 contrast.

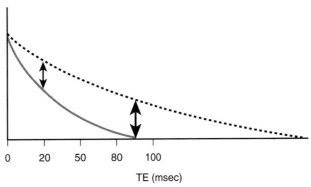

FIGURE 2. M_{xy} decay (transverse magnetization). By using a short TE (~20 msec), differences in T2 contrast in the image are minimized. These differences in T2 contrast would be more significant if a longer TE (~100 msec) were used.

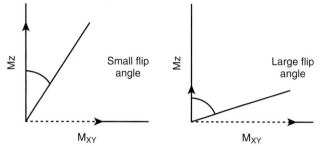

FIGURE 3. A larger flip angle "tips" most of the protons into the transverse plane *(dashed arrow)* with a small amount of longitudinal magnetization remaining. Similar to SE sequences, the signal differences between tissues are then dependent on tissue-specific T1 relaxation times.

This is opposed to conventional SE sequences, which apply a 180° refocusing pulse to rephase protons. In GRE acquisitions, the flip angle often plays a role in changing T1 contrast. Small flip angles allow the longitudinal magnetization to recover more rapidly. As such, the TRs used are typically short (< 200 msec), as are the TEs (< 10 msec to minimize T2 contrast).

T1 weighting in GRE sequences is maximized by using an excitation pulse with a large (~ 50° to 80°) flip angle, a short TR (~ 100 msec), and a short TE (< 10 msec). Both the flip angle and the TR have the greatest influence on T1 weighting, with the effect of the flip angle illustrated in Figure 3. Using large flip angles places an emphasis on T1 contrast as signal intensity produced depends on tissue specific T1 relaxation times. With small flip angles, different tissues retain most of their longitudinal magnetization (Fig. 3, *solid arrows*); because of this, the longitudinal magnetizations of tissues (and thus signal intensity) are similar on a T1W sequence, which reduces T1 contrast (see Fig. 3).

Strengths of GRE sequence over conventional SE include faster image acquisition (due to shorter TRs) and decreased RF power deposition (due to the lack of a 180° refocusing pulse). In exchange, signal is sacrificed; GRE suffers from irretrievable signal loss due to magnetic field inhomogeneities and susceptibility effects (T2*) because it does not apply a refocusing pulse. Thus, GRE sequences are generally lower in signal-to-noise ratio compared to SE sequences.

An important consequence of the short TRs used in GRE is the residual transverse magnetization remaining prior to the next excitation pulse. If left alone, the transverse magnetization will contribute to the longitudinal component after the next excitation pulse is administered, which eventually alters image contrast. To resolve this issue, a spoiler mechanism is used prior to the start of the next TR to prevent buildup of a transverse magnetization steady state and makes the magnetization in the longitudinal direction the chief contributor to M_z at the next excitation pulse.

When extremely short acquisition times are needed, "ultra-fast" GRE sequences are used. These sequences acquire images in 1 second or less by using extremely short TRs (< 3 msec) and small flip angles. Since these parameters are generally unfavorable for the T1 weighting needed in contrast-enhanced sequences, an additional step is needed to boost T1 contrast. A preparatory pulse applied prior to the excitation pulse inverts the longitudinal magnetization, which introduces T1 weighting by emphasizing differences in tissue T1 relaxation; this concept is discussed further in Chapter 6.

Part III: Clinical Applications

The contrast of a T1W sequence provides an important overview of anatomy. The two tissues that produce the most predictable signal intensity on a T1W image are fat and free water. This is a reflection of each tissue's T1 relaxation time, which is short for fat (~250 msec at 1.5T) and long for water (~2500 msec at 1.5T). Normal solid organs (brain, muscle, liver, spleen, kidneys) have intermediate relaxation times, ranging from 490 msec (liver) to 970 msec (gray matter) at 1.5 Tesla (1.5T). The differences in T1 contrast are secondary to the varying ratios of extracellular water and macromolecules. For example, the normal pancreas produces the greatest signal intensity on a T1W image of the solid abdominal organs due to its high protein synthesis and intracellular paramagnetic agents. Bone marrow demonstrates variable signal intensity depending on its ratio of red-to-yellow marrow.

Case 2

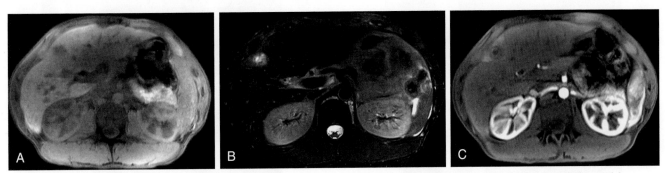

FIGURE 2A. Axial T1W image of the upper abdomen with fat suppression. An ill-defined low T1 signal lesion is seen in the anterior right hepatic lobe.

FIGURE 2B. Axial T2-weighted (T2W) image with fat suppression. The lesion is predominantly high in T2 signal; perilesional high T2 signal extends peripherally from the lesion.

FIGURE 2C. Axial postcontrast T1W image. The lesion demonstrates peripheral rim enhancement; there is parenchymal enhancement surrounding the focus, consistent with hyperemia or edema.

Diagnosis: Hepatic abscess.

Case 3

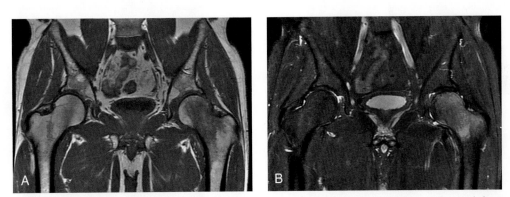

FIGURE 3A. Coronal T1W image of the pelvis. Homogeneous low T1 signal of the left femoral head and neck is present. The signal abnormality is slightly lower compared to muscle.

FIGURE 3B. Coronal T2W image with fat saturation: The left femoral head and neck are high in T2 signal.

Diagnosis: Idiopathic transient osteoporosis of the hip.

Discussion

Most lesions are low signal compared to normal parenchyma on T1W images, typically because of increased extracellular water content which prolongs T1 relaxation. Identifying this signal abnormality on a T1W image should alert you to focus on more fluid-sensitive images, such as found on a T2-weighted (T2W) sequence, or on gadolinium-enhanced T1W sequences. This is seen in the small hepatic abscess (Case 2), which exhibits the typical signal pattern of many lesions: low on T1, high on T2, and enhancement on postcontrast T1W images.

In Case 3, the low signal intensity of the left femoral head and neck is due to bone marrow edema, which results in prolongation of the normal T1 relaxation time of the marrow spaces and produces a low-signal abnormality on the T1W sequence. As expected, the extra free water within the marrow produces hyperintense signal on the corresponding fat-suppressed T2W image (see Fig. 3B).

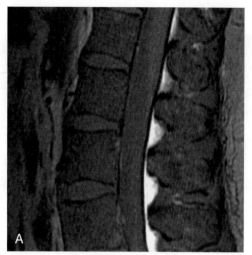

FIGURE 4A. Sagittal T1W image of the lumbar spine. There is diffuse marrow abnormality of the vertebral bodies in the lower thoracic and lumbar spine; the marrow is lower in signal intensity compared to the adjacent normal intervertebral discs.

Diagnosis: Metastatic breast cancer.

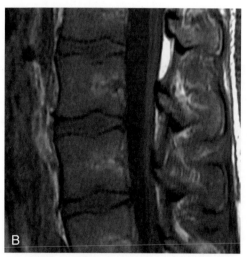

FIGURE 4B. Sagittal T1W image of the lumbar spine. Intermediate marrow signal is seen in all vertebral bodies. The signal intensity of the marrow is of slightly higher intensity compared to the adjacent discs.

Diagnosis: Red marrow hyperplasia.

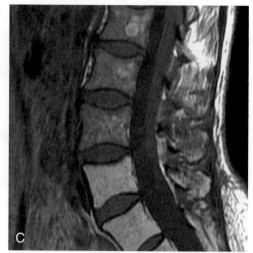

FIGURE 4C. Sagittal T1W image of the lumbar spine. Intermediate bone marrow signal, greater in intensity compared to the adjacent discs, in the upper three vertebral bodies is consistent with red marrow. Homogeneous high signal intensity is demonstrated in the lower lumbar vertebral bodies.

Diagnosis: Postradiation fatty marrow replacement of the lower lumbosacral spine with red marrow hyperplasia of the upper lumbar spine.

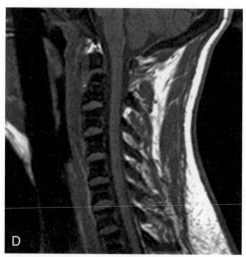

FIGURE 4D. Sagittal T1W image of the cervical spine. Diffuse low signal intensity of the cervical spine is demonstrated. Type II dens fracture "incidentally" noted.

Diagnosis: Osteopetrosis.

Discussion

The signal intensity of normal bone marrow is determined by the ratio of active (red marrow) and inactive (yellow marrow) cellular components. Yellow marrow consists of nearly 80% fat cells, which is responsible for the high signal on both T1W and fast SE T2W sequences. Red marrow consists of 40% fat, 40% water, and 20% proteins, which explains its intermediate signal intensity. As aging progresses, the ratio of fat cells to water normally increases.

T1W sequences are the most valuable in evaluating the status of bone marrow, particularly in the lumbar spine. In general, if the marrow process is *higher* in signal compared to the adjacent normal disc on a T1W sequence, then it indicates the presence of red marrow (see Fig. 4B). Figure 4C shows the geographic changes in marrow composition in a patient with prior radiation changes to the spine, with the radiated lower lumbosacral marrow completely replaced by fat, while the vertebral bodies not included in the radiation portal showed evidence of red marrow hyperplasia.

T1W sequences are also important for detection of infiltrative and focal marrow processes; if the marrow signal is *lower* compared to the adjacent normal disc, then is it is either an infiltrative process, such as metastatic breast cancer (see Fig. 4A), or a marrow replacement process, as is seen in diseases such as myelofibrosis and osteopetrosis (see Fig. 4D).[11]

CASE 5

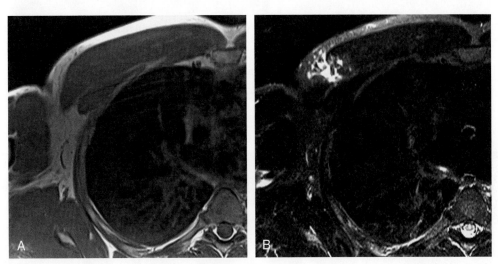

FIGURE 5A. Axial T1W image of the right chest. No signal or morphologic abnormality is identified.

FIGURE 5B. Axial short tau inversion recovery (STIR) image of the right chest, same level. Focal increased STIR signal abnormality of the lateral aspect of the right pectoralis major muscle is now evident.

Diagnosis: Full-thickness right pectoralis major muscle tear.

Discussion

Lesions that exhibit similar T1 relaxation times compared to surrounding normal tissues may go virtually undetected on a T1W image. This is illustrated in Case 5, where the fluid and hemorrhage filling the full-thickness pectoralis muscle tear are obviously seen on the short tau inversion recovery (STIR) image (see Fig. 5B). However, on the T1W image (see Fig. 5A), the fluid-filled tear is isointense to the adjacent normal musculature, with no focal morphologic abnormality appreciated.

Case 6

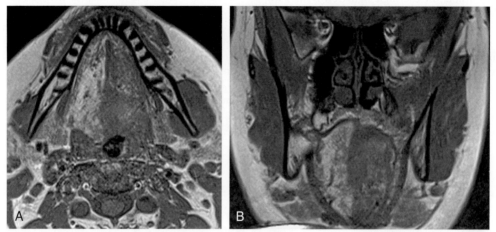

FIGURES 6A AND 6B. Axial (A) and coronal (B) T1W images of the oropharynx demonstrate high-signal fat replacing the musculature of the right half of the tongue. Note the sharp demarcation between the atrophic changes of the right side of the tongue as compared to the normal left half.

Diagnosis: Fatty atrophy of the right tongue due to ipsilateral hypoglossal nerve dysfunction.

Case 7

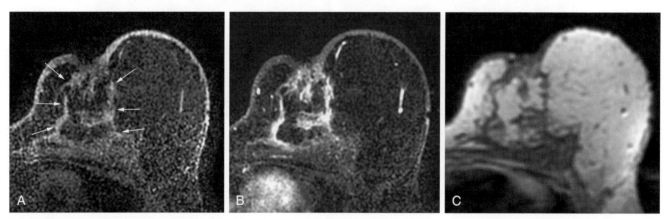

FIGURE 7A. Axial T1W image of the breast with fat suppression. Irregular bands of soft tissue are noted in the medial left breast *(arrows)*. Overlying distortion and skin thickening are also present.

FIGURE 7B. Axial fat-suppressed postcontrast T1W image demonstrates enhancement of the irregular tissue bands with nonenhancement centrally.

FIGURE 7C. Axial T1W SE image without fat suppression. The irregularly enhancing soft tissue is low in T1 signal and surrounds a large area of high-signal fat.

Diagnosis: Biopsy-proven fat necrosis.

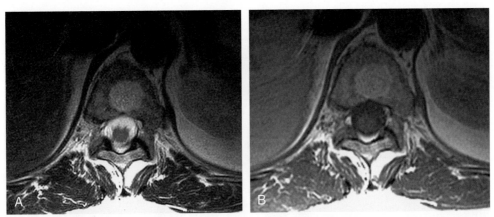

FIGURE 8A. Axial fast SE T2W image of the lower thoracic spine without fat suppression. A high-signal round lesion is present in the vertebral body.

FIGURE 8B. Axial T1W image at the same level. The lesion is hyperintense compared to the vertebral marrow and nearly isointense to intra-abdominal fat.

Diagnosis: Intraosseous hemangioma.

Discussion

While the low signal intensity exhibited by most lesions on a T1W sequence is helpful, it is nonspecific and is seen in a wide range of both benign and aggressive processes. Conversely, causes of intrinsic *high* T1 signal are far fewer in number and can help you narrow the differential to a handful of diagnoses, most of which are typically benign. The remaining cases of this chapter will provide an overview of the various causes of and principles behind T1 bright lesions.

The most common tissue that exhibits intrinsic high T1 signal is fat. As discussed earlier in this chapter, the high signal intensity produced by fat on a T1W sequence is because of its short T1 relaxation time. Companion Cases 6 through 8 illustrate clinical scenarios in which this common tissue is found in uncommon places.

Anatomic information on MRI is best evaluated on T1W sequences. In Case 6, atrophy and complete replacement with fat of the right half of the tongue is clearly displayed, particularly when comparing it to the normal left half. This patient had idiopathic ipsilateral hypoglossal nerve dysfunction.

Irregularly enhancing tissue is frequently an ominous finding in breast MRI. The presence of high-signal-intensity fat within the confines of the irregular tissue (see Fig. 7C), however, suggests fat necrosis (Case 7). Identifying this on the non–fat-suppressed T1W image sequence is critical in suggesting this benign diagnosis. Given the aggressive appearance of this area in the breast, as well as the patient's history of breast cancer, a biopsy was performed, which confirmed the diagnosis.

Increased signal within a vertebral body lesion on a T2W image (Case 8) may be a cause for concern as a number of aggressive bone lesions are potential considerations. However, recognizing bright T1 signal within the lesion confirms the presence of intralesional fat, and is consistent with a benign intraosseous hemangioma.[12]

Case 9

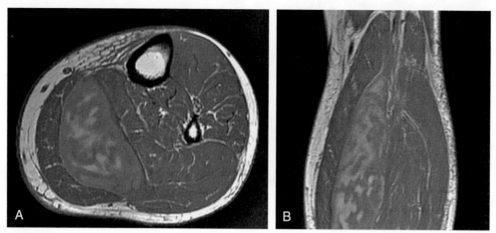

FIGURE 9A. Axial T1W image of the calf. A large, oval mass is located between the medial head of the gastrocnemius and the soleus muscle. The mass demonstrates intrinsic heterogeneous high T1 signal intensity.

FIGURE 9B. Coronal T1W image of the upper calf. The mass conforms to intermuscular fascial planes of the medial gastrocnemius and soleus muscles.

Diagnosis: Plantaris tendon rupture with subacute hemorrhage.

Case 10

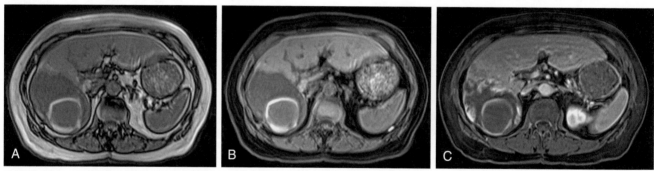

FIGURE 10A. Axial T1W opposed phase GRE image of the upper abdomen. A large low-T1-signal right hepatic lobe mass is demonstrated; a round mass with high-T1-signal rim and low-T1-signal center is present within the posterior aspect of the lesion.

FIGURE 10B. Axial fat-suppressed T1W image. The high-T1-signal rim persists and is unchanged.

FIGURE 10C. Axial postcontrast T1W image with fat saturation, portal venous phase. The mass demonstrates peripheral nodular enhancement.

Diagnosis: Giant hemangioma with internal hemorrhage.

Discussion

Aside from fat, two of the most frequent tissues that exhibit high signal on a T1W image include subacute blood clot (methemoglobin) and proteinaceous fluid; the remaining cases in this chapter discuss these tissues plus a number of less frequently encountered causes.

Methemoglobin is a breakdown product in subacute hemorrhage. As the oxidation of hemorrhage progresses, the integrity of the red blood cell membrane is lost; nearby free water protons then freely diffuse across the membrane and interact with the five unpaired electrons of the methemoglobin iron. These protons experience a shortening of their normal T1 relaxation times, which appears as high signal intensity on a T1W sequence. Of the four hemoglobin breakdown products (oxyhemoglobin, deoxyhemoglobin, methemoglobin, and hemosiderin), methemoglobin is the only one that causes high T1 signal.

Identifying the high signal within the "mass" seen in the calf musculature on the T1W image (Case 9) confirms the subacute hemorrhagic component of this lesion. On the coronal T1W image, the "mass" seems to respect muscular fascial planes. With its characteristic location and appearance, and combined with the clinical history of acute onset of pain, the findings were consistent with a plantaris tendon rupture.

Case 10 is an example of a giant hepatic hemangioma with intratumoral hemorrhage. The high-signal methemoglobin ring surrounds an intermediate- to low-signal center of blood products. This case also demonstrates how multiple sequences are valuable in coming to a definitive conclusion in MRI; the persistently increased signal on a fat-suppressed T1W image (see Fig. 10B) confirms the nonfat nature of the high-T1-signal rim, and the addition of intravenous gadolinium (see Fig. 10C) demonstrates the peripheral nodular enhancement of the surrounding hepatic mass, a pattern typical of hemangiomas.

CASE 11

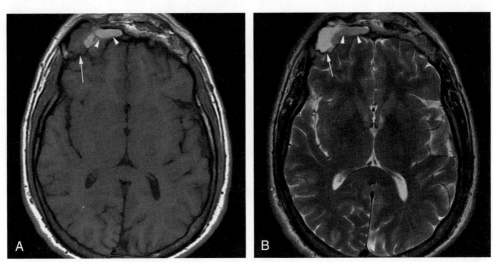

FIGURE 11A. Axial T1W image at the level of the third ventricle. A lobulated lesion in the right frontal sinus is demonstrated. Compared to white matter, the lesion is high in T1 signal intensity compared to the brain medially *(arrowheads)*, while the lateral aspect of the lesion is intermediate to low in T1 signal intensity *(arrow)*.

FIGURE 11B. Axial T2W image at the same level. The right frontal lesion demonstrates the reverse pattern of signal changes seen on the T1W image, with the lesion exhibiting intermediate to low T2 signal intensity medially *(arrowheads)* and high T2 signal intensity laterally *(arrow)*.

Diagnosis: Right frontal sinus mucocele.

Discussion

The T1 shortening effect of macromolecules (proteins) is different than that exhibited in paramagnetic agents. A protein binds free water protons onto its surface via hydrophilic side chains, creating a layer of bound water protons; this is referred to as the ***hydration layer effect.*** Now bound, the water protons' motional frequency is decreased, making energy transfer to the lattice more efficient and leading to T1 shortening.

Case 11 demonstrates how varying concentrations of proteins affect both T1 and T2 signal intensity. The mildly expansile focus centered in the right frontal sinus represents a mucocele. The obstructed sinus drainage leads to the accumulation of inspissated secretions; as the protein concentration increases, so does the T1 signal intensity. This is what we see within the mucocele, which is of greater signal intensity medially as compared to laterally because of its greater protein concentration.[14]

These findings are confirmed by the signal changes of the mucocele on the corresponding T2W image (see Fig. 11B). The signal changes on the T2W image reflect the *decreased* concentration of free water protons in the areas of *increased* protein. The mechanism by which proteinaceous fluids cause decreased T2 signal is complex; however, the combination of hydration layer effects, as well as the decreased free water concentration, likely play significant roles.

Case 12

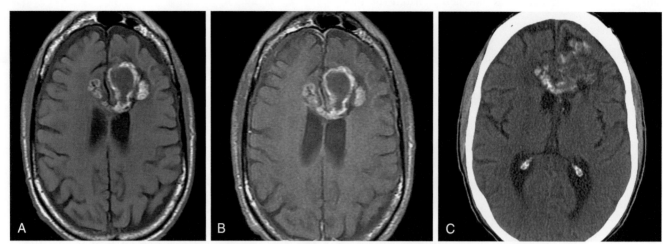

FIGURE 12A. Axial T1W image demonstrates an irregular lesion with intrinsic high T1 signal that crosses the anterior corpus callosum.

FIGURE 12B. Axial postcontrast T1W image at the same level demonstrates persistent high signal intensity of the corpus callosum.

FIGURE 12C. Axial noncontrast CT image of the brain; irregular hyperdensity of the bifrontal mass consistent with calcification.

Diagnosis: Treated glioblastoma multiforme with underlying mineralizing microangiopathy.

Case 13

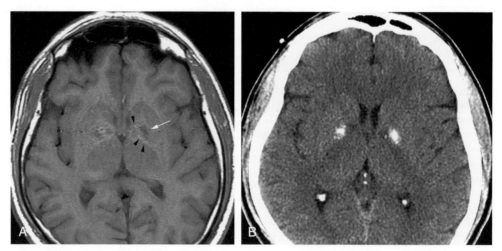

FIGURE 13A. Axial T1W image demonstrates focal hypointense T1 signal in the bilateral basal ganglia *(white arrow);* the low-signal foci are surrounded by subtle high signal intensity *(black arrowheads).*

FIGURE 13B. Axial computed tomography image demonstrates dense foci in the bilateral basal ganglia.

Diagnosis: Senescent basal ganglia calcifications.

Discussion

Because of the lack of mobile proton density and susceptibility effects, dense calcifications (such as those found in cortical bone) are of low signal intensity on all pulse sequences. However, there are certain situations in which calcium produces high signal on a T1W image.

A surface relaxation phenomenon is the mechanism of T1 shortening exhibited by ionic calcium, which is similar to the hydration layer effect of macromolecules (proteins).[14] The calcium salts form a crystalline lattice in which free water protons settle, causing a decrease in the T1 relaxation time of those protons. The larger the surface area of the lattice, the more bound free water protons and the greater the T1 signal intensity.

In the brain, high T1 signal from calcium salt deposits occurs in the setting of mineralizing microangiopathy, a recognized sequela of radiation and chemotherapy.[10] Case 12 shows the importance of recognizing this paradoxical finding; the irregular area of calcification also appears as high signal on the postcontrast T1W sequences, which could be mistaken for enhancement. Careful comparison between the noncontrast and postcontrast T1W sequences is necessary to confirm that each foci of increased T1 signal is indeed matched. The corresponding computed tomography (CT) scan (see Fig. 12C) confirms the presence of calcifications.

As the concentration of calcium rises above a certain percentage (30% to 40%), the lack of mobile proton density and susceptibility effects become the dominant factors in determining signal intensity of calcium. This leads to the more-familiar low signal intensity of calcium on all pulse sequences. The bilateral basal ganglia calcifications (Case 13) are denser centrally on the CT image and are correspondingly low signal on the T1W image; however, the subtle high T1 signal peripherally is in part due to a lower concentration of calcium.[9]

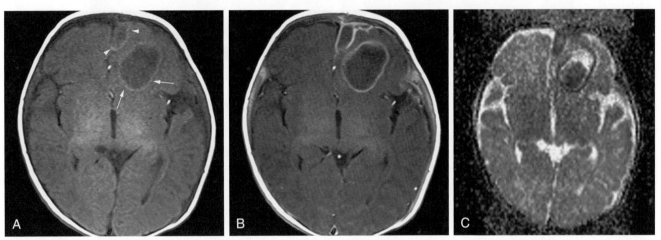

FIGURE 14A. Axial T1W image at the level of the third ventricle. A low-signal left frontal mass is outlined by a thin rind of high-T1-signal tissue *(arrows)*. An additional curvilinear high-T1-signal focus is present along the left anterior parafalcine region *(arrowheads)*.

FIGURE 14B. Axial postcontrast T1W image at the same level. The low-signal left frontal and left parafalcine masses demonstrate peripheral rim enhancement. Also note thickened enhancement of the anterior falx.

FIGURE 14C. Axial apparent diffusion coefficient (ADC) map demonstrates restricted diffusion centrally as well as within the rim.

Diagnosis: Left frontal abscess with left parafalcine subdural empyema.

Discussion

Free radical production from the respiratory burst of macrophages during phagocytosis is frequently observed in abscess formation (Case 14). The imaging appearance on MRI is described as a high-T1-signal capsule around the low-signal abscess center.[3] The signal changes are due to the accumulation of methemoglobin as well as the paramagnetic effects of the free radicals themselves.

Along with myelin breakdown products, macrophages and free radicals are thought to be responsible for high T1 signal often seen in the rim of active demyelination in multiple sclerosis plaques.[4]

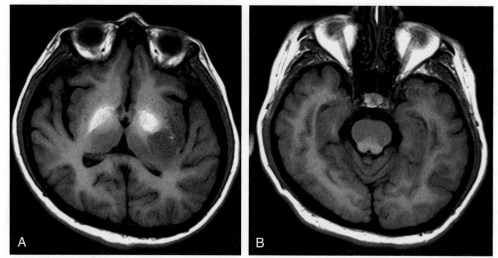

FIGURE 15A. Axial T1W image of the brain. Symmetrical high-T1-signal areas within the globus pallidi are demonstrated. Round low-T1-signal focus in the posterior basal ganglia is consistent with acute hemorrhage.

FIGURE 15B. Axial T1W image of the pons, same patient. High T1 signal intensity of the pontine tegmentum and anterior pituitary gland are noted.

Diagnosis: Manganese deposition secondary to long-term total parenteral nutrition (TPN).

Discussion

Manganese (Mn) is an ion found normally in foods and is a supplementary addition in total parenteral nutrition (TPN) formulations. It is primarily excreted via the hepatobiliary system and, to a variable extent, the pancreatic and renal systems. Like gadolinium, manganese is paramagnetic and was previously available as a T1-shortening chelate (Mn-DPDP, **mangafodipir trisodium,** Teslascan) used primarily in hepatobiliary and pancreatic imaging. (Effective September 2004, Teslascan is no longer commercially available in the United States.)

Accumulation of excess Mn blood levels can cause neurologic symptoms similar to those seen in parkinsonism. The two most common clinical settings of Mn toxicity are chronic liver disease and long-term TPN (Case 15). Bypass of the normal regulatory mechanisms used to normalize manganese levels occurs in TPN.[8] Other potential sites of intracranial manganese deposition include the pontine tegmentum and anterior pituitary (see Fig. 15B), as well as the midbrain and corpus callosum.[8]

Other causes of high T1 signal in the basal ganglia include a number of atypical processes, such as hypoxic ischemic encephalopathy, Japanese encephalitis, calcium deposition (hyperparathyroidism, hypoparathyroidism), neurofibromatosis 1, and diabetic hyperglycemia.[1,5]

Case 16

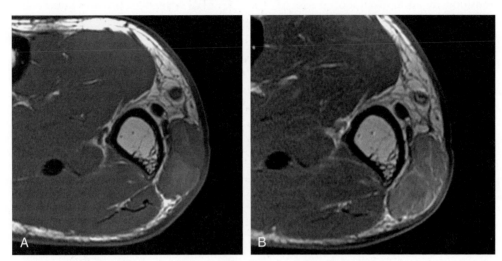

FIGURE 16A. Axial T1W image of the right thumb. An oval mass lateral to the cortex of the right thumb first metacarpal is mostly isointense to muscle but contains areas of intrinsic high T1 signal internally. A well-defined fat plane separates the mass from the metacarpal cortex.

FIGURE 16B. Axial postcontrast T1W image; the mass demonstrates heterogeneous internal enhancement.

Diagnosis: Metastatic melanoma.

Case 17

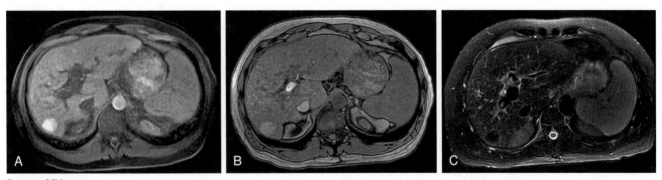

FIGURE 17A. Axial postcontrast T1W image with fat suppression of the upper abdomen, arterial phase. Round high signal lesion is present in the posterior right hepatic lobe.

FIGURE 17B. Axial T1W opposed phase GRE image at the same level. The lesion demonstrates high T1 signal.

FIGURE 17C. Axial T2W image with fat saturation. The lesion is homogeneously low signal.

Diagnosis: Dysplastic nodule in the setting of cirrhosis.

Discussion

High T1 signal may be the result of multiple factors, as illustrated in these companion cases. Melanoma (Case 16) is classically described as a T1-hyperintense lesion due to the paramagnetic effects of melanin free radicals *and* subacute blood products (methemoglobin). An alternative mechanism was proposed by Enochs et al., who demonstrated melanin's high affinity and binding capacity for other paramagnetic metal ions, including manganese and zinc.[2]

Dysplastic nodules (Case 17) are premalignant lesions in the cirrhotic liver. These nodules frequently demonstrate high T1 signal, with glycogen and fat implicated as causative factors. The most important differential diagnosis of a high-T1-signal nodule in a cirrhotic liver is a well-differentiated hepatocellular carcinoma; seeing homogeneous low signal on a T2W image (see Fig. 17C) provides additional imaging support for a dysplastic nodule.[13]

1. T1 represents the efficiency of energy transfer from a resonating proton to its lattice following energy deposition by an RF excitation pulse.
2. Molecules that move at a motional frequency similar to the Larmor frequency quickly transfer energy to the lattice, and results in a short T1 relaxation time and increased signal on a T1W image. An example is a medium-sized molecule such as fat.
3. Small molecules (bulk water) and large molecules (proteins) exhibit motional frequencies much different than the Larmor frequency, resulting in inefficient energy transfer to the lattice and long T1 relaxation times.
4. MR images have a different mix of contrasts (T1, T2, and proton density); operator-adjustable parameters are manipulated to promote a particular weighting, which emphasizes differences of one particular tissue contrast while minimizing the others.
5. In SE sequences, a moderate TR (~ 600 msec) and a shortest possible TE (< 10 msec) produces a T1W image. In GRE sequences, an excitation pulse with a large flip angle, a short TR, and the shortest possible TE produces a T1W image.
6. In a T1W sequence, tissues with short T1 relaxation times produce high signal (fat, gadolinium-enhanced tissues, proteinaceous fluid), while tissues with long T1 times produce low signal (free water, cerebrospinal fluid).
7. T1W sequences provide good anatomic information and are used to evaluate enhancing tissues following intravenous gadolinium chelate administration.
8. Most pathologic tissues are low signal on non-contrast T1W images due to T1 relaxation prolongation from increased extracellular water concentration.
9. T1 shortening refers to the reduction of normal T1 relaxation of tissues due to the effects of external agents, causing them to produce high signal on a T1W sequence.
10. Paramagnetic agents exhibit unpaired electrons that produce a strong, local magnetic field and induce both T1 and T2 relaxation of nearby protons. Examples of paramagnetic agents include gadolinium chelates, methemoglobin, and melanin.
11. The hydration layer effect refers to the binding of water protons to the surface of macromolecules (proteins); this slows down the motional frequency of water protons, making energy transfer to the lattice more efficient and leading to a reduction in its T1 relaxation.
12. Other less common agents of T1 shortening include ionic calcium, manganese, and free radicals.

References

1. Caruso RD, Postel GC, McDonald CS, Sherry RG: High signal on T1-weighted MR images of the head: a pictorial essay. *Clin Imaging* 25:312-319, 2001.
2. Enochs WS, Petherick P, Bogdanova A, et al: Paramagnetic metal scavenging by melanin: MR imaging. *Radiology* 204:417-423, 1997.
3. Haimes A, Zimmerman R, Morgello S, et al: MR imaging of brain abscesses. *AJR Am J Roentgenol* 152:1073-1085, 1989.
4. Janardhan V, Suri S, Bakshi R: Multiple sclerosis: hyperintense lesions in the brain on nonenhanced T1-weighted MR images evidenced as areas of T1 shortening. *Radiology* 244:823-831, 2007.
5. Lai P, Chen C, Liang H, Pan H: Hyperintense basal ganglia on T1-weighted MR imaging. *AJR Am J Roentgenol* 172:1109-1115, 1999.
6. Bonneville F, Cattin F, Marsot-Dupuch K, et al: T1 signal hyperintensity in the sellar region: spectrum of findings. *RadioGraphics* 26:93-113, 2006.
7. Mengiardi B, Pfirrmann CWA, Gerber C, et al: Frozen shoulder: MR arthrographic findings. *Radiology* 233:486-492, 2004.
8. Uchino A, Noguchi T, Nomiyama K, et al: Manganese accumulation in the brain: MR imaging. *Neuroradiology* 49:715-720, 2007.
9. Henkelman RM, Watts JF, Kucharczyk W: High signal intensity in MR images of calcified brain tissue. *Radiology* 179:199-206, 1991.
10. Shanley DJ: Mineralizing microangiopathy: CT and MRI. *Neuroradiology* 37:331-333, 1995.
11. Helms CA, Major NM, Anderson MW, , et al: *Musculoskeletal MRI*, 2nd ed. Philadelphia: Elsevier Saunders, 2008.
12. Vilanova JC, Barceló J, Smirniotopoulos G, et al: Hemangioma from head to toe: MR imaging with pathologic correlation. *RadioGraphics* 24:367-385, 2004.
13. Siegelman ES: *Body MRI*. Philadelphia: Elsevier Saunders, 2005.
14. Tchoyoson Lim CC, Dillon WP, McDermott MW: Mucocele involving the anterior clinoid process: MR and CT findings. *AJNR Am J Neuroradiol* 20:287-290, 1999.

Chapter 2

T2 Contrast

Scott M. Duncan and Timothy J. Amrhein

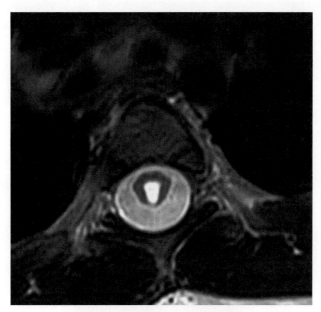

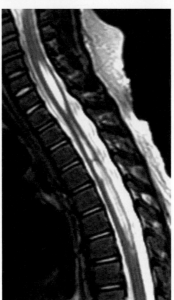

1. What type of sequence is this? How do you know?

2. What TR and TE parameters would you use to obtain T2 weighting with a spin echo sequence?

3. What tissues have long T2 relaxation times? Do they appear bright or dark on T2-weighted images?

4. What is the normal maximal diameter for the central canal?

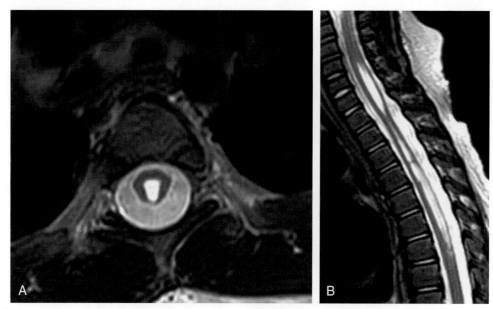

FIGURE 1A. Axial T2-weighted image of the thoracic spine demonstrates a large T2-hyperintense space involving the central canal and surrounding white matter.

FIGURE 1B. Sagittal T2-weighted image of the thoracic spine. Vertically oriented central hyperintensity extends throughout the cervical and thoracic cord.

1. These are T2-weighted sequences. This can be discerned because structures composed predominantly of water are bright (hyperintense) on T2-weighted sequences. Such structures include the cerebrospinal fluid in brain and spine images, the gallbladder or fluid in the abdomen, the bladder in the pelvis, and intra-articular synovial fluid in the extremities.

2. To achieve T2 weighting on a spin echo image, one would use a long time to repetition (TR) and an intermediate to long time to echo (TE).

3. Tissues that contain mostly water have long T2 relaxation times and they appear hyperintense (bright) on T2-weighted images. This is in contrast to tissues with long T1 relaxation times, which appear dark on T1-weighted sequences.

4. In adults, the central canal is often not identified as it is below the resolution of the scan. A canal diameter greater than 3 mm is considered to be abnormal.

Diagnosis: Syringohydromyelia.

Part 1: Basic Spin Principles and T2 Relaxation

After a radiofrequency (RF) pulse tips the net (or main) magnetization into the transverse plane, it will gradually lose phase coherence as individual protons will experience a dephasing process as a result of spin-spin interactions. This phenomenon is known as T2 or transverse relaxation (or decay). At the same time, the magnetization will also return to its original state via T1 or longitudinal relaxation (or recovery). This chapter focuses on the T2 or transverse relaxation.

An RF pulse generates a magnetic field oriented in the transverse (or *xy*) dimension. During its application, the net magnetization along the longitudinal direction will be tipped into the transverse plane. Immediately after this rotation, all protons naturally would have the same phase and thus phase coherence.[1] Once the RF pulse is turned off, there is progressive loss of phase coherence. This occurs because individual protons begin to precess at slightly different frequencies due to different local microenvironments and spin-spin interactions. The resultant slight differences in precession frequencies among protons causes phase dispersion, signal cancellation, and loss of transverse magnetization. It is important to note that transverse relaxation or decay is therefore due to loss of order (i.e., phase dispersion) rather than the loss of magnetization.

Why does this phase dispersion occur if all of the hydrogen protons are exposed to the same external magnetic field? It occurs because there are inherent inhomogeneities within the magnetic field that lead to differing magnetic microenvironments and subsequently slightly different proton precession frequencies. There are two separate causes of magnetic field inhomogeneity: inhomogeneities within the external magnetic field (T2′) and microscopic interactions between adjacent protons (T2). The combined loss of signal resulting from both of these causes is called T2* decay. The dephasing effects from the external magnetic field have a much larger contribution to T2* decay than do the T2 effects. Unfortunately, inhomogeneities that arise from the external magnetic field are independent of the patient and therefore provide little information about the patient. Fortunately, the loss of phase coherence from these static inhomogeneities can be reversed, for example, by a 180° refocusing pulse. (This point will become more important when we discuss spin echo imaging.) Loss of phase coherence arising from T2 effects is not reversible but does provide information about the

FREE INDUCTION DECAY

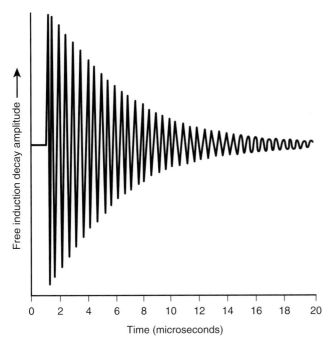

FIGURE 1. Free induction decay.

microenvironment that the proton is experiencing, aiding in tissue characterization.

Let's further explore the concept of T2*. A magnetic resonance (MR) signal can only be detected when the magnetization is in the transverse plane. When an RF pulse is applied, the magnetization vector is "tipped" into the transverse plane while still rotating about the z-axis at the Larmor frequency. The resultant MR signal appears as a sinusoidal wave, peaking when the vector is pointed toward the detector and reaching a trough when the vector is pointed 180° away from the detector. Further, remember that immediately after the RF pulse is turned off, phase dispersion occurs, causing a rapid and continuous fall in signal. The resultant waveform, called free induction decay (FID), is a combination of this declining magnetization and the 360° rotating signal. As shown in Figure 1, the FID appears as an oscillating waveform that rapidly falls to zero. The FID describes the detected MR signal, which experiences a rapid exponential loss at the rate of T2*.

The component of T2* that does provide information about the patient is the T2 relaxation. T2 relaxation occurs at an exponential rate analogous to T2* relaxation, except at the rate of T2. As mentioned previously, the T2 relaxation time is governed by individual protons' local environment and spin-spin interactions, resulting in phase dispersion. In general, all molecules are influenced by their local magnetic microenvironment, which fluctuates over time. Larger molecules have relatively slowly varying magnetic fields. As a result, this more static magnetic field variation results in some areas with stronger local magnetic fields and other areas with weaker local magnetic fields. These differences result in different precessing frequencies among the protons, causing significant dephasing. Smaller molecules (such as water), in contrast, are rapidly moving, leading to an averaging of the magnetic field variability (i.e., the smaller molecules experience a mixture of both

stronger and weaker magnetic fields that is averaged out over time). This leads to increased homogeneity of the experienced magnetic field, resulting in less phase dispersion and therefore longer T2 relaxation times. Unlike T1 relaxation times, T2 relaxation times are less dependent on magnetic field strength. T2 relaxation times for most tissues within the body range from 30 to 60 msec. The T2 relaxation time for cerebrospinal fluid, which is mostly free water, is 1000 msec.

T2-weighted (T2W) images are well suited for the detection and assessment of most pathologic processes, as pathology often results in increased water content, causing T2 hyperintensity relative to the isointense signal of normal soft tissue.

Part II: T2 Contrast and Pulse Sequence Considerations

Two general categories of sequences are employed to produce images weighted by transverse relaxation times: spin echo (SE) sequences and gradient-recalled echo (GRE) sequences. Pure T2W images can only be obtained with SE sequences. GRE sequences can produce T2*-weighted images, but are unable to produce purely T2W images for reasons that will be explained later.

Spin Echo

SE imaging involves an initial 90° RF pulse that tips the longitudinal magnetization into the transverse plane and aligns the phases. This is then followed by a 180° pulse that realigns the spins. Remember, when the initial 90° RF pulse is turned off, the protons immediately begin to dephase. Subsequently, a 180° RF pulse (also known as a "refocusing pulse") is used to reverse the precession direction of the protons (i.e., instead of rotating clockwise, they begin to rotate counterclockwise about the z-axis or vice versa). This has the intended effect of reversing the phase dispersion caused by static magnetic field inhomogeneities. The reversal occurs because the protons continue to precess at the same rate that they did in developing different phases; however, they now do so in the reverse direction. Thus, over the same amount of elapsed time a faster precessing proton that was able to change phase in relation to its slower precessing counterparts now precesses faster than the slower proton, but in the opposite direction, and effectively "catches back up" with the slower precessing proton. By this process, the transverse magnetization that was lost due to magnetic field inhomogeneities will be recovered (Figure 2). Therefore, any loss of signal in an SE sequence is from phase dispersion due to microscopic fluctuations in the magnetic field caused by the local molecules (i.e., pure T2 relaxation).

In SE sequences, there are two main parameters that affect the "weighting" of an image (i.e., T1, T2, or proton density weighting): the time to repetition (TR) and the time to echo (TE). In generating an image, the protons within a patient are repeatedly exposed to RF pulses in order to fill each line of K-space. During the first excitation, all of the longitudinal magnetization is "tipped" into the transverse plane. Over time, the longitudinal magnetization returns (or recovers) at a tissue-specific rate, which is based on its T1 relaxation time. If the TR is shorter than the time it takes to fully recover longitudinal magnetization (i.e., another 90° RF pulse is introduced prior to complete longitudinal magnetization recovery), then there will be less signal available to "tip" into the transverse plane with the next pulse. Given a short TR, substances with short T1 relaxation times will recover more longitudinal

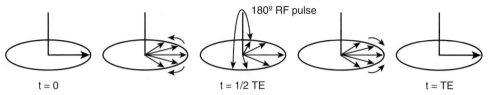

FIGURE 2. Effect of 180° refocusing pulse on phase dispersion. Once the initial 90° RF pulse is turned off, the protons begin to dephase. The 180° refocusing pulse reverses the phase dispersion and results in rephasing of the protons, which occurs maximally at TE (= 2τ in this figure). *Adapted from Clare S: Principles of magnetic resonance imaging. In Functional MRI: Methods and Applications. Doctor of Philosophy Thesis, October 1997, University of Nottingham, UK. Available at http://users.fmrib.ox.ac.uk/~stuart/thesis/chapter_2/section2_4.html.*

magnetization and will therefore appear hyperintense (bright), whereas substances with long T1 relaxation times will not recover signal prior to the next excitation pulse and will be hypointense (dark). In contradistinction, if the TR is long, then both tissues will fully recover their longitudinal relaxation and the T1 relaxation time will not significantly affect the final signal.

The TE is defined as the time between the first 90° RF pulse and the time of signal acquisition. As was previously described, SE sequences employ a 180° pulse to realign dephased spins and remove signal loss from magnetic field inhomogeneities. To acquire maximal signal in an SE image, the 180° RF pulse is placed at one half of the TE. In other words, the spins that *dephase* during the first half of the TE are subsequently *rephased* during the second half of the TE, which results in maximal signal at the time of signal acquisition. All signal loss is therefore secondary to the inherent T2 relaxation of the tissue (fluctuations in the local magnetic field secondary to the structures of the local molecules). An intermediate to long TE allows enough time for tissues with short T2 relaxation times to lose some signal (and appear hypointense), while tissues with long T2 relaxation times still retain most of their signal (and appear hyperintense). However, if the programmed TE is very short, not enough time will have elapsed to allow for any significant T2-related decay and no tissue will experience any significant transverse decay; therefore, there will be no contrast between different types of tissues.

As you can see from the description above, manipulation of the TR provides separation of tissues based on their T1 relaxation times and changing the TE results in tissue separation based on inherent T2 relaxation properties. The TE and TR can therefore be adjusted to maximize signal based upon either the T1 or the T2 relaxation properties of a tissue. This preferential bias toward one relaxation parameter versus another is referred to as "weighting." With T2W images, one minimizes the T1 relaxation effects on signal production by lengthening the TR, and maximizes the T2 relaxation effects by choosing an intermediate to long TE. As a memory aid, one might consider that T"1" is a smaller number than T"2"and thus has

smaller TRs and TEs. For a typical T2W image, the TR is greater than 2000 msec and the TE is greater than 100 msec.

Gradient-Recalled Echo

GRE sequences involve a single "excitation" RF pulse that transfers some of the longitudinal magnetization into the transverse plane, where it can be used to acquire signal. A significant difference between GRE sequences and standard SE sequences is the absence of a 180° refocusing pulse. Without this additional pulse, the phase dispersion caused by inhomogeneities in the main magnetic field is not corrected. Therefore, the loss of signal in a GRE sequence is due to T2* effects. As was previously described, these T2* effects are significantly influenced by the inhomogeneity in the external magnetic field and do not provide exclusive information about the relaxation properties of the tissue being imaged.

Recently, steady-state GRE sequences have been used that produce more weight on T2 and not T2* contrast. In steady-state imaging, both the longitudinal and transverse magnetization enter a steady state. In spoiled gradient imaging, the residual transverse magnetization after the echo has been recorded is usually spoiled by use of a spoiler gradient before the next TR. However, in steady-state imaging, the residual transverse magnetization is added back to the longitudinal magnetization, resulting in higher signal to noise ratio. The amount of residual transverse magnetization is based on the T2 time. Substances with long T2 times will have more residual magnetization to add back to the longitudinal magnetization, which can be used in subsequent excitations. Additionally, molecules with short T1 times will have recovered more longitudinal magnetization before the next TR, resulting in more magnetization in subsequent excitations. Thus, the steady-state sequences are T2/T1 weighted. In other words, substances that have long T2 times (water) and short T1 times (fat) will be bright on these sequences.[1] These sequences are commonly used in cardiac imaging and in imaging the base of the skull, where high-resolution thin-slice T2W images are used. Further discussion about steady-state imaging and its role in cardiac imaging is provided in Chapter 10.

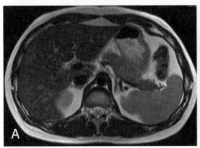 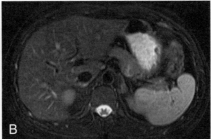 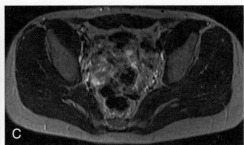

FIGURE 2A. Axial T2W fast spin echo (FSE) image of the abdomen: normal, with bright fat signal.

FIGURE 2B. Axial T2W FSE image with fat saturation of the abdomen: normal, with dark fat signal.

FIGURE 2C. Axial T2W SE image of the pelvis: normal, with intermediate gray signal of fat.

Diagnosis: Normal fat appearance on FSE, fat saturation (fat-sat) FSE, and SE sequences.

Physics Discussion

As was mentioned in the beginning of the chapter, T2W images have a relatively long TR to allow the longitudinal magnetization to recover. In order to shorten the total scan time, multiple 180° refocusing pulses can be applied (and thus multiple echoes collected) during a single TR interval. The number of refocusing pulses applied during a single TR interval is called the echo train length or turbo factor. Imaging time reduction is directly proportional to the echo train length (i.e., for an echo train length of 9, the imaging time is reduced by a factor of 9). These sequences are known as turbo or fast spin echo (FSE) sequences. The number of additional echoes depends on the length of the TR. Sequences with longer TRs, such as T2W images, can fit 8 or more TEs into each TR. Blurring occurs in sequences with short TEs, such as T1-weighted (T1W) and proton density images, so only a short echo train length of 3 to 7 can be used. Because of its much improved image time, the FSE technique has completely replaced conventional SE imaging for T2W imaging. In fact, most residents and young attendings have never seen an SE T2W imaging sequence in clinical practice.

The FSE sequences allow T2W images of the abdomen to be obtained in a single breath hold. This is not possible with the SE technique and is why the SE image shown in Case 2 is of the pelvis. Imaging the abdomen with an SE sequence would have resulted in blurring secondary to respiratory motion artifact unless a respiratory triggering or gating method is applied.

One consequence of the FSE technique is the relatively increased signal intensity of fat in comparison with a conventional SE image (this is one reason why T2W sequences are often fat-saturated or inversion recovery sequences). As you may recall, fat has a relatively short T2 relaxation time secondary to its large molecular size, which results in rapid loss of transverse magnetization. Further, fat molecules are subject to signal loss secondary to a phenomenon called J-coupling, which is a very complex topic and applies more to nuclear magnetic resonance spectroscopy than to MR imaging. Macromolecules, such as lipids, share electrons between their nuclei via the electron cloud, causing a slight alteration in the local magnetic fields of different nuclei on the same molecule. This, in turn, results in a change in the precessional frequencies of these different nuclei leading to a rapid dephasing that occurs in addition to the normal T2 dephasing. This phenomenon is referred to as J-coupling and explains why fat appears with low to intermediate signal on T2W SE sequences. Why, then, does fat appear *brighter* when using FSE techniques? The answer lies in the multiple refocusing pulses employed in an FSE sequence, which do not allow sufficient time for J-coupling dephasing to occur. This prolongs the overall T2 relaxation of fat and leads to the relatively higher signal of the fat on the FSE T2W image in comparison with the conventional SE T2W image.

Case 3

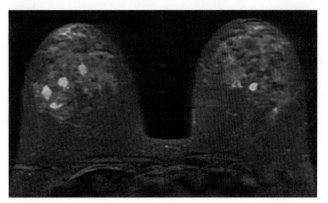

FIGURE 3. Axial T2W FSE image with fat saturation (fat-sat): multiple bilateral T2-hyperintense lesions within the breasts consistent with simple cysts.

Diagnosis: Multiple bilateral simple breast cysts.

Discussion: The criteria for diagnosing a simple cyst within the breast on magnetic resonance imaging (MRI) are similar to those in ultrasound. The cyst is usually homogeneously hyperintense (fluid bright) on a T2W image and should demonstrate a smooth contour. On a T1W image, the cyst is usually uniformly hypointense and should exhibit no internal enhancement after the administration of contrast. A thin rim of peripheral enhancement is acceptable.[2,3]

Case 4

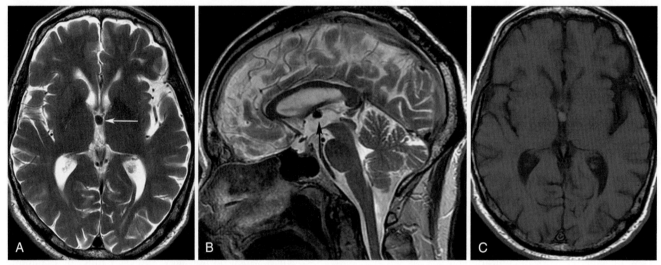

FIGURE 4A. Axial T2W image. A small homogeneous T2-hypointense mass is seen in the region of the foramen of Monro *(arrow)*.

FIGURE 4B. Sagittal T2W image. The T2-hypointense mass is redemonstrated in the region of the foramen of Monro *(arrow)*.

FIGURE 4C. Axial T1W image. The mass exhibits T1 hyperintensity.

Diagnosis: Colloid cyst.

Discussion: There are many different appearances of cysts on MRI. Colloid cysts are typically T2 hyperintense. However, in this case the concentration of internal protein and paramagnetic material is high, which results in T2 hypointensity and

T1 hyperintensity. Colloid cysts have a very characteristic location at the foramen of Monro, which greatly aids in their diagnosis.[4] As with other cysts, colloid cysts should be homogeneous and should not exhibit central enhancement.

Case 5

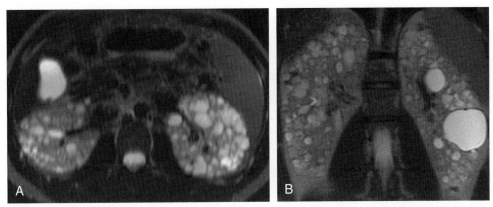

FIGURE 5A. Axial T2W fat-sat FSE image.

FIGURE 5B. Sagittal half-Fourier single-shot turbo spin echo (HASTE) T2W image. Both images demonstrate innumerable heterogeneous T2-hyperintense foci within the bilateral kidneys.

Diagnosis: Autosomal dominant polycystic kidney disease.

Discussion: The cysts in this case have a heterogeneous appearance. Many exhibit fluid-bright T2 hyperintensity, others are intermediate in signal, and a few are T2 hypointense (dark). The heterogeneity reflects variable protein and blood product content within the different renal cysts.

Physics Discussion

True cysts occur throughout the body and typically have a characteristic appearance on MRI regardless of their location. In general, cysts appear fluid bright on T2W images (T2 hyperintense) and dark on T1W images (T1 hypointense). Additionally, true simple cysts should contain a thin wall and be devoid of internal enhancement on postcontrast T1W images. However, the imaging characteristics of cysts can vary secondary to changes in their internal composition. The main determinants of a cyst's MR signal characteristics include the internal protein concentration, the presence of internal paramagnetic material (most commonly in the form of blood products), and the concentration of free water within the cyst.[5] Cysts that contain mostly free water and little protein or other material will demonstrate the "typical" fluid-bright T2-hyperintense signal and T1-hypointense signal. However, as the concentration of protein and/or paramagnetic material increases within the cyst, it will become more and more T1 hyperintense. Cysts typically maintain their T2 hyperintensity until the internal concentration of protein and/or paramagnetic materials increases over 50%. When this occurs, the short T2 relaxation times of the large protein macromolecules (and paramagnetic substances) will dominate, resulting in the cyst appearing dark (hypointense) on T2W images. This phenomenon is most clearly exemplified in Case 4, the colloid cyst.

CASE 6

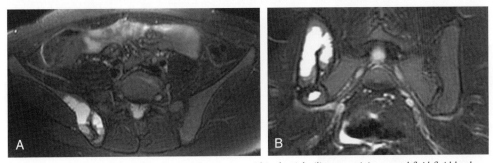

FIGURE 6A. Axial T2W fat-sat FSE image of the pelvis. A cystic mass is seen within the right ilium containing several fluid-fluid levels.

FIGURE 6B. Coronal T2W fat-sat FSE image of the pelvis. The expansile cystic mass within the right iliac bone is redemonstrated.

Diagnosis: Aneurysmal bone cyst.

Discussion: Fluid-fluid levels on an MR image of an expansile lytic bone lesion were once thought to be pathognomonic for an aneurysmal bone cyst. However, multiple lesions have since been shown to contain fluid levels, including telangiectatic osteosarcomas and chondroblastomas. Fluid-fluid levels occur secondary to dependent stagnant blood products that layer within these dilated spaces.[4] The blood products shorten the T2 relaxivity of the lesion and result in areas of relative T2 hypointensity.

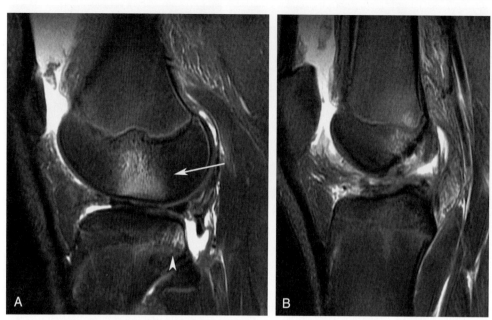

FIGURE 7A. Sagittal T2W fat-sat FSE image along the lateral aspect of the knee. Increased signal within the bone marrow of the lateral femoral condyle *(arrow)* as well as within the posterolateral aspect of the tibial plateau *(arrowhead)* is consistent with a "pivot shift" contusion pattern.

FIGURE 7B. Sagittal T2W fat-sat FSE image focused over the intercondylar notch. Conspicuous absence of discernable anterior cruciate ligament (ACL) fibers is consistent with an ACL tear.

Diagnosis: Pivot shift marrow contusion pattern with associated ACL tear.

Discussion: This case demonstrates T2 hyperintensity within the bone marrow of the lateral femoral condyle and the posterolateral tibial plateau consistent with edema. This contusion pattern occurs after the ACL has been torn, which allows the tibia to move anteriorly in relation to the femur, resulting in contact between the posterior aspect of the lateral tibial plateau and the lateral femoral condyle.

Physics Discussion

T2 hyperintensity within the bone marrow is consistent with extracellular edema. There are multiple etiologies for bone marrow edema, including trauma (contusions and fractures), neoplasms, and infection.

CASES 8, 9, AND 10: COMPANION CASES

Case 8

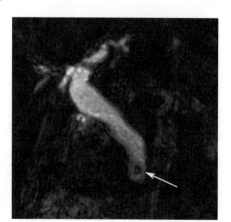

Diagnosis: Common bile duct stones resulting in biliary ductal dilation.

Discussion: The MRCP image well delineates the hypointense bile duct stones within the distal common bile duct. There is resultant marked biliary duct dilation.

FIGURE 8. Coronal magnetic resonance cholangiopancreatography (MRCP) image through the common bile duct. There is a rounded focus of hypointensity within the common bile duct *(arrow)* resulting in moderate to severe biliary duct dilation.

Case 9

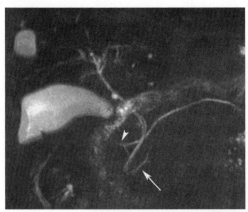

FIGURE 9. MRCP maximum intensity projection (MIP). Nondilated pancreatic and biliary ducts are seen. Note that the ducts of Wirsung *(arrow)* and Santorini *(arrowhead)* empty into the duodenum at different locations.

Case 10

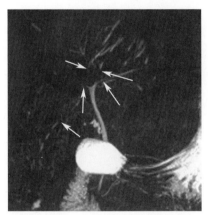

FIGURE 10. MRCP MIP. Focal areas of narrowing *(arrows)* are seen within the central intrahepatic bile ducts. Note also the prominent intrahepatic biliary dilation within the left hepatic lobe.

Diagnosis: Primary sclerosing cholangitis (PSC).

Discussion: Focal areas of alternating stricture and dilation of the biliary system are characteristic of PSC. Realizing that the central intrahepatic ducts are not visible secondary to severe narrowing and that the peripheral intrahepatic ducts are dilated within the left hepatic lobe is critical to establishing this diagnosis. Remember, the biliary ductal system should always increase in caliber moving centrally toward the hilum. The reverse is occurring in this case.

Physics Discussion

MRCP has become an increasingly utilized technique for the evaluation of the biliary system, particularly within the last 10 years. It has several obvious advantages over endoscopic retrograde cholangiopancreatography in that it is noninvasive, is less expensive, often provides better and more detailed delineation of the anatomy, and can provide additional information about extraductal pathology. While MRCP images may appear to be the result of a drastically different type of MR sequence

Diagnosis: Pancreas divisum.

Discussion: Pancreas divisum occurs when the duct of Santorini, which drains the body and tail of the pancreas, fails to fuse with the duct of Wirsung, which drains the head of the pancreas. It is the most common anatomic anomaly of the pancreas and occurs in 5% to 14% of the population.[6] While the clinical significance of this finding is debatable, many patients with this anatomic variant are reported to have increased rates of abdominal pain and pancreatitis. MRCP well demonstrates a duct crossing the common bile duct (in between the duodenum and the common bile duct) to empty into the duodenum. Identification of this anomalous "crossing duct sign" allows one to make the diagnosis of a pancreas divisum.

and technique, they are, in actuality, simply a heavily T2W sequence. The resultant images exhibit extreme contrast with very little in the way of intermediate shades of gray. How is this type of image produced? Recall that lengthening the TE of a sequence allows the protons more time to lose their transverse magnetization secondary to pure T2 relaxation. Standard T2W sequences employ an intermediate to long TE time that allows for the differences in the T2 relaxation times between different tissues to become more apparent. Care is taken with these sequences to assign a TE that is not too long because this will result in loss of the entirety of the transverse magnetization within the imaged tissues and subsequently absence of signal. With MRCP images, the TE is drastically lengthened so that the transverse magnetization from short T2 molecules (essentially everything in the body except water) is nearly completely lost, resulting in absence of signal. Since water has a very long T2 relaxation time, it is able to retain most of its transverse magnetization and continues to appear hyperintense. As bile is mostly composed of water, it too has a long T2 relaxation and produces considerable signal despite the very long TE. This is the basis for an MRCP image, which essentially eliminates all signal except that within the biliary system.

The above explanation of the MRCP technique applies to an SE-based sequence. However, MRCP can also be performed using a steady-state GRE sequence, which has both T1 and T2 weighting. Because GRE MRCP is T1 and T2 weighted, not only will water appear bright (because of its T2 properties) but fat and blood can also appear bright (because of their T1 properties).

The advent of gadolinium-based contrast agents with significant biliary excretion (such as gadoxetate disodium [Eovist]) allows for a new methodology in the MR evaluation of the biliary system. With these new agents, the contrast is excreted into the biliary system, allowing for the acquisition of an MR cholangiogram on delayed images. This can be conceptualized as analogous to an evaluation of the collecting system via computed tomographic urography and renally excreted iodinated contrast. However, it is important to recognize that evaluation of the pancreatic system is not possible with this method as the contrast agent will only be present within the bile. This technique demonstrates considerable promise, particularly for the purposes of problem solving and for further

evaluation when a traditional T2W MRCP image is nondiagnostic secondary to patient motion. Further, imaging with biliary-excreted contrast agents can provide physiologic information about the biliary system not otherwise available with traditional imaging techniques.[7]

CASES 11, 12, AND 13: COMPANION CASES

Case 11

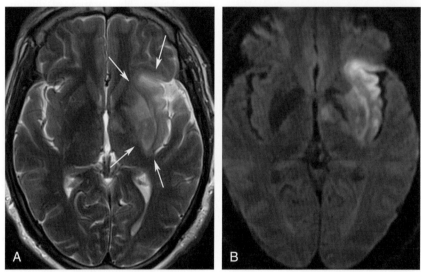

FIGURE 11A. Axial T2W FSE image. Increased T2 signal is identified within the left insula, internal capsule, and basal ganglia *(arrows)*.

FIGURE 11B. Axial diffusion-weighted image. Hyperintense signal is seen corresponding to the areas of T2 hyperintensity on the prior image. This is suggestive of restricted diffusion, but should be confirmed by comparison to an apparent diffusion coefficient (ADC) map.

Diagnosis: Right middle cerebral artery (MCA) territory acute stroke.

Discussion: This case represents a classic right MCA distribution acute stroke. Increased T2 signal within the area of

infarct arises 6 to 24 hours after the acute occlusion and peaks at 3 to 7 days.[8] The edema can persist for 6 to 8 weeks even after the blood-brain barrier has been restored.

Case 12

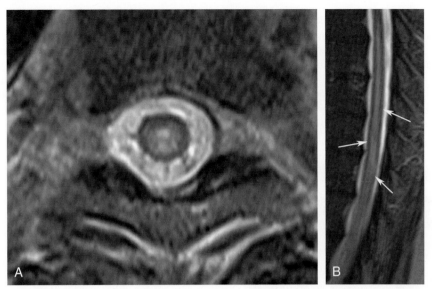

FIGURE 12A. Axial T2W FSE image of the thoracic spinal cord. T2 hyperintensity is seen within the central portion of an expanded cord.

FIGURE 12B. Sagittal T2W image of the thoracic spine. T2 hyperintensity and cord expansion *(arrows)* extends from the midthoracic cord inferiorly.

Diagnosis: Spinal cord ischemia and infarct.

Discussion: The involvement of the central gray matter of the cord and the long craniocaudal extent of the abnormality suggests cord ischemia. In ischemia, the gray matter is primarily involved because of its increased energy requirements.

However, in severe cases one may note additional involvement of the white matter. The T2 hyperintensity is a result of cytotoxic edema in an manner analogous to infarctions in the brain.

Case 13

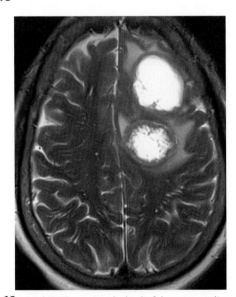

FIGURE 13. Axial T2W image at the level of the corona radiata. Two T2-hyperintense masses are identified within the left frontal lobe. T2 hyperintensity consistent with edema is present in the adjacent white matter.

Diagnosis: Vasogenic edema secondary to multiple brain metastases from lung cancer.

Discussion: The two most common subtypes of edema within the brain are cytotoxic and vasogenic edema. While there are often components of both types in a disease process, one usually predominates. It is very important to be able to distinguish between these two patterns of edema as they suggest different etiologies and therefore different diagnoses. To understand the pattern of edema, is it important to review the pathologic cause of each type of edema.

Cytotoxic edema occurs when there is a breakdown of cellular metabolism, the most common cause of which is infarction. After the initial insult, the sodium-potassium pump stops working appropriately, resulting in an influx of water into the intracellular space due to ion imbalances and resultant osmosis. Thus, cytotoxic edema is secondary to an intracellular accumulation of water. As opposed to vasogenic edema, cytotoxic edema occurs maximally in the gray matter because of the increased energy demand in comparison with the white matter, but also occurs in the white matter.[9] In addition, since it is most often due to infarct, the edema is usually wedge shaped and extends all the way to the cortex. To summarize, cytotoxic edema, as the result of an ischemic infarct, involves both gray and white matter, is usually wedge shaped, and extends to the cortex.

In contradistinction, vasogenic edema is due to breakdown of the blood-brain barrier, and results in extracellular edema, as opposed to intracellular edema. The result is that vasogenic edema primarily occurs within the white matter tracts where the extracellular space is less rigid than in the gray matter. The most common causes are tumors, trauma, and ischemic injury.[9]

Both cytotoxic and vasogenic edema can occur in the setting of a cerebral infarct. Initially, because of the lack of oxygen and energy, there is a resultant cytotoxic edema. However, prolonged deprivation leads to cellular death (including death of the cells that establish the blood-brain barrier), which causes a breakdown of the blood-brain barrier tight junctions and a superimposed vasogenic edema.[9] This vasogenic edema is the major component that results in the significant swelling that can occur a few days after a stroke, leading to mass effect and herniation.

CASE 14

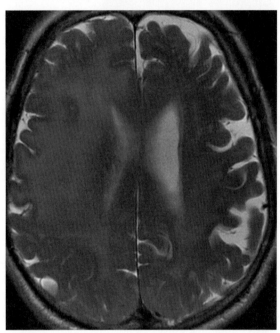

FIGURE 14. Axial T2W image at the level of the corona radiata. Diffuse T2 hyperintensity is seen throughout the right cerebral hemisphere with thickening of the gyri.

Diagnosis: Gliomatosis cerebri.

Discussion: Gliomatosis cerebri is a diffusely infiltrative glioma that occupies most of one cerebral hemisphere. As in Case 14, there is relative preservation of the underlying neural architecture. Characteristically, MR images demonstrate an area of diffuse T2 hyperintensity involving predominantly the white matter with some involvement of the gray matter as well. These areas typically do not enhance after the administration of contrast. While the pattern and appearance are similar to vasogenic edema, the findings actually represent diffuse tumor involvement.

Physics Discussion

This case provides an excellent opportunity to further elucidate the physics behind T2 hyperintensity as well as point out a common misunderstanding in MR neuroradiology. Anaplastic astrocytomas and glioblastoma multiforme lesions (GBMs) exhibit adjacent T2 hyperintensity that is often erroneously described as vasogenic edema. While the appearance of this "edema" is very similar to the vasogenic edema identified in the setting of other intracranial pathology (such as in the metastatic lesions in Case 13), pathologic evaluation of these areas often demonstrates a combination of both edema and tumor cells. Thus, in the setting of an astrocytoma, *any* adjacent T2 hyperintensity is assumed to represent tumor infiltration. Consider the underlying physics: any process that results in T2 relaxation prolongation will cause hyperintensity on a T2W image. Avoid the common pitfall of assuming that all areas of T2 hyperintensity represent edema alone.

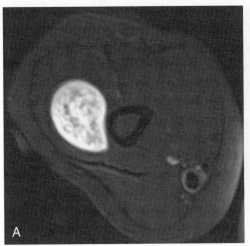 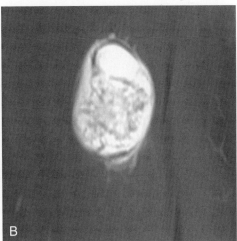

FIGURES 15A AND 15B. T2W fat-sat FSE images of the distal humerus in the axial (A) and coronal (B) planes. A T2-hyperintense mass is seen adjacent to the humerus.

Diagnosis: Peripheral nerve schwannoma.

Physics Discussion

Peripheral nerve tumors exhibit characteristic T2 hyperintensity. Identifying a solid lesion with these signal characteristics in the soft tissues of an extremity can help to narrow one's differential diagnosis to synovial cell sarcoma and a peripheral nerve sheath tumor. Further identifying an association between the lesion and an adjacent nerve is essentially diagnostic of a peripheral nerve tumor. Differentiating between a schwannoma and a neurofibroma (types of peripheral nerve tumors) is often not possible. However, schwannomas are considered to be typically located eccentric to the nerve, while neurofibromas are often centered on the nerve.[10] The etiology of the T2 hyperintensity found in peripheral nerve tumors is multifactorial and includes a combination of cystic changes, generalized increased vascularity of these tumors, and intrinsic high water content.

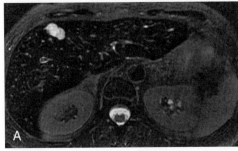 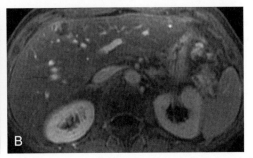

FIGURE 16A. Axial T2W fat-sat image of the liver. A homogeneously T2-hyperintense lesion is seen within the anterior aspect of the right hepatic lobe.

FIGURE 16B. Axial postcontrast T1W fat-sat image of the liver. Note the peripheral nodular enhancement of the lesion.

Diagnosis: Hepatic hemangioma.

Physics Discussion

Similar to schwannomas, hemangiomas demonstrate fluid-bright T2 hyperintensity. Additionally, hemangiomas often exhibit a characteristic peripheral nodular enhancement on postcontrast T1W images, which establishes their diagnosis (see Fig. 16B). The T2 hyperintensity occurs secondary to slow-flowing blood coursing through dilated vascular spaces within the mass.[11] Blood contains intrinsic long T2 relaxation times (with resultant T2 hyperintensity) secondary to its high free water component. The slow velocity of the blood within the hemangioma prevents signal loss from flow voids (discussed further in Chapter 10).

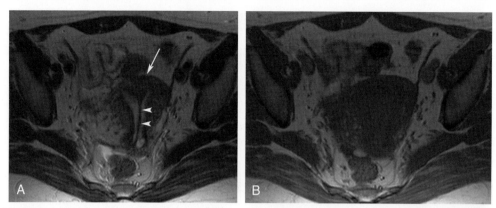

FIGURE 17A. Axial T2W image of the pelvis. The uterus has two separate cavities separated by a thin black septum *(arrowheads)*. Note that the uterine fundal contour is convex *(arrow)*.

FIGURE 17B. Axial T1W image of the pelvis. The uterus is homogeneously gray, precluding accurate evaluation of uterine anatomy.

Diagnosis: Septate uterus.

Discussion: Differentiating a septate uterus from a bicornuate uterus can be difficult. However, the distinction is important as it changes both the treatment options and the prognosis for pregnancy. A septate uterus is secondary to failure of resorption of the septum after fusion of the müllerian ducts. A bicornuate uterus is secondary to failure of complete fusion of the müllerian ducts. Bicornuate uteri will have endometrium and myometrium separating the two cavities, while septate uteri will have only a separating fibrous septum. Patients with bicornuate uteri have fewer problems with infertility. If one is unable to distinguish distinct endometrial and myometrial tissue separating the two cavities, then evaluating the fundal contour may be helpful. The fundal contour is convex in a septate uterus (as in this case) and concave in a bicornuate uterus.[12]

Physics Discussion

T2W images provide an excellent evaluation of the female pelvis as they clearly demarcate the zonal anatomy of the uterus.[13] The central endometrium is T2 hyperintense secondary to the presence of mucinous glands and a highly vascularized stroma. The junctional zone, or inner myometrium, is dark on T2W images as it contains densely organized smooth muscle fibers and a paucity of free water. This morphology results in shortening of the T2 relaxation time and a decrease in resultant signal. The outer myometrial layer exhibits a relative T2 hyperintensity secondary to a higher free water content as well as to the presence of less densely packed smooth muscle fibers.[12]

It is often difficult to identify the type of pulse sequence used to produce a female pelvic MR image, particularly when only a single image is offered (such as in a case conference setting). When this situation arises, an evaluation of the uterus may be particularly helpful in determining the sequence type. The uterus is characteristically homogeneously gray in signal on T1W sequences (see Fig. 17B). In contradistinction, if the trizonal anatomy of the uterus is identifiable, then the sequence is T2W.

Case 18

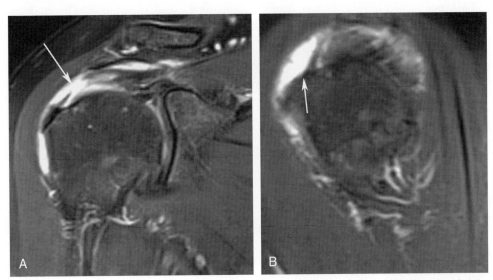

FIGURE 18A. Coronal oblique T2W image of the shoulder. T2 hyperintensity is seen completely disrupting the supraspinatus tendon *(arrow)* with mild retraction of the tendon.

FIGURE 18B. Sagittal oblique T2W image of the shoulder. Fluid-bright T2 hyperintensity is seen in the expected location of the supraspinatus tendon *(arrow)*.

Diagnosis: Full-thickness tear of the supraspinatus tendon (rotator cuff tear).

Discussion: Fluid-bright T2-hyperintense signal replaces the supraspinatus tendon, which is retracted. Findings are diagnostic for a full-thickness tear of the rotator cuff.

Case 19

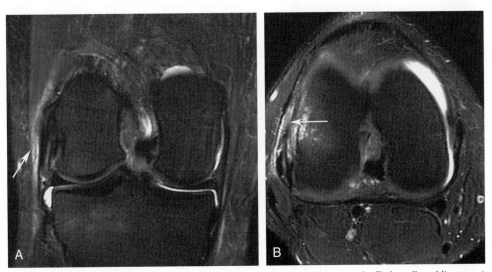

FIGURE 19A. Coronal T2W fat-sat image of the knee. T2 hyperintensity is seen in the tissues adjacent to the fibular collateral ligament *(arrow)*.

FIGURE 19B. Axial T2W fat-sat image of the knee at the level of the femoral condyles. T2 hyperintensity is seen adjacent to and within the fibular collateral ligament *(arrow)*.

Diagnosis: Fibular collateral ligament sprain.

Discussion: The T2 hyperintensity within the soft tissues immediately adjacent to the fibular collateral ligament is edema. Additionally, note the increased T2 signal within the substance of the fibular collateral ligament, which implies internal injury and a more severe sprain.

Physics Discussion

Tendons and ligaments both consist of large ordered collagen fibers containing very little internal water and therefore very few freely mobile protons. As a result of this relative paucity of mobile protons, variations in the magnetic field cannot be readily dispersed and rapid loss of transverse magnetization occurs as a result of dephasing. This produces the dark (almost black) signal identified in these structures on T2W images. This facilitates the detection of pathology, which typically manifests as edema and T2 hyperintensity. For this reason, MRI has a very high sensitivity and specificity for ligament and tendon pathology. Fluid-bright T2 hyperintensity within both tendons and ligaments represents fluid intercalation within their substance and implies fiber disruption, or a tear. Descriptions of the subtypes of tendon injury and tears are beyond the intended scope of this chapter, but can be found in many excellent clinically oriented musculoskeletal MRI books.

CASE 20

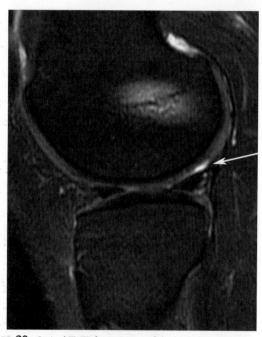

FIGURE 20. Sagittal T2W fat-sat image of the knee through lateral femoral condyle. A focal area of T2 hyperintensity is seen along the posterior aspect of the lateral femoral condyle *(arrow)*.

Diagnosis: Partial-thickness cartilage defect.

Physics Discussion

Evaluating for cartilage abnormalities is an integral component in the interpretation of musculoskeletal MRI. While several viable options exist, T2W MR sequences are excellent for detecting cartilage pathology. Cartilage irregularities and defects represent loss of normal cartilage, which is replaced by intra-articular fluid. Therefore, these defects are hyperintense on T2W sequences and are rather conspicuous secondary to their excellent contrast with the adjacent intermediate- to low-signal cartilage.[14] Cartilage actually contains an abundance of water molecules. However, they are bound within the rigid molecular structure of the cartilage molecule, precluding their free mobility. This prevents dispersion of the magnetic field variations and results in a persistence of the inhomogeneities that cause dephasing and signal loss. While this principle results in signal loss, the bound water molecules still exhibit relatively long T2 relaxation times in comparison to other tissues in the body (just less than those of free water). Therefore, the combination of these effects leads to the resultant intermediate to low signal of cartilage on T2W images.

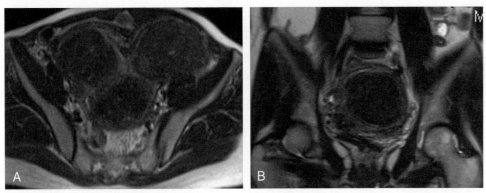

FIGURE 21A. Axial T2W image of the pelvis. Multiple low-signal masses are seen throughout the uterus.

FIGURE 21B. Coronal T2W image of the pelvis. The dominant low-signal intrauterine mass is redemonstrated.

Diagnosis: Uterine leiomyomas.

Physics Discussion

Similar to the junctional zone, leiomyomas contain numerous tightly packed smooth muscle cells and very little free water/intercellular space. This results in an abundance of large molecules and a tissue structure that contains short T2 relaxation times, producing low signal on T2W images. It should be noted, however, that fibroids may contain some areas of internal T2 hyperintensity if they have undergone degeneration/necrosis.

The densely packed cells can also occur in neoplasms such as central nervous system lymphoma. In addition to the sparse intercellular matrix, there is also a high nuclear-to-cytoplasmic ratio. This results in a relative paucity of free intracellular water, which results in short T2 relaxation times and low signal throughout the mass. Other densely packed tumors include GBMs, medulloblastomas, and pineoblastomas.

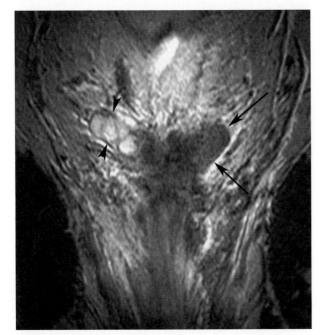

FIGURE 22. Coronal T2W image through the seminal vesicles. The expected normal T2 hyperintensity, as visualized within the right seminal vesicle *(arrowheads),* has been replaced by T2 hypointensity within the left seminal vesicle *(arrows).*

Diagnosis: Prostate adenocarcinoma invasion into the left seminal vesicle.

Physics Discussion

Prostate MRI is not typically used for the diagnosis of prostate cancer, but rather for staging the disease. MRI is used to determine tumor resectability. Findings that preclude surgical intervention include invasion into the periprostatic fat, invasion into the seminal vesicles, the presence of lymph node involvement, and the presence of osseous metastatic disease. Normal seminal vesicles are T2 hyperintense secondary to the physiologic fluid that they produce and contain. However, invasion with prostate adenocarcinoma causes a fibrotic reaction that replaces the seminal vesicle and manifests as T2 hypointensity. The low signal is secondary to the relative paucity of free water and to the presence of macromolecules in the fibrotic tissue, both of which cause shortening of the T2 relaxation time.

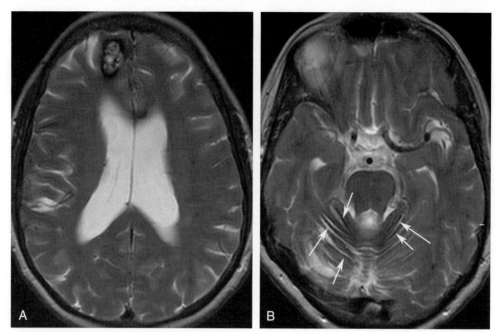

FIGURE 23A. Axial T2W FSE image of the brain at the level of the lateral ventricles. A heterogeneous mass is identified within the right frontal lobe that contains a thick rim of black signal.

FIGURE 23B. Axial T2W FSE image of the brain at the level of the cerebellum. There is a thin rim of black signal outlining the cerebellar fovia *(arrows)*.

Diagnosis: Cavernoma with superficial siderosis.

Physics Discussion

Hemorrhage has a complex appearance on MR based upon its age. It can be either hyper- or hypointense on both T1W and T2W images, but is a common cause of T2 hypointensity. Cavernous malformations, or cavernomas, are dilated endothelial cell–lined spaces without interposed normal brain. Cavernomas have a propensity to hemorrhage and often contain blood degradation products of varying stages. This can result in heterogeneous internal MR signal. However, cavernomas often demonstrate a characteristic thin rim of dark signal on T2W MR images. This finding occurs because macrophages and microglial cells collect iron from blood breakdown products and transport them to the periphery of the lesion. These iron aggregates are stored as hemosiderin and are extremely paramagnetic. As is described in more detail in Chapter 8, paramagnetic substances significantly alter the local magnetic field, which results in rapid loss of transverse magnetization and the absence of signal production (i.e., a very short T2 relaxation time). This characteristic peripheral rim of dark signal is well demonstrated in Figure 23A.

The second image (see Fig. 23B) exhibits findings suggestive of multiple prior hemorrhages within the cavernoma. A subtle lining of T2 hypointensity is identified along the folia of the cerebellum, which is suggestive of diffuse hemosiderin deposition. This finding is termed *superficial siderosis* and is the result of multiple repeated hemorrhages within the subarachnoid space. With repeated hemorrhages and over time, the hemosiderin blood products accumulate dependently within the subarachnoid space (often along the cerebellar folia, as in this example). Superficial siderosis can be the sequela of any etiology of repeated subarachnoid hemorrhage, including cavernomas, arteriovenous malformations, chronic warfarin therapy, and alcoholism.[15]

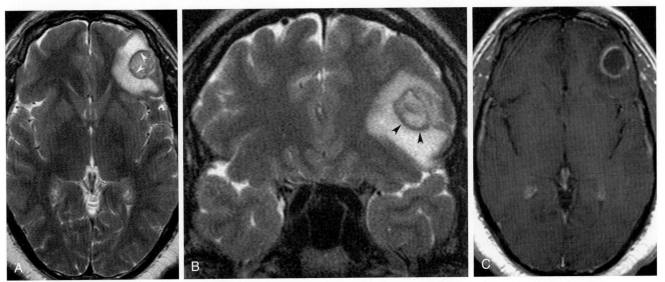

FIGURES 24A AND 24B. Axial (A) and coronal (B) T2W FSE images of the brain. There is an intermediate-signal mass with a subtle rim of T2 hypointensity (*arrowheads*, B).

FIGURE 24C. Axial postcontrast T1W image of the brain. The mass demonstrates a peripheral rim of enhancement.

Diagnosis: Brain abscess with thin T2-hypointense rim.

Physics Discussion

The differential diagnosis for an intra-axial rim-enhancing mass is lengthy and nonspecific. There is, however, an MRI finding that can narrow the differential diagnosis. Brain abscesses often exhibit a peripheral rim of low signal intensity on T2W images representing their capsule. A proposed etiology for this hypointensity is the high concentration of oxygen free radicals secondary to macrophages entering the capsule. These free radicals are highly paramagnetic, which causes magnetic susceptibility and considerable effective shortening of the T2 relaxation time (with concomitant low T2 signal). Of note, acute abscesses do not demonstrate this peripheral T2-hypointense rim as they have not yet formed a capsule.

Physics

1. T2 relaxation reflects the process in which the transverse magnetization loses phase coherence, which is an exponential decay at the rate of T2.
2. Loss of transverse magnetization is primarily due to phase dispersion (loss of phase coherence) among the precessing protons.
3. Loss of phase coherence is due to inhomogeneities in the main magnetic field and the spin-spin interactions in the protons' local microenvironment; together these create T2* effects.
4. Free induction decay (FID) is the oscillating waveform that occurs when the RF pulse is turned off and reflects the decaying transverse magnetization. T2* effects determine the rate at which FID occurs.
5. T2 is the loss of magnetization solely due to proton spin-spin interactions within the protons' microscopic environment.
6. Quantitatively, the T2 time for a tissue is the time at which 63% of the original signal is lost during the exponential T2 decay.
7. Since T2 reflects time to loss of signal, tissues with long T2 times will be bright and tissues with short T2 times will be dark on T2W images.
8. Macromolecules have short T2 times (T2 hypointense). Water has a long T2 time (T2 hyperintense).
9. A T2W sequence has a long TR and an intermediate-to-long TE.
10. Gradient sequences can produce a T2*-weighted sequence, but cannot produce a purely T2W image as they do not employ a 180° phase refocusing pulse.
11. Image acquisition times can be reduced in SE sequences by applying multiple 180° RF excitation pulses per each TR. This allows for the collection of multiple lines of K-space during each TR and is called a turbo or fast spin echo (FSE) sequence.
12. The decrease in image acquisition time is proportional to the number of RF pulses that occur during each TR. This is called the turbo factor or echo train length.
13. Fat appears brighter on T2W FSE images than on T2W SE images because the repeated RF pulses disrupt J-coupling.
14. MRCP is a heavily T2W sequence that allows enough time for phase dispersion to occur in just about all tissues except those containing abundant free water (such as bile).
15. Tissues that are highly ordered, have a paucity of water, or have tightly packed cells are T2 hypointense.
16. Paramagnetic substances such as blood degradation products and oxygen free radicals are also hypointense on T2W images secondary to magnetic susceptibility effects.

Clinical

1. The central canal of the spinal cord is usually not identifiable and is considered pathologic if greater than 3 mm.
2. Cysts are typically bright on T2W images, but can be isointense to hypointense on T2W images with greater concentrations of protein and blood product content.
3. Fluid-fluid levels within a lytic bone lesion were classically thought to be pathognomonic for an aneurysmal bone cyst; however, several benign and malignant bone lesions can exhibit this MR finding.
4. Identification of a "crossing duct sign" on MRCP is diagnostic of a pancreas divisum.
5. The two most common causes of edema within the brain are cytotoxic and vasogenic.
6. Cytotoxic edema results from increased intracellular water secondary to dysfunction of the sodium-potassium pump. The most common etiology for cytotoxic edema is an infarct.
7. Vasogenic edema occurs secondary to breakdown of the blood-brain barrier and is most commonly secondary to malignancy.
8. The T2 hyperintensity often identified around gliomas does not represent vasogenic edema alone, but may also represent tumor extension.
9. Peripheral nerve sheath tumors are characteristically hyperintense on T2W images.
10. Hepatic hemangiomas are typically T2 hyperintense with peripheral nodular enhancement on postcontrast images.
11. T2W images are excellent for evaluating the zonal anatomy of the uterus. The endometrium is hyperintense, the junctional zone is hypointense, and the outer myometrium is hyperintense.
12. Ligament and tendon injuries are well demonstrated on T2W images secondary to the strong contrast between the hyperintense edema and the hypointense normal ligament or tendon.
13. T2 hypointensity within the seminal vesicle is suggestive of fibrotic prostate tumor invasion.
14. The hypointense peripheral rim exhibited by cerebral abscesses on T2W images can help to narrow an otherwise extensive differential diagnosis.

References

1. Lee VS: *Cardiovascular MRI: Physical Principles to Practical Protocols.* Philadelphia: Lippincott Williams & Wilkins, 2005, p 402.
2. El Yousef SJ, Duchesneau RH, Alfidi RJ, et al: Magnetic resonance imaging of the breast: work in progress. *Radiology* 150:761-766, 1984.
3. Dash N, Lupetin AR, Daffner RH, et al: Magnetic resonance imaging in the diagnosis of breast disease. *AJR Am J Roentgenol* 146:119-125, 1986.
4. Edelman RR: *Clinical Magnetic Resonance Imaging*, 3rd ed. Philadelphia: Elsevier Saunders, 2006.
5. Runge VM: *Clinical MRI.* Philadelphia: Saunders, 2002.
6. Kamisawa T, Tu Y, Egawa N, et al: MRCP of congenital pancreaticobiliary malformation. *Abdom Imaging* 32:129-133, 2007.
7. Gupta RT, Brady CM, Lotz J, et al: Dynamic MR imaging of the biliary system using hepatocyte-specific contrast agents. *AJR Am J Roentgenol* 195:405-413, 2010.
8. Brant WE, Helms CA: *Fundamentals of Diagnostic Radiology.* Philadelphia: Lippincott, Williams & Wilkins, 2007.
9. Klatzo I: Pathophysiological aspects of brain edema. *Acta Neuropathol* 72:236-239, 1987.
10. Goodwin RW, O'Donnell P, Saifuddin A: MRI appearances of common benign soft-tissue tumours. *Clin Radiol* 62:843-853, 2007.
11. Bartolozzi C, Lencioni R, Donati F, Cioni D: Abdominal MR: liver and pancreas. *Eur Radiol* 9:1496-1512, 1999.
12. Kennedy AM, Gilfeather MR, Woodward PJ: MRI of the female pelvis. *Semin Ultrasound CT MR* 20:214-230, 1999.
13. Proscia N, Jaffe TA, Neville AM, et al: MRI of the pelvis in women: 3D versus 2D T2-weighted technique. *AJR Am J Roentgenol* 195:254-259, 2010.
14. Bredella MA, Tirman PF, Peterfy CG, et al: Accuracy of T2-weighted fast spin-echo MR imaging with fat saturation in detecting cartilage defects in the knee: comparison with arthroscopy in 130 patients. *AJR Am J Roentgenol* 172:1073-1080, 1999.
15. Offenbacher H, Fazekas F, Schmidt R, et al: Superficial siderosis of the central nervous system: MRI findings and clinical significance. *Neuroradiology* 38:S51-S56, 1996.

Chapter 3
Proton Density

Kimball L. Christianson, Rodney D. Welling, Allen W. Song, and Christopher D. Lascola

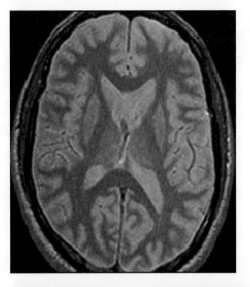

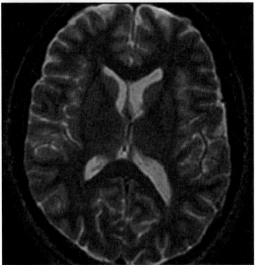

1. What are the two sequences above?

2. What are the imaging characteristics that help distinguish these sequences?

3. Which sequence has greater SNR?

4. What are some clinical applications where proton density images may be most helpful?

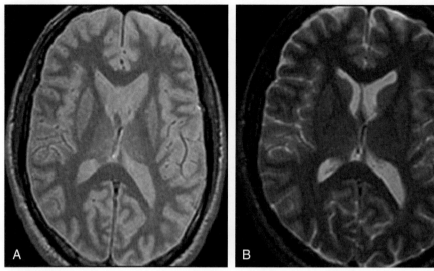

FIGURE 1A. Axial PDW image.

FIGURE 1B. Corresponding T2W image.

1. Axial proton density–weighted (PDW) image on the left, and corresponding T2-weighted (T2W) image on the right.

2. Intrinsic contrast between gray matter, white matter, and cerebrospinal fluid (CSF) is diminished as compared to the adjacent T2W image; CSF is intermediate and isointense to gray matter; overall signal intensity of the image is greater than the corresponding T2W image.

3. Proton density (PD).

4. PD images have a signal-to-noise ratio (SNR) that is higher than any comparable T1-weighted or T2W image. PDW imaging is particularly helpful for imaging complex tissues with limited SNR, such as in the posterior fossa, neck, and spine. In some musculoskeletal applications, differences in PD within tissue elements is inherently high so that PDW imaging provides both excellent contrast and superior SNR.

Physics Discussion

As discussed in Chapter 2, magnetic resonance (MR) image contrast is not exclusively due to differences in T1 or T2 characteristics, but rather varies along a spectrum of two parameters, time to repetition (TR) and time to echo (TE). Different combinations of TR and TE produce three major types of tissue contrast: T1 weighted, T2 weighted, and proton density weighted. T1-weighted (T1W) imaging enhances the T1 effect and minimizes T2 weighting by shortening TR and TE. T2-weighted (T2W) imaging enhances the T2 effect and minimizes T1 weighting by lengthening both TE and TR. Proton density–weighted (PDW) imaging minimizes both T1 and T2 by *lengthening* TR and *shortening* TE.

By reducing the contribution from T1 and T2, signal intensity in PDW imaging becomes proportional to the number of protons in each tissue (i.e., "proton density"). In "true" PDW imaging, pure water will have the most signal since its proton

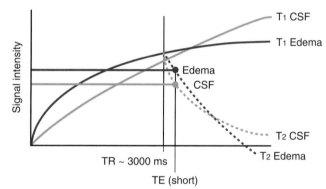

FIGURE 1. Modified PDW imaging sequence for brain and spine imaging. Composite graph of T1 recovery and T2 decay illustrates how a PD sequence is modified to enhance sensitivity for detecting pathology (edema) in central nervous system tissues. TR is shortened from its "true" (i.e., infinitely long) PDW imaging time, increasing the relative contribution of T1 contrast between edema and CSF. Edema is now brighter than CSF. TR remains relatively long, however, and TE is still short, thus preserving the advantage of increased SNR that PDW imaging provides.

density (PD) is higher than that of any tissue. In practice, however, sequence parameters for PDW imaging are modified so that T1 and/or T2 contributions are moderately increased to optimize contrast within the tissue of interest.

In brain, for example, PDW imaging sequences are designed to depict edema as brighter than cerebrospinal fluid (CSF), even though CSF has a higher PD. TR is shortened to reintroduce more T1 contribution and take advantage of the differences in T1 relaxation between edema and CSF (Fig. 1). Although CSF has higher PD, edema has a shorter T1 recovery. For PDW imaging in the brain, TR is shortened to a time when T1 contrast between CSF and edema is present, and signal intensity related to T1 recovery is still higher for edema (see Fig. 1).

One may wonder what utility remains for PDW imaging, given the near-universal adoption of fast spin echo (FSE) sequences, especially those with inversion recovery preparatory pulses (e.g., fluid-attenuated inversion recovery [FLAIR], short tau inversion recovery [STIR]) that provide excellent contrast in brain and bone. Indeed, PDW images demonstrate little intrinsic contrast, since variations in PD between different tissue elements is often small (< 10%). Before FSE became commonplace, PDW imaging did not add imaging time because PD images were acquired "free" during conventional spin echo (CSE) T2W sequences. PD signal was collected at an intermediate TE within the same TR. With FSE, PDW imaging must instead be run as an entirely separate sequence.

PD images are still useful because their signal-to-noise ratio (SNR) is higher than any comparable T1W or T2W image. High SNR is achieved because longitudinal recovery is maximized and transverse decay minimized. PDW imaging is most helpful in those settings where SNR is at a premium, and the advantages of higher SNR outweigh any disadvantages related to lower intrinsic tissue contrast. These settings include deep, complex tissues with significant magnetic field inhomogeneity, such as the posterior fossa, neck, and spine. In some musculoskeletal applications, intrinsic differences in PDs between tissue elements (e.g., bone/soft tissue) are high enough that PDW imaging provides both excellent contrast and high SNR.

CASES 2 AND 3: COMPANION CASES

Case 2

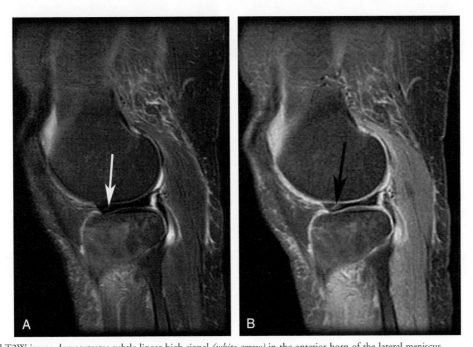

FIGURE 2A. Sagittal T2W image demonstrates subtle linear high signal *(white arrow)* in the anterior horn of the lateral meniscus.

FIGURE 2B. This same area of linear high signal is better visualized on the PDW image and is clearly seen to extend to the articular surface *(black arrow)*.

Diagnosis: Oblique tear of the anterior horn of the lateral meniscus.

Case 3

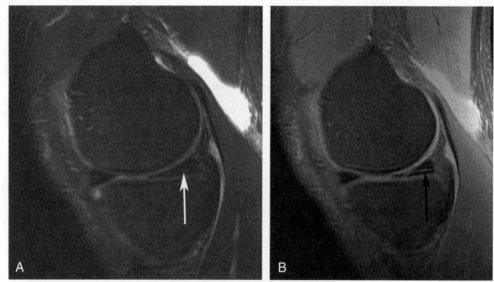

FIGURE 3A. Sagittal T2W image demonstrates very subtle linear high signal *(white arrow)* in the posterior horn of the lateral meniscus.

FIGURE 3B. On the sagittal PDW image, the signal is much better appreciated and clearly extends to the articular surface *(black arrow)*.

Diagnosis: Oblique tear of the posterior horn of medial meniscus.

Discussion

Both of these cases demonstrate meniscal tears. A meniscal tear is defined as abnormal signal in a meniscus that extends to the articular surface. In each case, the meniscal tears can be seen on both the T2W image (long TE) and the PDW image (short TE); however, recognition of the tear and visualization of tear extent to the articular surface is much better seen on the PDW image. The meniscus is best evaluated with short-TE sequences (T1, PD, and gradient-recalled echo). PDW imaging is often used because of its higher SNR. In recent years, FSE-PD sequences have been implemented in evaluating the meniscus, with the primary advantage being faster imaging times. The disadvantages of using FSE-PD sequences includes increased blurring of the image and the brighter appearance of fat on FSE imaging compared with CSE. There is controversy in the literature over whether FSE techniques perform as well as CSE techniques in evaluating meniscal pathology.[1-4]

Case 4

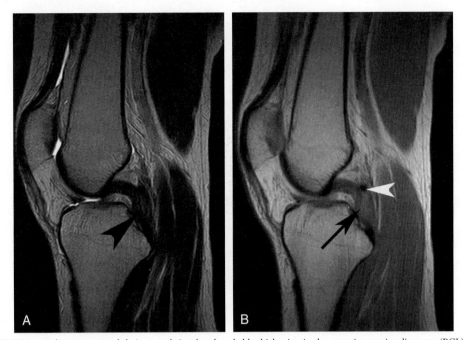

FIGURE 4A. Sagittal T2W image demonstrates subtle increased signal and probable thickening in the posterior cruciate ligament (PCL) *(black arrowhead)*.

FIGURE 4B. Sagittal PDW image demonstrates more pronounced increased signal within the PCL *(black arrow)* as well as thickening of the PCL. The *white arrowhead* denotes the posterior meniscofemoral ligament (ligament of Wrisberg) just posterior to the PCL, which is very low in signal.

Diagnosis: Tear of the posterior cruciate ligament.

Case 5

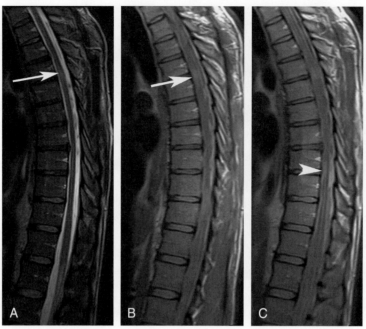

FIGURE 5A. Sagittal T2W image demonstrates ill-defined high T2 signal within the spinal cord *(white arrow)* at the T5/T6 level.

FIGURES 5B AND 5C. Sagittal PDW image (B) demonstrates the same finding as the T2W image *(white arrow);* however, on the sagittal PDW image there is a second high-signal lesion seen at the T9/T10 level *(white arrowhead,* C) that was not seen on the T2W image.

Diagnosis: Neuromyelitis optica.

Case 6

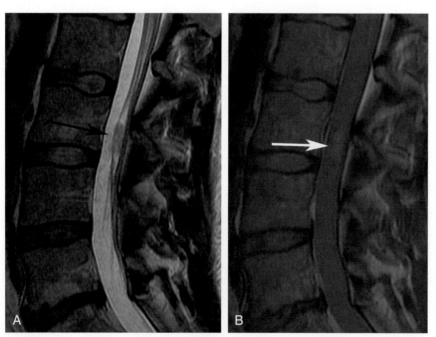

FIGURE 6A. Sagittal T2W image demonstrates a subtle low-T2-signal intradural, extramedullary lesion *(black arrow)* at the level of the cauda equina.

FIGURE 6B. The same lesion *(white arrow)* appears more conspicuous on the sagittal PDW image because it is higher in signal than the surrounding background.

Diagnosis: Schwannoma.

50

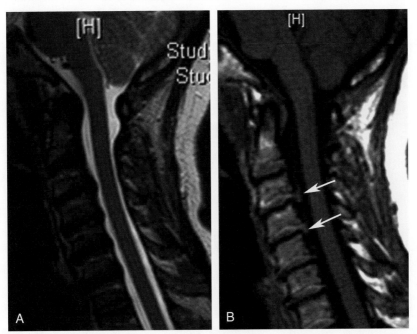

FIGURE 7A. Sagittal T2W image demonstrates disc bulges at C3/C4 and C4/C5. The disc material itself is similar in signal intensity to the surrounding bone and ligaments.

FIGURE 7B. Sagittal PDW image again demonstrates the disc bulges seen at C3/C4 and C4/C5. However, on this PDW image the disc material is easily distinguished from the cortical bone and ligament *(arrows)*.

Diagnosis: Degenerative disc disease.

Discussion

PDW images minimize but do not eliminate contributions from T1 and T2, so that most contrast reflects variations in the numbers of protons within tissues. In many settings, the number of protons within tissue will not vary significantly, and contrast with PDW imaging is low. In some tissues, however, intrinsic differences in PD are high, allowing PDW imaging to provide images that not only offer optimal SNR but also decent contrast. PDW imaging is particularly useful in the cervical spine, where overall SNR is poor due to location and tissue complexity, and the inherent differences in PD between different elements (bone, disc, ligament, paravertebral soft tissues) are high.[2,5]

In Case 4, understanding that on a short-TE sequence (PDW imaging) the PCL should be uniformly dark in signal makes the bright signal within the expanded tendon very noticeable. The stark contrast between the very-low-signal posterior meniscofemoral ligament (ligament of Wrisberg) and the bright-signal PCL emphasizes this point.

In Cases 5 and 6, the decrease in tissue contrast between the CSF and the spinal cord results in the increased conspicuity of the very subtle demyelinating plaque within the cord and the schwannoma.

PDW imaging can be helpful in the cervical spine, because the soft intervertebral disc material can often be difficult to resolve against cortical bone and ligaments in this region. Case 7 illustrates how PDW imaging can be helpful in contrasting the low-signal-intensity structures in the cervical spine, such as the cortical bone, from the higher signal intensity disc, thereby allowing for a more accurate estimate of the severity of the degenerative disc disease.[6]

Case 8

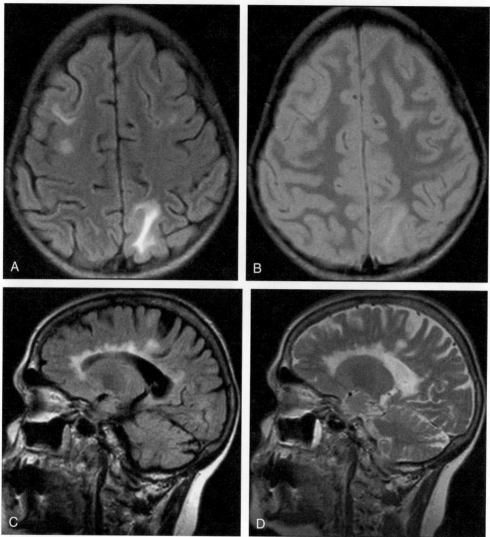

FIGURE 8A. Axial FLAIR image demonstrates increase T2 prolongation in the right centrum semiovale and left subcortical, posterior parietal white matter.

FIGURE 8B. Axial PDW image. The white matter changes are seen but less conspicuous.

FIGURE 8C. Sagittal FLAIR image demonstrates significant increased T2 signal within the periventricular white matter.

FIGURE 8D. Sagittal PDW image. The abnormal periventricular white matter signal is clearly present but less conspicuous.

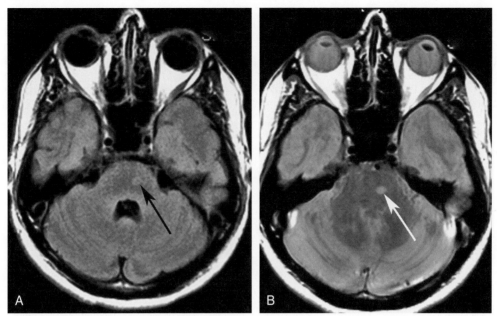

FIGURE 9A. Axial FLAIR image demonstrates a very subtle high-signal-intensity focus in the left aspect of the pons *(black arrow)*.

FIGURE 9B. Axial PDW image. The same hyperintense focus in the pons is much more conspicuous *(white arrow)*.

Diagnosis: Multiple sclerosis (MS).

Discussion

MS plaques are high in signal on T2W imaging. The cortex, subcortical white matter, and periventricular white matter are areas where MS plaques can be difficult to detect on T2W imaging. This is because the bright CSF and cortical signal can obscure small white matter lesions. Both FLAIR and PD pulse sequences are especially helpful in detecting MS plaques in the periventricular white matter because the CSF is lower in signal, allowing the MS plaques to stand out as hyperintense lesions. FLAIR imaging is superior to PD in the evaluation of MS plaques in the cortical and subcortical white matter, as shown in Case 8.[7-9] However, several studies have shown that PD is better than FLAIR in detection of MS plaques in the posterior

fossa.[7,8] (Note that these studies compared CSE-PD, not FSE-PD, with FLAIR.)

Several factors likely contribute to decreased sensitivity of FLAIR in the posterior fossa. SNR is often significantly diminished because of flow artifacts, dense adjacent bone containing multiple aerated compartments, and the distance and geometry of the posterior fossa in relation to the head coil. Moreover, even though inversion recovery sequences such as FLAIR improve soft tissue contrast, they do so at the expense of losing more signal intensity, thus further compounding any SNR problem. In the supratentorial brain where signal is abundant, the superior contrast from FLAIR usually triumphs. In the posterior fossa, where SNR is less consistent, optimized SNR with PDW imaging may be a better option.

References

1. Rubin D, Kneeland JB, Listerud J, et al: MR diagnosis of meniscal tears of the knee: value of fast spin-echo vs conventional spin-echo pulse sequences. *AJR Am J Roentgenol* 162:1131-1135, 1994.

2. Kaplan PA, Dussault R, Helms CA, Anderson MW: *Musculoskeletal MRI*. Philadelphia: Elsevier Saunders, 2001.

3. Blackmon GB, Major NM, Helms CA: Comparison of fast spin-echo versus conventional spin-echo MRI for evaluating meniscal tears. *AJR Am J Roentgenol* 184:1740-1743, 2005.

4. Wolff AB, Pesce LL, Wu JS, et al: Comparison of spin echo T1-weighted sequences versus fast spin-echo proton density-weighted sequences for evaluation of meniscal tears at 1.5 T. *Skeletal Radiol* 38:21-29, 2009.

5. Edelman RR, Hesselink J, Zlatkin M: *MRI Clinical Magnetic Resonance Imaging*, 2nd ed. Philadelphia: Saunders, 1996.

6. Mitchell DG, Cohen M: *MRI Principles*, 2nd ed. Philadelphia: Elsevier Saunders, 2004.

7. Filippi M, Yousry T, Baratti C, et al: Quantitative assessment of MRI lesion load in multiple sclerosis. *Brain* 119:1349-1355, 1996.

8. Gawne-Cain ML, O'Riordan JI, Thompson AJ, et al: Multiple sclerosis lesion detection in the brain: a comparison of fast fluid-attenuated inversion recovery and conventional T2-weighted dual spin echo. *Neurology* 49:364-370, 1997.

9. Miller DH, Grossman RI, Reingold SC, et al: The role of magnetic resonance techniques in understanding and managing multiple sclerosis. *Brain* 121:3-24, 1998.

Chapter 4

Gadolinium-Based Contrast Agents

Kimball L. Christianson, Allen W. Song, and Elmar M. Merkle

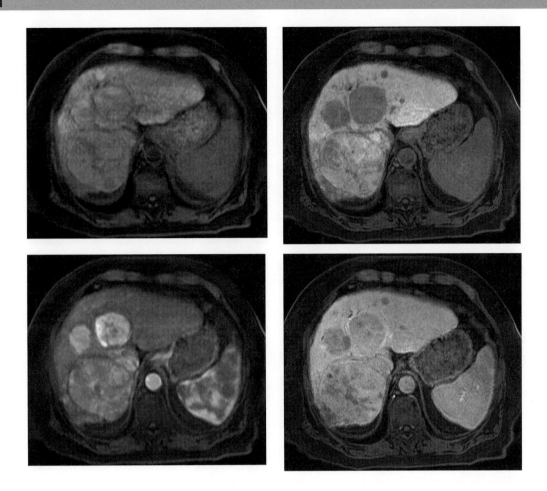

1. What is the most likely diagnosis?

2. How is the administration of a contrast agent helpful in establishing this diagnosis?

3. How does gadolinium result in increased T1 signal?

4. What is relaxivity?

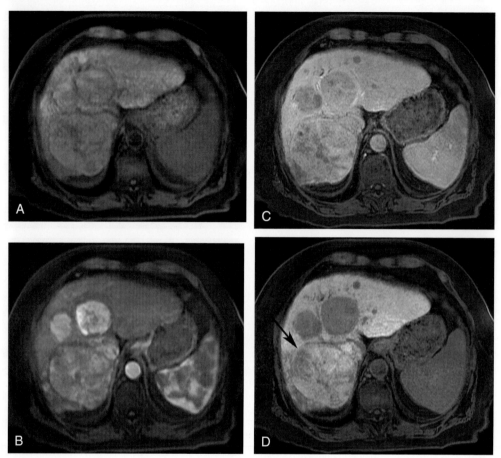

FIGURES 1A, 1B, AND 1C. Fat-suppressed three-dimensional (3D) gradient-recalled echo (GRE) T1-weighted (T1W) precontrast (A) and postcontrast (B and C) images demonstrate hyperenhancement of multiple large liver masses in the arterial phase (B) with rapid washout of contrast seen on the portal venous phase (C).

FIGURE 1D. Of note, some tumor components *(black arrow)* take up the hepatocyte-specific contrast agent gadoxetate disodium, while most of the lesions do not, during the hepatocyte phase.

1. Multifocal hepatocellular carcinoma (HCC).

2. In a cirrhotic patient, a lesion that is rapidly enhancing on the arterial phase with early washout on the later phases is very characteristic of HCC.

3. Gadolinium is a paramagnetic element with seven unpaired electrons. These unpaired electrons spin and create an oscillating magnetic field. When these electrons spin at the proper frequencies, the result is shortening of the T1 relaxation time. Unlike computed tomography, where the iodine molecule itself generates the contrast we see, in magnetic resonance imaging we do not see the gadolinium; we see its effects on the surrounding protons.

4. Relaxivity is a measurement of the efficiency of a contrast agent to shorten T1 and T2 relaxation times.

Diagnosis: Multifocal HCC in a patient with cirrhosis.

Physics Discussion

Gadolinium is a paramagnetic element that generates a small and positive magnetic field only when placed in an external magnet (e.g., a magnetic resonance imaging [MRI] scanner).

This small magnetic field alters the uniformity of the main magnetic field of the scanner to generate useful imaging contrast. Paramagnetic properties arise from unpaired electrons in the element that can realign their orbits in the presence of the external magnetic field. Because gadolinium has seven unpaired electrons, it is highly paramagnetic.

Paramagnetic agents, such as gadolinium chelates, shorten the T1 and T2 relaxation times of adjacent molecules. One important measure of the effectiveness of a contrast agent in shortening relaxation times is **relaxivity.** In general, the higher the relaxivity of a contrast material, the greater the decrease in proton relaxation time. At low contrast medium concentrations, the T1 relaxation effect predominates as a result of the fast inherent transverse relaxation in tissue. The result is increased signal on T1-weighted (T1W) images. However, at higher concentrations of contrast medium, the T2 relaxation is so short that T2 effects predominate and low signal results.

Paramagnetic gadolinium chelates are believed to increase relaxivity through two primary mechanisms. First, water molecules can transiently bind to the gadolinium chelate and undergo a chemical exchange that enhances relaxation. This is called inner-sphere relaxation. The second mechanism is called

Table 4-1 Relaxivities of Common Commercially Available MR Contrast Agents

| Trade Name | Generic Name | RELAXIVITIES OF CONTRAST AGENTS IN PLASMA AT 37°C | | | |
| | | 1.5 T | | 3 T | |
		R1	R2	R1	R2
Magnevist	Gadopentetate dimeglumine	4.1	4.6	3.7	5.2
Gadovist	Gadobutrol	5.2	6.1	5.0	7.1
ProHance	Gadoteridol	4.1	5.0	3.7	5.7
Multihance	Gadobenate dimeglumine	6.3	8.7	5.5	11
Omniscan	Gadodiamide	4.3	5.2	4.0	5.6
Optimark	Gadoversetamide	4.7	5.2	4.5	5.9
Eovist	Gadoxetate disodium	6.9	8.7	6.2	11
Ablavar	Gadofosveset trisodium	19	34	9.9	60

Adapted with permission from Rohrer M, Bauer H, Mintorovitch J, et al: Comparison of magnetic properties of MRI contrast media solutions at different magnetic field strengths. *Invest Radiol* 40:715-724, 2005.

outer-sphere relaxation and describes the enhanced relaxation created by the interaction of the surrounding protons with the dipole moment created by the paramagnetic ion.[1]

The relaxivity of a contrast agent varies by magnetic field strength. The relaxivity of contrast agents decreases as the magnetic field strength increases (Table 1).[2]

Contrast Agents

Contrast agents can be divided into extracellular agents, agents that are both extracellular and hepatobiliary, and blood pool agents.

Extracellular Agents

These are the most commonly used and least expensive magnetic resonance (MR) contrast agents. The most common trade names include Magnevist, Omniscan, ProHance, Optimark, and Gadovist. Gadolinium chelates have pharmacokinetics similar to iodine. Excretion is almost entirely through the kidneys.

Combined Agents

These are contrast agents that demonstrate both extracellular and hepatobiliary behavior. Examples include Multihance and Eovist.

Multihance has several important differences from the purely extracellular gadolinium chelates. First, Multihance demonstrates weak binding to plasma proteins, resulting in prolonged time within the intravascular space. Prolonged intravascular time allows for more T1 shortening to take place and in turn allows for lower doses to be administered while achieving the same T1 shortening. This fact has made Multihance the default agent for contrast-enhanced MR angiography (MRA) for many institutions (please note: this is an off-label indication!). Second, hepatocytes take up 2% to 5% of Multihance through an organic anionic transport mechanism otherwise used by bile salts, organic anions, and bilirubin.[3] Finally, the hepatocytes excrete Multihance into the biliary canaliculi through the canalicular multispecific organic anionic transport mechanism (cMOAT; aka multidrug-resistance–associated protein [MRP]). The hepatocyte uptake allows for the acquisition of T1W datasets during the hepatocyte phase, which usually takes place 40 to 120 minutes postinjection.

Eovist is another paramagnetic contrast agent with both extracellular and hepatobiliary excretion. In contrast to Multihance, 50% of Eovist is excreted into the biliary system and 50% is excreted through the kidneys. Like Multihance, Eovist binds weakly to plasma proteins primarily through the addition of the EOB ligand, which decreases its tumbling rate, resulting in increased time within the blood pool, higher relaxivity, and a lower administered dose if desired. Because of the markedly higher hepatocyte uptake, the acquisition of hepatocyte-phase images and/or T1W MR cholangiography datasets can be performed much earlier, usually within the first 20 minutes postinjection. This has significant implications on patient workflow as the patient does not need to come back to the MR suite for delayed imaging.

Blood Pool Agents

Ablavar is currently the only contrast agent that is U.S. Food and Drug Administration (FDA) approved for contrast-enhanced MRA. It has several properties that make it unique. The extracellular contrast agents have short plasma half-lives (about 80 to 100 minutes). Ablavar is unique in that it binds reversibly to albumin at a high rate, enabling the contrast agent to remain in the intravascular space for a much longer period (plasma half-life about 15.5 hours). The relaxivity of Ablavar is about four times higher at 1.5T when compared to extracellular contrast agents, allowing a much smaller dose to be administered. Use of the other contrast agents in contrast-enhanced MRA depends heavily on perfectly timing the arterial phase. Ablavar potentially allows for increased flexibility in imaging the vasculature because its vascular contrast lasts for approximately 1 hour.[4]

Adverse Effects of Contrast Agents

Unbound gadolinium is toxic. This is in part related to the fact that the gadolinium ion (Gd^{3+}) is roughly the same size as the calcium ion and can act as an antagonist at calcium receptors in the body. This can have a deleterious effect wherever calcium plays an important role, such as in respiration and muscle contraction. It can also result in deleterious effects to the liver and spleen and act in enzyme inhibition. The chelates that are bound to gadolinium significantly reduce its toxicity.

Nephrogenic Systemic Fibrosis

Nephrogenic systemic fibrosis (NSF) is a rare fibrosing disorder that appears to be associated with renal failure and gadolinium use. Clinical symptoms of NSF include swelling and eventual

SUMMARY OF AVAILABLE GADOLINIUM-BASED CONTRAST AGENTS				CASE REPORTS ASSOCIATED WITH NSF*	
Trade Name	Compound Name	Class	FDA Approved (Y/N)/Year	FDA-Reported Cases	Approximate # of Doses (in millions)
Omniscan	Gadodiamide	Linear, nonionic	Y/1993	382 (12/2009)	13
Optimark	Gadoversetamide	Linear, nonionic	Y/1999	35 (12/2009)	4.7
Multihance	Gadobenate dimeglumine	Linear, ionic	Y/2004	10 (2008)	
Magnevist	Gadopentetate dimeglumine	Linear, ionic	Y/1998	195 (12/2009)	23
Eovist	Gadoxetate disodium	Linear, ionic	Y/2008	0	
Ablavar	Gadofosveset trisodium	Linear, ionic	Y/2008	0	
Prohance	Gadoteridol	Macrocyclic, nonionic	Y/1992	9 (2008)	
Dotarem	Gadoterate meglumine	Macrocyclic, nonionic	N	0	
Gadavist	Gadobutrol	Macrocyclic, nonionic	Y/2011	0	

*The most current data within the last two columns comes from the ACR Manual on Contrast Media, Version 7, 2010, which specifically mentions the number of FDA-reported cases associated with Omniscan, Optimark, and Magnevist as of December, 2009.
Data from Juluru K, Vogel-Claussen J, Macura K, et al: MR imaging in patients at risk for developing nephrogenic systemic fibrosis: protocols, practices, and imaging techniques to maximize patient safety. *RadioGraphics* 29:9-22, 2009; and Penfield J, Reilly R: Nephrogenic systemic fibrosis risk: is there a difference between gadolinium-based contrast agents? *Semin Dialysis* 21:129-134, 2008.

induration and fibrosis of the lower extremities, upper extremities, and lower abdomen. In severe cases the vital organs and muscles can become involved, which can be life threatening. As was previously mentioned, free Gd^{3+} is highly toxic. There may be an association between free Gd^{3+} and the development of NSF. In order to avoid the toxic effects, Gd^{3+} water-soluble chelates were made that demonstrate high affinity for the Gd^{3+} cation.

Stability describes the tendency of a Gd^{3+} cation to remain bound to its chelates. Stable chelates characteristically are ionic and have a cyclic morphologic structure. Conversely, chelates that are nonionic and have a linear configuration are less stable. In terms of stability, the configuration of the molecule is more important than the ionic state. The vast majority of cases of NSF have been reported with Omniscan, which is nonionic and has a linear morphologic structure (Table 2).[5,6]

Current risk factors for the development of NSF include intravenous administration of gadolinium-based contrast agents (GBCAs) in patients with acute and chronic renal failure.[5] The risk of developing NSF is increased with higher doses of contrast. Renal failure is hypothesized to increase toxicity by two mechanisms. First, the delay in excretion of gadolinium chelates due to renal failure results in prolonged retention in the body. This increases the chance that the gadolinium chelates will dissociate and release free Gd^{3+}. The second mechanism is referred to as transmetallation. Transmetallation is a process by which another metal in the body replaces the chelated Gd^{3+} cation and free Gd^{3+} molecule is released.[7]

In order to minimize the risk of NSF related to exposure to GBCAs, the FDA recently issued the following recommendations[8]:

• Not use three of the GBCA drugs—Magnevist, Omniscan, and Optimark—in patients with AKI or with chronic, severe kidney disease (GFR <30 ml/min/1.73 m²). These three GBCA drugs are contraindicated in these patients.

• Screen patients prior to administration of a GBCA to identify those with AKI or chronic, severe, kidney disease. These patients appear to be at highest risk for NSF.

• Use clinical history to screen patients for features of AKI or risk factors for chronically reduced kidney function.

  • Features of AKI consist of rapid (over hours to days) and usually reversible decrease in kidney function, commonly in the setting of surgery, severe infection, injury, or drug-induced kidney toxicity. Serum creatinine levels and estimated GFR may not reliably assess kidney function in the setting of AKI.

  • For patients at risk of chronically reduced kidney function (such as patients over age 60 years, patients with high blood pressure, or patients with diabetes), estimate the kidney function (GFR) through laboratory testing.

• Avoid use of GBCAs in patients suspected or known to have impaired drug elimination unless the need for the diagnostic information is essential and not available with non-contrasted MRI or other alternative imaging modalities.

• Monitor for signs and symptoms of NSF after a GBCA is administered to a patient suspected or known to have impaired elimination of the drug.

• Do not repeat administration of any GBCA during a single imaging session.

• Record the specific GBCA and the dose administered to a patient.

• When administering a GBCA, do not exceed the recommended dose. Prior to any re-administration, allow sufficient time for elimination of the GBCA from the body. GBCA elimination half lives are prolonged in patients with renal impairment; for a GBCA that involves significant hepato-biliary elimination, liver dysfunction may also prolong elimination time.

• For patients receiving hemodialysis, physicians may consider the prompt initiation of hemodialysis following the administration of a GBCA in order to enhance the contrast agent's elimination from the body. The usefulness of hemodialysis in the prevention of NSF is unknown.

- Advise patients with kidney disease to contact a healthcare professional if any of the following symptoms occurs after receiving a GBCA: burning, itching, swelling, scaling, hardening and tightening of the skin; red or dark patches on the skin; stiffness in joints with trouble moving, bending or straightening the arms, hands, legs or feet; pain in the hip bones or ribs; or muscle weakness.

- Report any adverse events with GBCAs to FDA's MedWatch program.

The most current recommendations regarding GBCAs from the American College of Radiology (ACR) Manual on Contrast Media are as follows[9]:

1. Patients with end-stage renal disease on chronic dialysis:

    a. If no residual renal function consider CT with iodinated contrast.

    b. If contrast enhanced MRI must be performed avoid using group I agents (Omniscan, Optimark and Magnevist).

    c. Use lowest dose possible.

    d. Perform MRI as closely before dialysis as possible.

    e. Inform patient and referring physician of risks; both should agree with decision to proceed.

2. Patients with CKD 4 or 5 (eGFR <30 ml/min/1.73 m^2) not on chronic dialysis:

    a. More problematic as iodinated contrast may worsen renal function.

    b. Avoid contrast media if possible.

    c. If study is performed use lowest possible dose.

    d. Avoid using group I agents.

    e. Try to avoid re-administration of contrast agents for several days to a week.

3. Patients with CKD 3a (eGFR of 45–59 ml/min/1.73 m^2)

    a. Risk of NSF extremely low.

    b. Use lowest possible dose to ensure diagnostic study.

    c. Group I agent should only be used after appropriate risk-benefit assessment.

4. Patients with CKD 3b (eGFR of 30–44 ml/min/1.73 m^2)

    a. Risk of NSF also very low but not zero.

    b. eGFR values can fluctuate from one day to the next. Therefore, patients with eGFR approaching 30 may have similar risk as CKD 4 or 5 patients and the above recommendations should be considered.

5. Patients with CKD 1 or 2 (eGFR 60–119 ml/min/1.73 m^2)

    a. Not at increased risk for NSF.

    b. All contrast agents can be administered to these patients.

This book includes the up-to-date warnings at the time of publication. However, as the warnings change periodically, attention to the most current recommendations is advised.

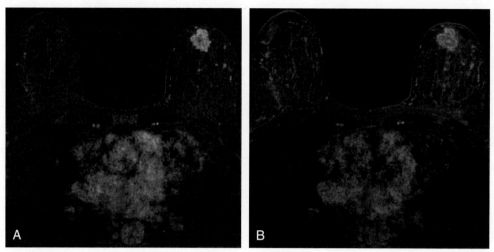

FIGURES 2A AND 2B. These postcontrast subtraction images demonstrate an irregular, immediately hyperenhancing mass (A) in the left breast with rapid washout on the more delayed arterial phase (B).

Diagnosis: Breast carcinoma.

Clinical Discussion

Enhancement kinetics are used in MRI of the breast to help better characterize breast lesions. Three enhancement patterns plotted on a signal intensity–time curve have been described (Fig. 1):

- Type I is a pattern of steadily increasing or persistent enhancement. This type of enhancement pattern typically represents a more benign pattern of enhancement.

- Type II is a pattern of initial rapid enhancement that then plateaus. This enhancement pattern is associated with an intermediate risk of malignancy.

- Type III is a pattern of early initial enhancement with rapid washout. This pattern of enhancement is the most concerning for malignancy.[10]

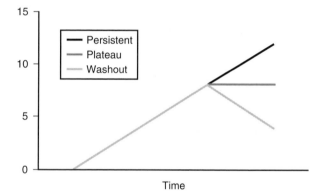

FIGURE 1 Graph demonstrating various potential enhancement curves of breast lesions.

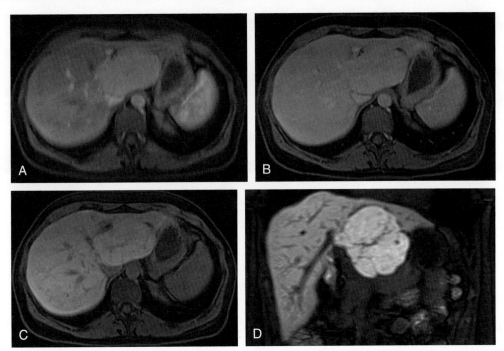

FIGURE 3A. 3D GRE volumetric interpolated breath-hold examination (VIBE) postcontrast (Eovist) arterial phase image demonstrates a large hyperenhancing mass in the left hepatic lobe. The mass is seen in A.

FIGURE 3B. The mass is isointense on the portal venous-phase image.

FIGURES 3C AND 3D. Hepatocyte-phase images in the axial (C) and coronal (D) planes demonstrate hyperenhancement of the mass.

Diagnosis: Focal nodular hyperplasia (FNH).

Clinical Discussion

There is a broad differential for a hyperenhancing mass with rapid fade in. However, the delayed images in this case demonstrate hyperenhancement consistent with biliary excretion. These findings in a noncirrhotic patient are consistent with FNH. The delayed images differ in that the flip angle on the axial image is 10° and it is 30° for the coronal image, which increases the T1 weighting. The coronal image clearly demonstrates hyperintensity of the mass secondary to biliary excretion, very suggestive of FNH. Eovist is helpful in liver lesion detection and characterization. It can aid in differentiating tumors that contain bile ducts (FNH and well-differentiated hepatocellular carcinoma [HCC]) from tumors that do not (poorly differentiated HCC, adenomas, metastases, and hemangiomas).

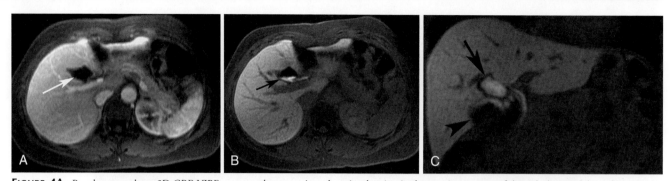

FIGURE 4A. Portal venous phase, 3D GRE VIBE sequence demonstrating a low-signal region in the anterior segment of the right hepatic lobe *(white arrow)*.

FIGURE 4B. Axial image acquired 20 minutes post contrast administration demonstrating biliary excretion of contrast into this low-signal area *(black arrow)*.

FIGURE 4C. Coronal image showing that this structure *(black arrow)* is separate from the gallbladder *(black arrowhead)* but that they both contain contrast.

Diagnosis: Focal ectasia of a biliary duct consistent with a choledochal cyst.

Clinical Discussion

These images demonstrate how Eovist is useful in certain biliary applications.

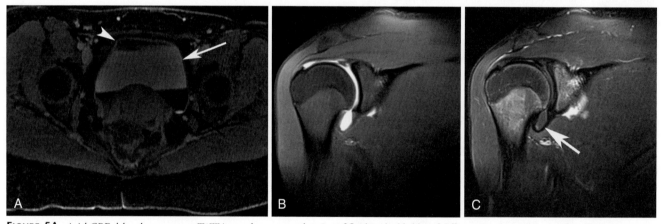

FIGURE 5A. Axial GRE delayed postcontrast T1W image demonstrates layering of fluid in the bladder of different signal intensities (parfait effect).

FIGURES 5B AND 5C. Coronal oblique fat-saturated T1W image (B) and coronal oblique T2 image (C) from an MR arthrogram. High-signal-intensity intra-articular fluid on the T1W image (B) is consistent with dilute gadolinium; there is probably a small tear of the superior labrum. On the T2-weighted (T2W) image (C), the intra-articular fluid *(white arrow)* is unexpectedly low in signal.

Diagnosis: Parfait effect.

Clinical Discussion

At high enough concentrations, gadolinium can cause a drop in signal because its T2-shortening properties predominate over its T1-shortening properties; this can be seen on both T1W and T2-weighted (T2W) sequences. The parfait effect is a normal phenomenon often seen in the renal pelvis or the urinary bladder of supine patients on delayed postcontrast T1W excretory-phase images (see Fig. 5A). A middle layer *(white arrow),* where the gadolinium concentration is diluted with urine, is hyperintense on T1 because the T1-shortening effects of gadolinium predominate at lower gadolinium concentrations (the gadolinium is mixing with urine). The top layer *(white arrowhead)* is hypointense because it contains only urine without gadolinium. The bottom layer *(black arrow)* is low in signal because of the higher concentration of gadolinium, in which case the T2-shortening effects predominate over the T1-shortening effects.[1]

In the case of the arthrogram, the concentration of gadolinium injected into the joint was 10 times greater than what is normally used. While the concentration of gadolinium was high enough to cause sufficient T2 shortening of the fluid on the T2W image, it was not high enough to cause noticeable signal loss on the T1W image.

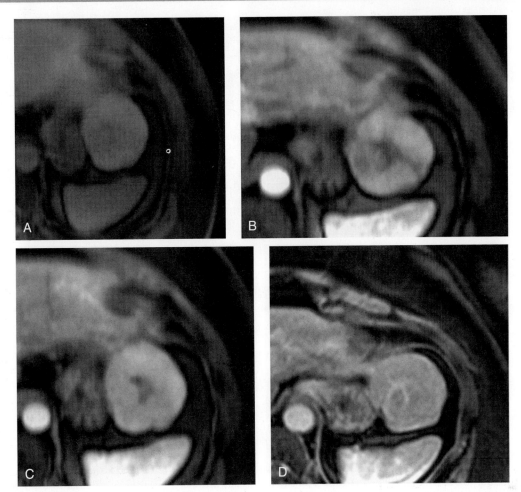

FIGURES 6A1 THROUGH 6D1. Precontrast fat-saturated T1 image (A) and fat-saturated T1 images in the arterial (B), portal venous (C), and equilibrium (D) phases after administration of an extracellular contrast agent with weak hepatobiliary effects demonstrate a lobulated left hepatic lobe mass that hyperenhances on arterial-phase images but is near isointense to liver on delayed phases, consistent with an FNH. Note the enhancement of the central scar on the equilibrium-phase image.

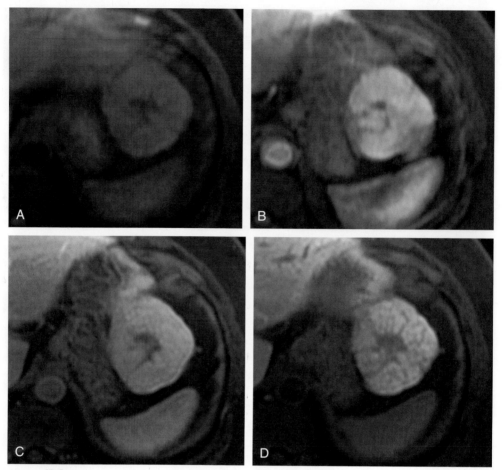

FIGURES 6A2 THROUGH 6D2. Same patient with examination performed 18 months later with a strong hepatocyte-specific contrast agent; no interval therapies were administered. The mass demonstrates similar enhancement characteristics compared to the prior study. However, while the signal of the liver and the mass are similar on the delayed phases, the signal intensities of both are greater compared to the prior study (use the spleen as an internal reference), and the central scar remains relatively hypointense throughout.

Diagnosis: Focal nodular hyperplasia.

Physics Discussion

Hepatocyte-specific contrast agents are oftentimes referred to as bimodal given their dual extracellular (perfusion) and liver imaging properties. As referenced earlier, two of the most commonly used agents are Gd-BOPTA (MultiHance) and Gd-EOB-DTPA (Eovist). This particular case illustrates the importance of knowing which specific contrast agent is being used as the lesion in question may show different enhancement characteristics that could potentially lead to diagnostic pitfalls.

Figures 6A1 through 6D1 show the typical enhancement pattern of FNH, with hyperenhancement on arterial-phase images, near isointensity to normal liver on delayed phases, and delayed enhancement of the central scar. Figures 6A2 through 6D2 in the same patient show a slightly different

enhancement pattern of the tumor, manifesting as apparent nonenhancement of the central scar on delayed images. The difference between the two was that MultiHance was used in Figures 6A1 through 6D1 and Eovist was used in Figures 6A2 through 6D2.

Remember that, while hepatocytes only take up 3% to 5% of MultiHance, that number is 50% of the uptake of Eovist; this, in concert with Eovist's increased T1 relaxivity effects, explains why a lower concentration of gadolinium can be administered (10 to 25 μmol/kg, as opposed to 0.1 mmol/kg for MultiHance). The apparent hypointensity of the central scar in the Eovist examination is likely the result of both relatively increased signal of the tumor parenchyma secondary to increased hepatobiliary uptake of Eovist and decreased concentration of gadolinium within the blood pooling in the central scar.

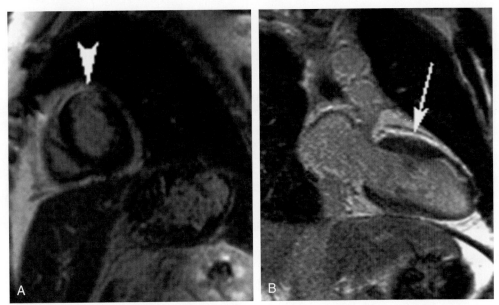

FIGURES 7A AND 7B. Short-axis (A) and vertical long-axis (B) delayed-enhancement MR images of the heart (segmented inversion recovery prepared fast GRE sequence). Both images demonstrate transmural hyperenhancement (*white arrowhead* in A and *white arrow* in B) within the anterior wall of the heart.

Diagnosis: Myocardial infarction in the left anterior descending coronary artery territory.

Physics Discussion

Myocardial delayed-enhancement images are produced by a 180° inversion recovery preparatory pulse followed by a GRE sequence. The inversion recovery pulse time to inversion (TI) is set to null the myocardium and enhance T1 relaxation, which increases the contrast between the myocardium and the region of enhancement. Delayed-enhancement imaging is helpful in demonstrating infarcted myocardium and in establishing whether there is viable myocardium that would benefit from reperfusion. It is postulated that delayed enhancement occurs in regions of acute myocardial infarction secondary to cell membrane breakdown, which allows gadolinium chelate to enter the cell. The gadolinium chelate remains within the ischemic tissue while it washes out of the nonaffected myocardium and leads to T1 shortening and increased signal. Delayed enhancement is also seen within areas of chronic myocardial infarction. The current thought is that fibrous tissue (infarct) has a greater area of interstitial space in which the gadolinium chelate can disperse when compared to the interstitial space surrounding normal packed cells. Viability is defined as myocardium in the region of ischemia that could survive if coronary revascularization is performed. Currently, if the hyperenhancement involves less than 50% of the myocardial wall, then remaining viable myocardium would benefit from coronary revascularization.

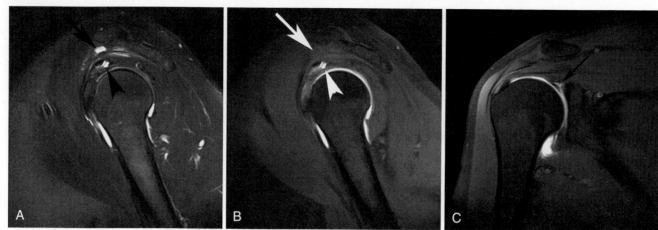

FIGURE 8A. Sagittal oblique T2W MR arthrogram image with fat saturation.

FIGURE 8B. Sagittal oblique T1W MR arthrogram image with fat saturation.

FIGURE 8C. Coronal oblique T2W MR arthrogram image with fat saturation.

Diagnosis: Supraspinatus tendon tear.

Physics Discussion

Figures 8A and 8B demonstrate high signal in the supraspinatus tendon *(black and white arrowheads)* consistent with a tear. The signal is bright on both T1W and T2W imaging, suggesting there is gadolinium within the tear. There is also high T2 signal within the subacromial/subdeltoid bursa *(black arrow in A),* which is low in signal on the T1W image *(white arrow in B)* consistent with fluid without gadolinium, suggesting this tear may be partial thickness. Gadolinium injected at a decreased concentration of 2 mmol/L (or 1 : 250) into the joint results in T1 shortening and increased signal (please note: this is an off-label indication!). This is the concentration of gadolinium typically given intravenously. The resultant signal increase in combination with joint expansion and fat suppression increases the sensitivity in detecting labral pathology. Figure 8C demonstrates this effect: the expansion of the joint aids in delineating the superior labral tear *(black arrow).* If gadolinium were injected into the joint without first being diluted, the joint space would display low signal because of the significant T2-shortening effects.[1]

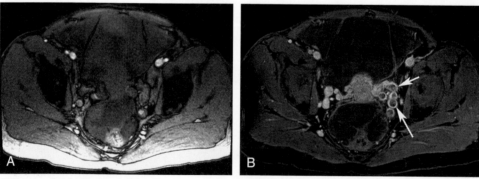

FIGURE 9A. Axial GRE image (bright blood technique) demonstrates normal external iliac veins with no evidence of deep vein thrombosis (DVT).

FIGURE 9B. Axial GRE VIBE image acquired about 10 minutes post gadofosveset trisodium (Ablavar) injection demonstrates numerous low-signal filling defects *(white arrows)* within dilated tubular structures within the left hemipelvis.

Diagnosis: Left internal iliac vein deep vein thrombosis (DVT).

Physics Discussion

Two-dimensional (2D) time-of-flight (TOF) imaging is an accurate, noninvasive way of evaluating for DVT. This technique's ability to evaluate the pelvic veins and inferior vena cava make it an especially useful tool when compared to ultrasound. However, these studies are sometimes difficult to interpret because of artifact, particularly inflow artifacts that simulate filling defects. TOF imaging is also hampered by its insensitivity to flow that is not perpendicular to the imaging plane. Also, slow-flowing blood is exposed to repetitive excitation pulses, becoming partially saturated and producing less signal. Both of these weaknesses are displayed in Figure 9A, where slow flow within a dilated tortuous left internal iliac vein produces signal that is isointense to the surrounding structures and is nondiagnostic.[11]

The postcontrast image in Figure 9B using gadofosveset trisodium as a contrast agent clearly demonstrates the numerous thrombi within the vein. Gadofosveset trisodium is particularly useful in evaluation for DVT given its long intravascular half-life, allowing for an extended imaging window and a high vascular signal-to-noise ratio resulting from a very high relaxivity, which allows for a much lower administered dose. Gadofosveset trisodium's increased flexibility in imaging the vasculature may also enable imaging of other sites, such as the pulmonary arteries. The potential to evaluate both the pulmonary arteries and the lower extremity veins in one exam would allow for a much more comprehensive workup of thromboembolic disease.[12]

KEY POINTS

1. Gadolinium is a paramagnetic element that results in T1 shortening (increased signal on T1W images).
2. Relaxivity is a measure of the efficiency of a contrast agent to decrease T1 and T2 relaxation times.
3. At low contrast medium concentrations, the T1 relaxation effect predominates as a result of the fast inherent transverse relaxation in tissue. The result is increased signal on T1W images. However, at high concentrations of contrast medium, the T2 relaxation is so short that low signal results.
4. The relaxivity of contrast agents decreases as the magnetic field strength increases.
5. Unlike CT, where the iodine molecule itself generates the contrast, in MRI gadolinium changes signal through its effects on the surrounding protons.
6. Extracellular contrast agents are the most commonly used.
7. The combined agents Multihance and Eovist are unique in that they are excreted in part by the hepatobiliary system. Multihance and Eovist have higher relaxivities because they exhibit low-level binding to plasma proteins and thus can stay in the blood pool longer.
8. Eovist can aid in differentiating tumors that contain bile ducts from tumors that do not.
9. Ablavar is FDA approved for contrast-enhanced MRA. It has a very long plasma half-life and very high relaxivity, which allows for a much lower administered dose and increased flexibility in imaging the vasculature.
10. Ionic, macrocyclic gadolinium chelates are the most stable and therefore thought to have the best safety profile in patients with renal failure.

References

1. Edelman RR, Hesselink JR, Zlatkin MB, Crues JV III: *Clinical Magnetic Resonance Imaging*. Philadelphia: Saunders Elsevier, 2006.
2. Rohrer M, Bauer H, Mintorovitch J, et al: Comparison of magnetic properties of MRI contrast media solutions at different magnetic field strengths. *Invest Radiol* 40:715-724, 2005.
3. Gandhi SN, Brown MA, Wong JG, et al: MR contrast agents for liver imaging: what, when, how. *RadioGraphics* 26:1621-1636, 2006.
4. Hadizadeh DR, Gieseke J, Lohmaier SH, et al: Peripheral MR angiography with blood pool contrast agent: prospective intraindividual comparative study of high-spatial-resolution steady-state MR angiography versus standard-resolution first-pass MR angiography and DSA1. *Radiology* 249:701-711, 2008.
5. Juluru KM, Vogel-Claussen J, Macura K, et al: MR imaging in patients at risk for developing nephrogenic systemic fibrosis: protocols, practices, and imaging techniques to maximize patient safety. *RadioGraphics* 29:9-22, 2009.
6. Penfield J, Riley R: Nephrogenic systemic fibrosis risk: is there a difference between gadolinium-based contrast agents? *Semin Dialysis* 21:129-134, 2008.
7. Morcos SK, Thomsen HS: Nephrogenic systemic fibrosis: more questions and some answers. *Nephron Clin Pract* 110:c24-c31, 2008; discussion, c32.
8. U.S. Food and Drug Administration: FDA Drug Safety Communication: New warnings for using gadolinium-based contrast agents in patients with kidney dysfunction. 2010. http://www.fda.gov.
9. ACR Committee on Drugs and Contrast Media: ACR Manual on Contrast Media, Version 7. American College of Radiology, 2010.
10. Macura KJ, Ouwerkerk R, Jacobs MA, Bluemke DA: Patterns of enhancement on breast MR images: interpretation and imaging pitfalls. *RadioGraphics* 26:1719-1734, 2006.
11. Mitchell D, Cohen M: *MRI Principles*, 2nd ed. Philadelphia: Elsevier Saunders, 2004.
12. Prince MR, Sostman HD: MR venography: unsung and underutilized. *Radiology* 226:630-632, 2003.

Chapter 5

Preparatory Pulses

Phil B. Hoang, Matthew P. Lungren, Allen W. Song, and Elmar M. Merkle

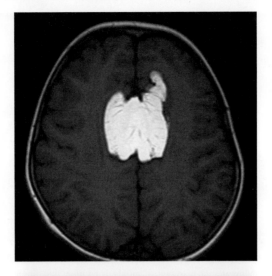

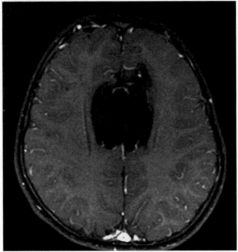

1. Name some common causes of high signal on a T1W image.

2. What are the two most common techniques to suppress fat signal?

3. Which of these techniques specifically suppresses signal from fat?

4. What is the diagnosis?

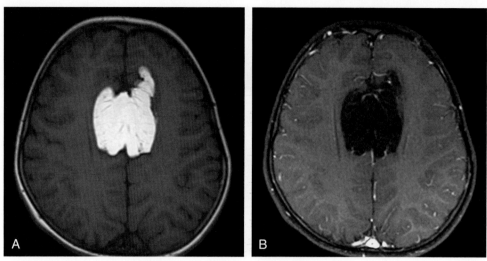

FIGURE 1A. Axial T1-weighted (T1W) image demonstrates the mass's interhemispheric position; thin, linear hypointense septa are noted.

FIGURE 1B. Axial postcontrast T1W image with fat saturation. Near-complete signal loss of the mass has occurred, with thin linear internal septations now evident.

1. Fat, subacute hemorrhage, proteinaceous fluid and melanin can all cause high T1 signal.

2. Frequency-selective fat saturation and short tau inversion recovery are the two most commonly used fat suppression techniques in MRI.

3. Frequency-selective fat saturation specifically suppresses signal from fat.

4. The diagnosis is a lipoma of the corpus callosum.

Preparatory Pulses Part I: Saturation Pulses

The common link between inversion recovery, spatial-selective presaturation, frequency-selective, and magnetization transfer sequences is the use of a radiofrequency (RF) pulse administered prior to the excitation pulse. This is referred to as the **preparatory pulse.** This chapter covers frequency-selective and spatial-selective presaturation pulses, while Chapter 6 reviews inversion recovery.

Frequency-selective saturation is a widely used and versatile technique. It is based on the assumption that a hydrogen proton resonates at a certain frequency based on its unique molecular environment. Protons in water and fat resonate at different frequencies when under the same external magnetic field because of the micromolecular environments unique to each tissue. These differences increase with increases in magnetic field strength. For example, protons in fat precess 74 Hz *slower* than protons in free water at 0.5T, 220 Hz slower at 1.5T, and 448 Hz slower at 3T. Frequency-selective saturation takes advantage of these differences in precessional frequencies, which allows signal suppression of either fat or water (Fig. 1).

Once the target protons are saturated (Fig. 2), they are dephased when a spoiler gradient is applied (Fig. 3). This spoiling of the protons' transverse magnetization suppresses their ability to produce signal. The excitation pulse is sent soon after. As mentioned before, water or fat signal may be suppressed if the appropriate RF saturation pulse is used.

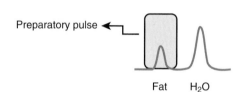

FIGURE 1. Frequency-selective saturation uses a *narrow-range RF preparatory pulse (gray box)* that matches the resonant frequency of the target protons, saturating them.

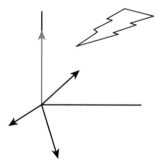

FIGURE 2. First, a frequency-selective *preparatory pulse (black bolt)* with a narrow range of frequencies **matching the resonant frequency of the target proton** is administered *(black arrow)*. The remaining protons *(gray arrow)* are unaffected and stay in net longitudinal magnetization.

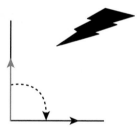

FIGURE 3. A *spoiler gradient (white bolt)* is subsequently applied, which dephases the protons magnetized by the preparatory pulse and **eliminates** their ability to produce signal. The excitation RF pulse is sent soon after and excites only the unspoiled protons.

The most common clinical use of frequency-selective saturation is to suppress the normally high signal intensity arising from fat on both fast spin echo T2-weighted (T2W) and contrast-enhanced T1-weighted (T1W) sequences. Benefits of frequency-selective saturation include its use to confirm or exclude the presence of fat within a high-T1-signal mass (see Case 1), as well as to suppress fat on postcontrast T1W sequences, which functions to increase tissue-lesion contrast and margin characterization.

Because the frequency-selective saturation pulse is broadcast at a narrow-range RF to specifically affect the target protons, the quality of signal suppression depends on a uniform magnetic field. The presence of magnetic field inhomogeneities typically results in poor signal suppression and, at times, inadvertent signal suppression of nontarget tissues.

Also, because fat has a short T1 relaxation time, it recovers a measure of its net longitudinal magnetization during the time between the preparatory and excitation pulses. This may require multiple fat saturation pulses to obtain the preferred signal loss, which contributes to RF energy deposition in the patient.

Frequency-selective techniques are typically not used at lower magnetic field strengths (< 1.0 Tesla) as there is an excessive overlap of resonant frequencies between water and fat protons; this leads to not only incomplete saturation of the desired protons, but also saturation of nontarget protons.

Another setting where a preparatory pulse is administered to affect tissue contrast is **magnetization transfer** (MT). MT refers to the transfer of longitudinal magnetization from restricted water protons to free water protons. This technique is based on the concept that restricted water protons are generally bound to macromolecules (e.g., proteins or lipids), and thereby subject to greater local field inhomogeneities. Free water protons, in contrast, exist in a comparatively uniform magnetic field environment. The different environments lead to different ranges of resonance frequencies of the water protons; free water will have a narrow resonance frequency range near 63 MHz (1.5T), while the range of resonance frequencies in bound water protons will be much broader owing to the inherent field inhomogeneities in their environment. Therefore, an "off-resonance" preparatory pulse will preferentially saturate bound water protons. What allows for variable soft tissue contrast, however, is the phenomenon by which magnetization is then transferred from bound water protons to available adjacent free water protons, leading to a saturation effect. The result is reduced signal from the free water protons in tissues where the magnetization transfer phenomenon is prevalent. Because the extent of signal decay depends on the exchange rate between free and bound water protons, MT can be used to provide an alternative contrast method to complement T1, T2, and proton density methods. The most accepted application is in magnetic resonance angiography, where MT markedly suppresses background tissue signal while leaving flowing blood unaffected. Magnetization transfer is also believed to be a nonspecific indicator of the structural integrity of the tissues, and has found promising applicability in highlighting specific tissue abnormalities in the brain (e.g., demyelination in multiple sclerosis).[6]

Spatial-selective presaturation is a technique used to suppress signal arising from regions of the body *outside* the imaging area of interest. A common clinical setting where spatial-selective presaturation is used is lumbar spine imaging, where reduction of phase-related motion artifact arising from peristalsing bowel is achieved with application of a saturation band placed over the abdomen.

CASES 2, 3, AND 4: COMPANION CASES

Case 2

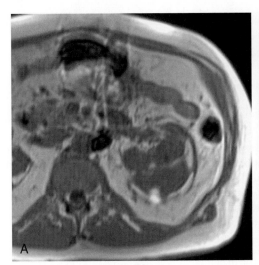 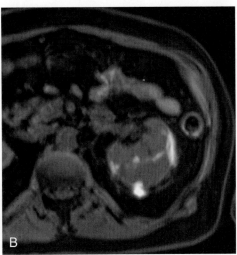

FIGURE 2A. Axial T1W image of the left hemiabdomen. Mixed-signal-intensity posterior left renal mass demonstrates peripheral margin of increased T1 signal intensity, which is isointense to fat.

FIGURE 2B. Axial T1W fat-saturated image. Subcutaneous and intra-abdominal fat signal is suppressed; the high T1 signal arising from the left renal mass persists.

Diagnosis: Subcapsular renal hematoma.

Case 3

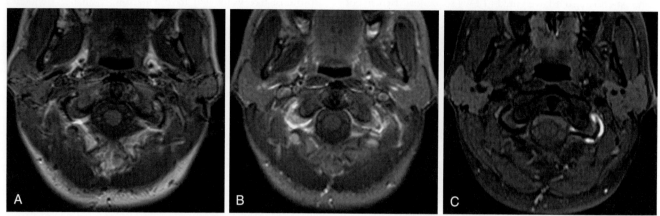

FIGURE 3A. Axial T1W image of the cervical spine at the level of the odontoid process. No abnormality is identified.

FIGURE 3B. Axial postcontrast T1W image. Again, no abnormality is seen.

FIGURE 3C. Axial postcontrast T1W image with fat saturation. High T1 signal abnormality in the periphery of the left vertebral artery is now evident.

Diagnosis: Left vertebral artery dissection with subacute thrombus in the false lumen.

Case 4

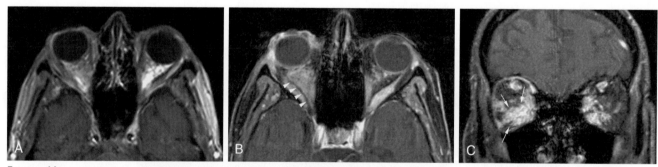

FIGURE 4A. Axial postcontrast T1W image of the orbits. No definite abnormality identified.

FIGURE 4B. Axial postcontrast T1W image with fat saturation at the same level. Enhancing right inferior intraorbital mass is now evident, which is outlined by a thin rim of low-signal intraconal fat laterally *(arrowheads)*.

FIGURE 4C. Coronal postcontrast T1W image with fat saturation of the orbits better demonstrates abnormal soft tissue filling the inferomedial orbit *(arrows)*.

Diagnosis: Metastatic breast cancer.

Discussion

Two important utilities of fat saturation are (1) suppression of high signal intensity fat to provide added contrast and (2) confirming the presence or absence of fat within a lesion. The left renal mass (Case 2) demonstrates high T1 signal peripherally, which is isointense compared to subcutaneous and intraabdominal fat. This raises the possibility of a fat-containing mass, such as an angiomyolipoma. However, given the lack of signal loss following administration of a fat saturation pulse (see Fig. 2B), a fat-containing mass is excluded. High T1 signal etiologies other than fat remain as potential etiologies, among which are subacute blood products as in this case of a subcapsular renal hematoma.

In Case 3, the subacute thrombus within the subintimal space of a left vertebral artery dissection is obscured by the high-signal-intensity fat near the vertebral arteries on the non–fat-suppressed T1W images; the use of a fat saturation pulse provided the needed "extra" contrast (see Fig. 3C) to reveal the abnormality.

Gadolinium-perfused tissues on postcontrast T1W sequences may demonstrate T1 relaxation times similar to that of fat. The distinction of enhancing lesions in a background of fat on a postcontrast T1W image *without* fat suppression can be challenging, as is shown in Case 4. The enhancing right intraconal mass on the axial non–fat-suppressed postcontrast T1W image (see Fig. 4A) was obscured by the similarly high-signal-intensity intraconal fat. Utilizing fat saturation (see Figs. 4B and 4C) to suppress signal from the intraconal fat provided the contrast needed to improve lesion detection.

Case 5

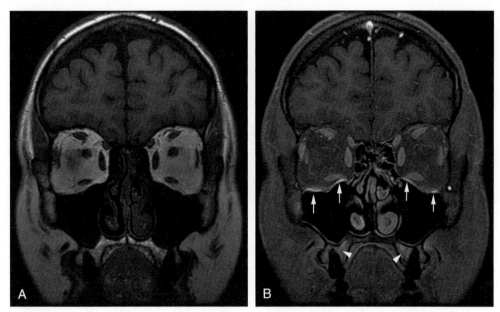

FIGURE 5A. Coronal T1W image of the orbits. Normal T1 high-signal orbital, marrow, and subcutaneous fat are demonstrated.

FIGURE 5B. Coronal postcontrast T1W image with fat saturation. There is near-homogeneous fat suppression of the orbital, marrow, and subcutaneous fat; high signal intensity is noted at the orbital floor *(arrows)* and within the marrow of the maxillae *(arrowheads)*.

Diagnosis: Poor fat saturation at air-bone interface of the orbits.

Case 6

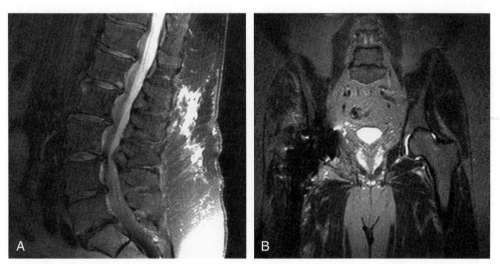

FIGURE 6A. Sagittal T2W image with fat saturation of the lumbar spine. Multilevel degenerative disc disease is evident. Notice the progressive decrease in signal intensity of the cerebrospinal fluid (CSF), with subtle progressive increase in signal intensity of the vertebral bodies of the fifth lumbar vertebral body and upper sacrum.

FIGURE 6B. Coronal short tau inversion recovery (STIR) image of the pelvis, same patient. Signal void of the right proximal femur and acetabulum compatible with orthopedic hardware.

Diagnosis: Poor fat saturation due to presence of right hip hardware with inadvertent CSF signal suppression inferiorly.

Case 7

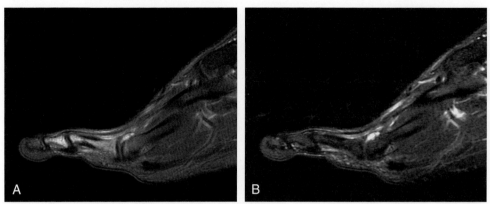

FIGURE 7A. Sagittal T2W image with fat saturation of the middle toe demonstrates diffuse high signal intensity of the middle and proximal phalanges. The signal intensity on the corresponding T1W image (not shown) was normal.

FIGURE 7B. Sagittal STIR image at the same level demonstrates no signal abnormality of the bones or soft tissues.

Diagnosis: Poor fat saturation mimicking bone marrow edema.

Discussion

Frequency-selective saturation operates under the assumption that all protons are precessing at the same frequency. The greater the main magnetic field homogeneity, the more uniform signal suppression is achieved. Unfortunately, field inhomogeneities are invariably present, particularly in areas of the body where there are significant differences in magnetic susceptibility between tissues (the subject of magnetic susceptibility is further explored in Chapter 8). This includes air-tissue interfaces (Case 5), orthopedic hardware (Case 6), and asymmetric body parts (Case 7).[7]

In orbital imaging (Case 5), fat saturation is necessary in order to depict abnormal enhancement on postcontrast T1W images. The differences in susceptibility at air-tissue borders lead to failure of fat suppression. This could make adjacent nonenhancing structures (e.g., ocular muscles or nerves) appear artifactually high in signal intensity on postcontrast images, which may be mistaken for abnormal enhancement.

Because of its ferromagnetic properties, orthopedic hardware (Case 6) causes variations in the local magnetic field,

resulting in alterations in the precessional frequencies of the neighboring tissues.[3] The presence of hardware can lead to failure of fat saturation and, possibly, inadvertent water suppression. The patient's right hip hardware (see Fig. 6B) altered the precessional frequencies of fat and water to the point that the saturation pulse meant to affect fat has instead suppressed signal from the CSF in the lower lumbar spine and sacrum (see Fig. 6A).

The high signal intensity of the phalanges could be misconstrued as edema (Case 7). However, given the lack of abnormality on the corresponding STIR image (see Fig. 7B), the "signal" abnormality was secondary to ineffective fat saturation in the setting of asymmetric body parts. Another area of the body where this failure in fat saturation frequently occurs is the axillae.

Cases 6 and 7 both illustrate how an alternative fat suppression technique, STIR, is more effective for fat suppression compared to its frequency-selective counterpart in the setting of magnetic field inhomogeneities. The principles behind the use of STIR (like fat saturation, a preparatory pulse technique) are further discussed in Chapter 6.

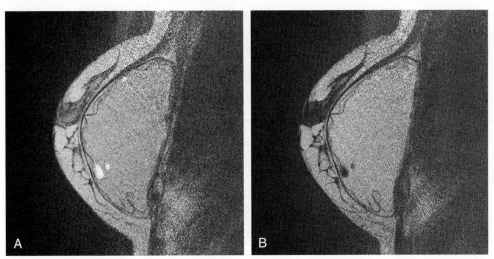

FIGURE 8A. Sagittal T2W image of the breast with subpectoral silicone implant. Multiple, thin curvilinear low-signal lines within the implant capsule are consistent with an intracapsular implant rupture. Multiple round and oval foci of higher signal intensity are demonstrated within the implant capsule.

FIGURE 8B. Sagittal T2W image with water saturation demonstrates signal intensity drop of those foci; note the lower signal intensity of the adjacent fibroglandular tissue.

Diagnosis: Intracapsular silicone implant rupture.

Discussion

This case demonstrates water suppression via the frequency-selective technique, which is used in breast implant integrity studies. The only difference between this and fat saturation is that the narrow-frequency RF preparatory pulse matches the resonant frequency of water protons (Fig. 4); the subsequent use of a spoiler gradient to dephase the transverse magnetization of the water protons is the same. Suppressing the normally high signal intensity from both water *and* fat on T2W images produces "silicone-only" images, which are key to evaluate extracapsular implant rupture with silicone leakage (see Chapter 6).

The diagnosis of an intracapsular breast implant rupture in Case 8 is not in doubt on the T2W image (see Fig. 8A). This case does illustrate the suppression of signal of the water droplets within the collapsed implant shell on the water saturation sequence (see Fig. 8B).

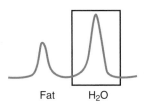

Fat H_2O

FIGURE 4. Water saturation. RF preparatory pulse *(box)* now matches water's resonant frequency.

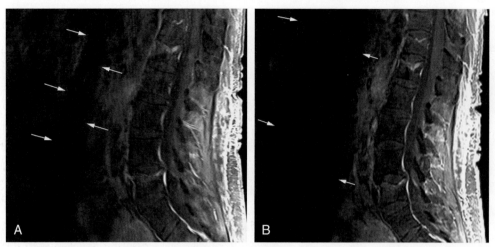

FIGURE 9A. Sagittal postcontrast T1W image with fat saturation of the lumbar spine. Despite the use of a saturation band *(arrows)*, marked bowel motion artifact causes heterogeneity and poor definition of the lumbar vertebral bodies and spinal canal.

FIGURE 9B. Sagittal postcontrast T1W image of the spine, same patient and level. A larger saturation band is evident in the anterior abdomen *(arrows)*. There is marked improvement in the resolution of the lumbar spine.

Diagnosis: Decreased motion artifact with the use of a larger saturation band over the anterior abdomen.

Discussion

Spatial-selective presaturation is a technique used to suppress unwanted signal arising from tissues within the imaging slice. Similar to fat and water saturation, spatial-selective presaturation uses a frequency-selective RF pulse followed by a spoiler gradient. Unlike fat/water saturation, the tissues targeted by the presaturation pulse are *outside* of the area of interest within the image.

Case 9 shows the common problem of motion artifact arising from peristalsing bowel loops in the abdomen, which produces a phase-related artifact that propagates posteriorly in the lumbar spine. The initial attempt at using a narrow saturation band (see Fig. 9A) placed over the abdomen was insufficient in reducing the signals arising from the bowel loops. This was recognized immediately by the technologist, who applied a wider saturation band covering virtually the entire width of bowel. This caused a marked reduction in the motion artifact, with subsequent improved resolution of the lumbar spine (see Fig. 9B).

1. Preparatory pulses are techniques that use an RF pulse administered prior to the excitation pulse.
2. Inversion recovery, frequency-selective saturation, spatial-selective presaturation, and magnetization transfer sequences utilize variations of preparatory pulses to affect tissue contrast.
3. Frequency-selective saturation is a common technique used to suppress signal from either fat or water protons. A preparatory pulse broadcast at the frequency that matches the resonant frequency of the target protons is used to magnetize those protons; a "spoiler" gradient is subsequently applied to dephase the magnetized protons, rendering them unable to produce signal.
4. The quality of frequency-selective saturation is dependent on the magnetic field strength and the presence of magnetic field inhomogeneities; the greater the field strength, the more specific the proton saturation.
5. Inhomogeneities within the external magnetic field cause variations of the target proton resonant frequency, resulting in incomplete signal suppression. Sources of inhomogeneities include air-bone interfaces (paranasal sinuses), orthopedic hardware, and asymmetric body parts (feet, axillae).
6. Preparatory pulses can be used with virtually any imaging sequence; the consequences of this include an increase in imaging time, increased RF energy deposition, and decrease in signal-to-noise ratio.
7. Frequency-selective saturation and inversion recovery sequences can be combined to accentuate signal from a particular tissue or to improve signal suppression from a particular tissue; this is used in breast imaging in the evaluation of silicone implants.
8. Spatial-selective presaturation pulses are administered outside of the area of interest in the body and are primarily used to reduce signal from protons responsible for motion-related artifacts (e.g., peristalsing bowel).
9. Magnetization transfer techniques use an off-peak RF pulse to magnetize bound water protons in macromolecules. These protons then transfer their magnetization to free water protons, leading to a saturation effect. The result is decreased signal in areas where this "magnetization transfer phenomenon" has occurred.

References

1. Mitchell DG, Cohen MS: *MRI Principles*, 2nd ed. Philadelphia: Elsevier Saunders, 2004.
2. Malghem J, Lecouvet FE, Francois R, et al: High signal intensity of intervertebral calcified disks on T1-weighted MR images resulting from fat content. *Skeletal Radiol* 34:80-86, 2005.
3. Lee MJ, Kim S, Lee SA, et al: Overcoming artifacts from metallic orthopedic implants at high-field-strength MR imaging and multi-detector CT. *RadioGraphics* 27:791-803, 2007.
4. Merkle EM, Nelson RC: Dual gradient-echo in-phase and opposed-phase hepatic MR imaging: a useful tool for evaluating more than fatty infiltration or fatty sparing. *RadioGraphics* 26:1409-1418, 2006.
5. Bogaert J, Dymarkoqwski S, Taylor AM: *Clinical Cardiac MRI: with Interactive CD-ROM*. New York: Springer, 2005.
6. Henkelman RM, Stanisz GJ, Graham SJ: Magnetization transfer in MRI: a review. *NMR Biomed* 14:57-64, 2001.
7. Delfaut EM, Beltran J, Johnson G, et al: Fat suppression in MR imaging: techniques and pitfalls. *RadioGraphics* 19:373-382, 1999.

Chapter 6

Inversion Recovery

Phil B. Hoang, Erica Berg, Allen W. Song, and Elmar M. Merkle

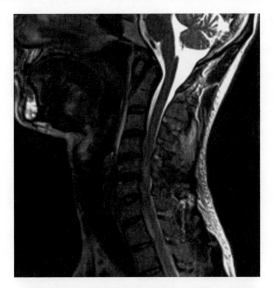

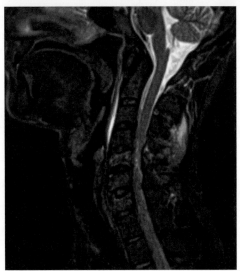

1. What weighting are these two images?

2. What is the normal signal intensity of fat on T2W FSE sequences?

3. What soft tissue was purposely suppressed in the image on the bottom?

4. We used STIR instead of FSFS in this instance. Why do you think this was done?

5. The patient had a history of trauma; what is the diagnosis?

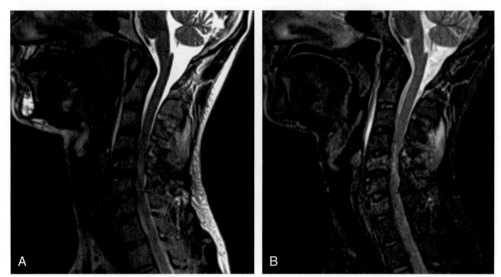

FIGURE 1A. Sagittal T2-weighted (T2W) fast spin echo (FSE) image of the cervical spine demonstrates mild height loss of the C5 vertebral body and high T2 signal in the prevertebral soft tissues. Cervical spinal canal stenosis is noted at this level with possible mild high T2 signal within the cord.

FIGURE 1B. Sagittal short tau inversion recovery (STIR) image at the same level. Prevertebral edema is more conspicuous, with edema now evident in the C5, C6, and C7 vertebral bodies. Persistent, abnormal high signal intensity of the posterior soft tissues is consistent with ligamentous injury. Possible mild high T2 signal in the spinal cord at this level is confirmed on the STIR.

1. Both of these images are T2 weighted.

2. Fat is high in signal on T2-weighted (T2W) fast spin echo (FSE) images.

3. Fat was purposely suppressed on these images.

4. Short tau inversion recovery (STIR) was used to avoid incomplete fat suppression, which occurs in the frequency-selective fat saturation (FSFS) technique due to the magnetic field inhomogeneities from the asymmetric tissues of the posterior neck.

5. The diagnosis is compression fractures of C5 to C7 with cord contusion and ligamentous injury.

Discussion

The high signal intensity of fat on T2-weighted (T2W) fast spin echo (FSE) sequences may obscure both osseous and soft tissue edema. Utilization of a fat suppression technique (see Fig. 1B) is necessary to reveal the urgent abnormalities in this case. Because of its ability to both suppress fat and increase the conspicuity of edema, short tau inversion recovery (STIR) was the preferred fat suppression technique.

Preparatory Pulses Part II: Inversion Recovery

Inversion recovery belongs to the family of preparatory pulse sequences. Chapter 5 reviewed both frequency-selective and spatial-selective presaturation pulses, and this chapter reviews inversion recovery. While the *use* of a preparatory pulse in inversion recovery is similar to frequency-selective techniques, the *principle* behind the desired signal nulling is different. Inversion recovery deploys a *nonspecific* preparatory pulse, which affects *all* protons and relies on different longitudinal recovery rates of different tissues to reach the desired signal nulling effect.

The preparatory pulse is often a 180° inversion pulse. All protons are flipped in polarity, going from positive ($+M_z$) to negative ($-M_z$) magnetization. Protons will begin to recover their net ($+M_z$) longitudinal magnetization as determined by their specific T1 relaxation times (Fig. 1).

Tissue-specific T1 recovery times form the basis for inversion recovery and enable signal suppression (or nulling) depending on the parameter selected; the most common tissues targeted are fat, cerebrospinal fluid (CSF), and myocardium. The null point is the position in time following the inversion preparatory pulse when the targeted protons produce minimal signal, and occurs when the tissue has recovered its equilibrium magnetization to the zero value.

The interval between the administration of the inversion pulse and the excitation pulse is known as the time to inversion (TI). The TI to null a particular proton pool can be calculated with the following formula: **$0.693 \times T1$, with T1 being the longitudinal relaxation time of that particular proton pool.** At 1.5T, the radiofrequency (RF) pulse is sent at 175 msec to suppress fat, and is somewhere between 2000 and 2500 msec for CSF. Since T1 relaxation times prolong with increasing magnetic field strengths, inversion times will also prolong.

Two inversion recovery techniques are in common clinical use and are primarily discussed in this chapter. The first is short T1 (or tau) inversion recovery (STIR), and the second is fluid-attenuation inversion recovery (FLAIR). Inversion recovery used in cardiac imaging is also briefly discussed.

STIR is used to both suppress the signal from fat and to increase contrast in tissues exhibiting long T1 relaxation and T2 decay times. **Contrast in STIR has been described as the "inverse" of T1, as tissues low in signal intensity on T1W sequences are correspondingly high in signal intensity on STIR.** In the setting of magnetic field inhomogeneities and

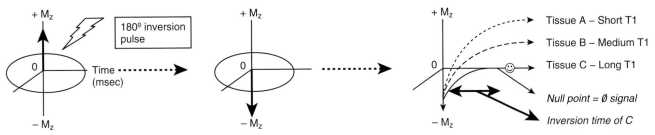

FIGURE 1. Following administration of the 180 degree inversion preparatory pulse, protons are flipped from positive ($+M_z$) to negative ($-M_z$) magnetization. Tissues begin recovering net longitudinal ($+M_z$) magnetization as determined by individual T1 relaxation times. The null point of a tissue (smiley face) is defined as the position in time following the inversion preparatory pulse when the tissue's net longitudinal magnetization is zero.

low field strengths, STIR is preferred over frequency-selective saturation for fat suppression. While STIR provides homogeneous fat suppression, it does so nonspecifically. As an unintended consequence, any tissue that exhibits a T1 relaxation time similar to fat will also suppress.

FLAIR is a staple in neuroimaging. The inversion time is set to eliminate signal from free water and simple fluids (i.e., CSF). Because of the long T1 relaxation time of free water, the TI is longer than what is used in STIR and is typically in the range of 2000 to 2500 msec at 1.5T. Nulling CSF signal improves lesion-parenchyma contrast, most notably for lesions within the CSF itself and lesions at the CSF-brain border. FLAIR is particularly important for depicting lesions that do not enhance following gadolinium administration. FLAIR techniques can also be applied on T1-weighted (T1W)

imaging, which has been utilized to accentuate faintly enhancing central nervous system lesions and to improve gray-white differentiation.

Cardiac imaging makes extensive use of inversion recovery to obtain the desired myocardial and vascular contrast. In the evaluation of myocardial viability, normal myocardial signal nulling improves detection of enhancing scar tissue. Inversion recovery uses *two* 180° inversion preparatory pulses to null signal from flowing blood; specifically, the first preparatory pulse nonselectively inverts all protons, while the second selectively inverts protons within the image slice, so that these protons are now back in equilibrium magnetization. This produces "black blood" images; this topic is further discussed in Chapter 10.

CASE 2

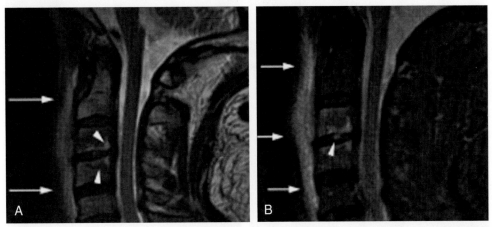

FIGURE 2A. Sagittal T2W FSE image of the upper cervical canal demonstrates areas of abnormal hyperintense signal involving the end plates adjacent to the C3/C4 disc *(arrowheads)*. There is also adjacent prevertebral soft tissue swelling and high-intensity signal *(arrows)*.

FIGURE 2B. Sagittal STIR image at the same level demonstrates increased conspicuity of the end plate and disc signal abnormalities *(arrowhead)*. More diffuse high signal involving the C3 and C4 vertebral bodies is now evident. Compare the signal intensity of the prevertebral soft tissue swelling *(arrows)* to that in A.

Diagnosis: Discitis-osteomyelitis.

Discussion

The abnormal high-signal edema of the C3 and C4 vertebral bodies is more conspicuous on STIR because the normal high signal from bone marrow is suppressed; note the low signal within the normal C2 and C5 vertebral bodies on the STIR image due to suppression of yellow marrow (see Fig. 2B). The prevertebral soft tissue swelling is also more striking on the STIR image.

This case illustrates an important point about STIR; tissues with long T1 relaxation times, such as the prevertebral soft tissue edema in Case 2, will produce hyperintense signal, and tissues exhibiting short T1 (fat) will be low in signal. This pattern is the opposite of that seen in conventional T1W images, and is the reason why the contrast in STIR is referred to as the *inverse* of T1.

Following the 180° inversion pulse, fat recovers its equilibrium longitudinal magnetization faster than tissues with longer T1 times. Once fat recovers to its null point, the excitation

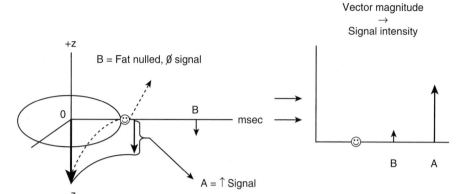

FIGURE 2. With a short TI *(solid lines)*, the protons (A) with the longest T1 (and thus farthest from their respective null points) will create the greatest amount of signal.

pulse is sent, rendering the fat unable to produce signal. The majority of protons in tissues with longer T1 times remain inverted, yet maintain a large vector with respect to their null points. In STIR, signal intensity depends on the *magnitude* (and not polarity) of the protons' longitudinal vector. In other words, it does not matter if the protons are pointing north ($+M_z$) or south ($-M_z$); rather, it is how far and how many of those protons are pointing north or south in relation to their respective null points that determines the signal intensity. The size of the protons' longitudinal vector influences signal intensity, not the direction of the protons (Fig. 2).

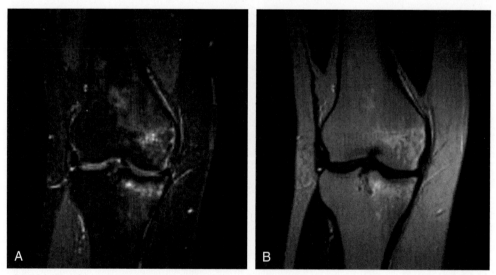

FIGURE 3A. Coronal STIR image of the knee. High-signal marrow edema is identified in the medial tibial plateau and medial femoral condyle. Fraying of the lateral meniscus free edge represents a degenerative radial tear.

FIGURE 3B. Coronal T2W FSE image at the same position. The edema is largely obscured by the high-signal-intensity marrow.

Diagnosis: Bone marrow edema.

Discussion

As mentioned in the Chapter 2, fat is high in signal intensity on a T2W FSE image. This is because of the use of multiple 180° refocusing pulses, which disturbs J-coupling effects normally seen in conventional T2W-spin echo sequences. As you recall, J-coupling refers to the spin-spin coupling of atomic nuclei in lipid molecules that results in shortening of T2 relaxation. This interruption of J-coupling affects the spin-spin interaction in fat, resulting in T2 prolongation and high signal intensity on a T2W sequence.

This can become problematic when evaluating bone marrow, where high-T2-signal edema may be masked by the similarly high-signal-intensity fat. In this setting, the use of fat suppression becomes a necessity. The benefit of fat suppression was previously illustrated in Cases 1 and 2; Case 3 demonstrates how high marrow signal on the T2W FSE image (see Fig. 3B) virtually obscures the edema in the medial knee, which was clearly depicted on the corresponding STIR image (see Fig. 3A).

Fat suppression using a frequency-selective fat saturation (FSFS) technique would have been just as effective in depicting the edema in Case 3 ... if only this study has been done at a higher main magnetic field strength (Case 3 was performed on a 0.6T magnet). Recall that the resonant frequencies of water and lipid protons are very similar at lower magnetic field strengths, resulting in a small chemical shift (approximately 74 Hz at 0.5T, 224 Hz at 1.5T, and 448 Hz at 3.0T). Had the narrow-bandwidth saturation pulse used to suppress fat been applied, the water protons precessing within the frequency range of the saturation preparatory pulse would have also been inadvertently suppressed (Fig. 3).[1]

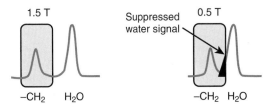

FIGURE 3. At higher field strengths, there is greater chemical shift (or separation) between water and lipid protons, which allow more precise fat suppression with FSFS. At *lower* field strengths, there is less chemical shift between water and lipid protons, with some overlap between protons at the ends of the frequency peaks *(black triangle)*; the narrow-frequency RF preparatory pulse would now suppress some water protons.

CASE 4

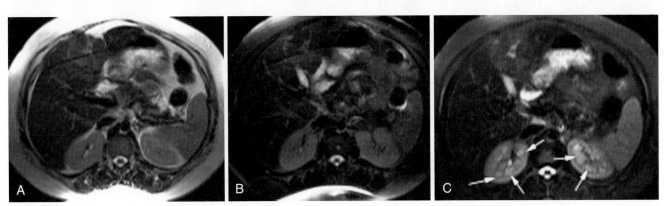

FIGURE 4A. Axial T2W FSE image of the upper abdomen. Note the signal contrast differences between the kidneys, liver, and spleen. The band of high signal intensity of the posterior body wall is consistent with wraparound artifact.

FIGURE 4B. Axial T2W image with FSFS at the same level. Outside of the suppression of signal from abdominal and subcutaneous fat, no significant differences in the contrast between the liver, spleen, and kidneys are evident.

FIGURE 4C. Axial STIR image at the same level. The kidneys and spleen have increased signal intensity relative to the liver. Also, note the increased signal arising from the renal pyramids *(arrows)*.

Diagnosis: Contrast differences between inversion recovery and fat saturation.

Discussion

At our institution, most T2W sequences in musculoskeletal and abdominal imaging are obtained with fat suppression, using either a frequency-selective saturation or inversion recovery pulse. The previous cases illustrate that, while the desired result may be the same between the frequency-selective and inversion recovery techniques (that is, fat suppression and increased lesion contrast), the principles behind these two are quite different. One important principle we discuss here, and as illustrated in Case 4, is the effect of inversion recovery on tissue contrast.

Recall that differences in signal intensity on an image are determined both by the tissue's relaxation characteristics (T1, T2, and proton density) and by operator-dependent factors (time to repetition [TR] and time to echo [TE] on spin echo sequences). Under normal physiologic circumstances, this will produce predictable tissue contrasts on conventional sequences; however, the introduction of an inversion pulse alters those expected contrast patterns, particularly when STIR is used for fat suppression on a T2W sequence.

In Case 4, no noticeable changes in tissue contrasts are evident when comparing the T2W FSE (see Fig. 4A) and T2W FSE with FSFS (see Fig. 4B), aside from the suppressed fat. However, when inversion recovery is used (see Fig. 4C), the subtle changes in contrast between the liver, spleen, and kidneys are more apparent. What is most striking in the STIR image is the increased corticomedullary contrast of the kidneys, which was not seen on the FSFS or non–fat-suppressed images. These differences in contrast between the two techniques are often evident even when the imaging parameters (TR and TE) are similar.

One other point this case displays is the ***additive*** effect of STIR on tissues with long T1 and T2 relaxation times. As the figures in Case 4 demonstrate, the inversion pulse "primes" tissues with long T1 relaxation times to produce more signal;

since these tissues also frequently exhibit long T2 relaxation times, greater signal is generated when a T2W sequence is applied. This is most beneficial for depicting pathologic tissues, which commonly exhibit both long T1 and long T2 relaxation times as a result of increased extracellular water content. As an example, the rather large focal nodular hyperplasia in the left hepatic lobe is best seen on the inversion recovery image compared to the other sequences because of greater lesion-parenchyma contrast in Case 4 (if you didn't notice it at first, look again).

CASE 5

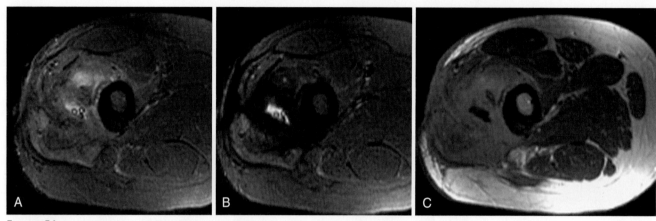

FIGURE 5A. Axial STIR image of the thigh. High-signal tissue in the deep lateral thigh adjacent to the femur extending to the subcutaneous soft tissues is demonstrated. Thickening of the posterior periosteum of the femur compatible with post-traumatic change is present. The three small round foci centrally in the soft tissue abnormality are surgical drains.

FIGURE 5B. Axial STIR image at the same level as A, following gadolinium administration. There is a complete dropout in signal intensity in the abnormal tissue; high signal intensity centrally is consistent with simple fluid.

FIGURE 5C. Axial postcontrast T1W image. The abnormal tissue enhances while the fluid collection centrally does not.

Diagnosis: Postoperative changes.

Discussion

Gadolinium is a paramagnetic agent that shortens both the T1 and T2 relaxation times of affected tissues. At the concentrations used in diagnostic imaging, the degree of T2 shortening is minimal and should not cause noticeable signal decreases in either T1W or T2W sequences (see Chapter 4).

The abnormal high-signal-intensity tissue in the lateral thigh seen in the first STIR image (see Fig. 5A) suppressed when a STIR sequence was repeated following gadolinium administration (see Fig. 5B). The postcontrast T1W image showed avid enhancement of the tissue (see Fig. 5C), meaning that it was perfused with gadolinium.

Can you guess what is going here? The drop in signal in the abnormal tissue on the postcontrast STIR image was due to inadvertent suppression. Gadolinium caused shortening of T1 relaxation of the tissue, which in turn led to a decrease in its inversion time. Because the inversion time of the abnormal tissue now closely approximates to that of fat, the addition of the STIR caused signal suppression. Because of this, FSFS is used for fat suppression purposes on postcontrast images.

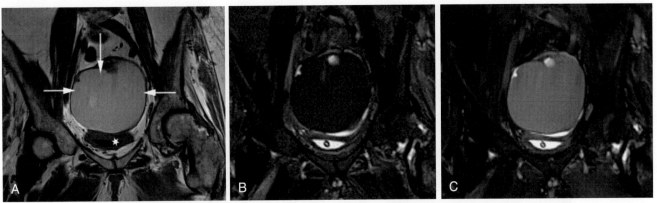

FIGURE 6A. Coronal T1W spin echo (SE) image of the pelvis. A round high-signal pelvic mass superior to the bladder is demonstrated *(arrows)*.

FIGURE 6B. Coronal STIR at the same level as A. Diffuse hypointense signal is demonstrated within the pelvic mass. High-signal nodular tissue is noted along the superior aspect of the mass.

FIGURE 6C. Coronal T2-FSE image with fat saturation. The mass is intermediate to high in signal intensity and is slightly hypointense to urine. *Images provided by Dr. Brad Restel, MD.*

Diagnosis: Hemorrhagic melanoma metastasis.

Discussion

The teaching points of this case are (1) not everything that is high in signal intensity on T1W spin echo (SE) and T2W FSE images is fat and (2) while STIR is primarily used to suppress fat, ***not*** everything with low signal intensity on STIR ***is*** indeed fat.

To quote "Nature Boy" Ric Flair, in Case 6 you have to stop and ask yourself, **"WOOOO!!!! What's caaaaaaausing all this?"** A high-T1-signal pelvic mass (see Fig. 6A) is low in signal intensity on the STIR (see Fig. 6B), but remained high in signal intensity on the fat-saturated T2W image (see Fig. 6C). If STIR was chosen as the sole fat suppression technique in this exam, the imaging pattern might have raised the possibility of a fat-containing mass, such as a lipoma. However, the *lack* of marked signal loss on the fat saturation image alerts you that this mass is definitively *NOT* fat containing (remember, fat saturation is *fat specific*) and triggers a search for an alternative diagnosis. This mass was a hemorrhagic metastatic lesion in a patient with melanoma.

The interesting aspect of this case is the appearance of the hemorrhagic pelvic mass, which appears low in signal on the STIR image but high in signal on the fat saturation T2W sequence. This, along with the increased T1 signal of the mass, confirms that the T1 relaxation time of this lesion was shortened by the effects of methemoglobin, a paramagnetic blood breakdown product seen in subacute hemorrhage. The methemoglobin caused a decrease in the inversion time of the mass, making it susceptible to inadvertent signal nulling by STIR.

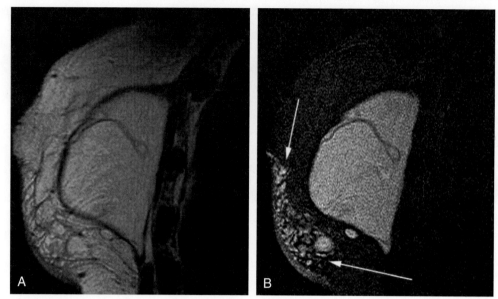

FIGURE 7A. Sagittal T2W image with water saturation (WS) demonstrates a retropectoral silicone breast implant with a curvilinear internal low-signal-intensity abnormality; high signal on both sides of the lines is consistent with an intracapsular implant rupture.

FIGURE 7B. Sagittal T2W image with WS *and* STIR. Homogeneous fat and water suppression again demonstrates intracapsular rupture. High-signal round and globular foci in the inferior breast tissues *(arrows)* are consistent with extracapsular silicone leakage/rupture. Note the progressive decrease in signal-to-noise ratio as signal from water and fat is suppressed.

Diagnosis: Extracapsular silicone implant rupture.

Discussion

In breast imaging, suppression of water and fat signal produces "silicone-only images," which are used both to evaluate silicone implant integrity and to search for signs of extracapsular silicone leakage. As in fat saturation, an excitation preparatory pulse specifically excites water protons; a "crusher" gradient then dephases the excited water protons, rendering them unable to produce signal when the excitation RF pulse is administered.

Lipid and silicone have similar signal intensities and precessional frequencies, and have a chemical shift of only 1.5 ppm (as opposed to 3.5 ppm between lipid and water); this equates to a resonance frequency difference of only 80 Hz at 1.5T. Given this small difference, fat saturation is not used in implant integrity studies as signal from silicone may inadvertently suppress the signal. For this reason, STIR is the preferred fat suppression modality and aids in the detection of implant rupture with extracapsular leakage of silicone (Case 7).

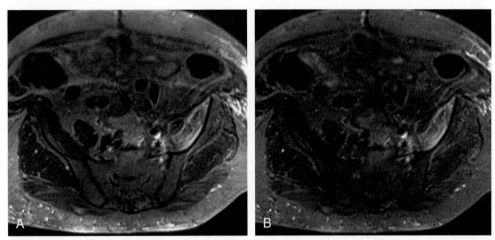

FIGURE 8A. Axial STIR image of the pelvis; TI = 110 msec, performed on a 1.5T strength magnet. Diffuse high signal of the left iliacus muscle is seen. Linear high signal in the left sacral ala is also demonstrated. Note the intermediate signal intensity arising from subcutaneous and intra-abdominal fat.

FIGURE 8B. Axial STIR image of the pelvis; TI = 150 msec. There is increased contrast between the linear signal abnormality of the left sacral ala and the background of fat. Diffuse edema in the left iliacus is again seen. The signal arising from fat is decreased, and there is increased contrast between the left sacral lesion and normal bone.

Diagnosis: Left sacral fracture and left iliacus muscle strain.

Discussion

Case 8 shows the effect of varying inversion times on image contrast. With the inversion time set at 110 msec, the signal intensity arising from fat is mildly suppressed but is sufficient to easily see the insufficiency fracture of the left hemisacrum and the edema in the left iliacus muscle. With the inversion time set closer to the inversion time of fat at 150 msec, there is increased signal suppression from fat and increased contrast between bone and fracture. However, the drawback of using a longer inversion time is a slightly increased imaging time.

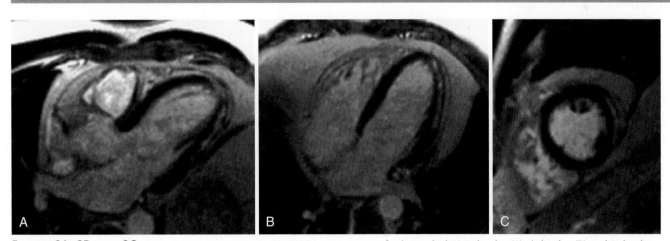

FIGURES 9A, 9B, AND 9C. Delayed postcontrast T1W IR-FLASH (inversion recovery fast low angle shot) 3-chamber (A), 4-chamber (B), and 2-chamber (C) views of the heart. Epicardial-to-midmyocardial enhancement is demonstrated in the basal inferior wall, mid to apical lateral wall, and apical anteroinferior walls; the subendocardial tissue is normal.

Diagnosis: Nonischemic pattern of delayed myocardial enhancement.

Discussion

Inversion recovery is the conventional method for the evaluation of myocardial scar (infarction) or fibrosis in contrast-enhanced cardiac imaging. The signal from *normal* myocardium is nulled instead of fat.

The technique begins with a nonselective 180° preparatory inversion pulse; this preparatory pulse introduces T1 contrast in the image as signal intensity is determined by tissue-specific T1 relaxation times. Because of its slightly higher concentration of gadolinium, myocardial scar regains its longitudinal magnetization at a faster rate compared to normal myocardium. By administering the excitation pulse at the null point of normal myocardium (approximately 300 msec), the myocardial scar will have since regained a significant portion of its equilibrium longitudinal magnetization and will create the greatest signal intensity.[2] This allows differentiation between "bright is dead" scar and normal myocardium. This subject is further discussed in Chapter 4.

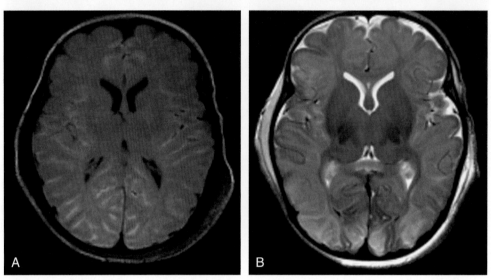

FIGURE 10A. Axial FLAIR image through the level of the basal ganglia. Diffuse hyperintense signal within the sulci as well as high signal dependently layering in the subdural spaces, compatible with both subarachnoid and subdural hematomas.

FIGURE 10B. Axial T2W FSE image at the same level. The abnormal signal seen on the FLAIR image is obscured by the hyperintense CSF signal. Myelination pattern is consistent with a newborn infant.

Diagnosis: Subarachnoid hemorrhage.

Discussion

Similar to STIR, FLAIR emphasizes differences in T1 contrast by using a nonselective inversion pulse and is frequently incorporated with long TE sequences to produce heavily T2W images. Unlike STIR, the inversion time in FLAIR is set to null the usually high-signal CSF; because of CSF's long T1 relaxation time, the TI is typically 2000 to 2500 msec. With this long TI, most tissues regain equilibrium longitudinal magnetization when the excitation pulse is administered, while the signal from CSF is normally suppressed (Fig. 4).

When high FLAIR signal in the CSF spaces is present, it frequently means something is present that is altering *both* the T1 and T2 relaxation times of CSF. In Case 10, the high FLAIR signal within the sulci and posterior convexities is due primarily to the presence of blood, which shortens the T1 relaxation time of CSF. This, in turn, alters the inversion time of CSF, resulting in lack of desired signal suppression. FLAIR is considered the most sensitive magnetic resonance imaging (MRI) sequence in detecting acute subarachnoid hemorrhage.[5] Other things to consider in the setting of high FLAIR signal in the CSF/subarachnoid spaces include meningitis and leptomeningeal spread of disease.

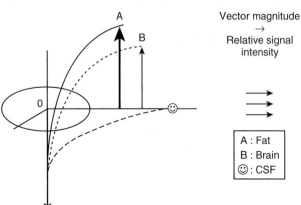

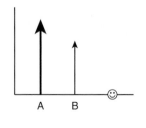

FIGURE 4. After administration of a nonselective 180° pulse, the long TI used to suppress CSF *(smiley face)* allows significant longitudinal relaxation of other tissues (A and B).

Vector magnitude
→
Relative signal intensity

A : Fat
B : Brain
☺ : CSF

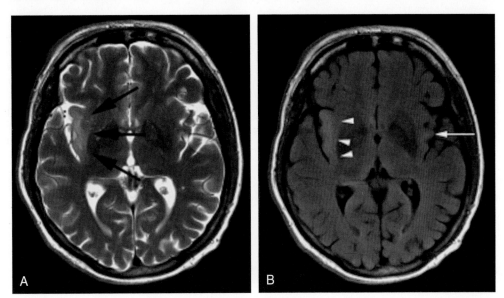

FIGURE 11A. Axial T2W FSE image at the level of the basal ganglia. Possible signal abnormality in the right insula is noted *(arrows)*.

FIGURE 11B. Axial FLAIR image, same level as A. Signal abnormality is confirmed in the right insula *(arrowheads)*; also, subtle FLAIR signal is present in the left insula *(arrow)*.

Diagnosis: Herpes encephalitis.

Discussion

Case 11 is a case of a young patient with altered mental status; the possible right insular signal abnormality on the T2W image is confirmed on FLAIR as the suppression of CSF results in improved contrast between normal and abnormal parenchyma. The FLAIR image also revealed a subtle abnormality in the contralateral insula, which was undetectable on the T2W image. The finding of bilateral, asymmetric parenchymal abnormalities in this patient with altered mental status raised the possibility of herpes encephalitis, which was confirmed on subsequent CSF studies.

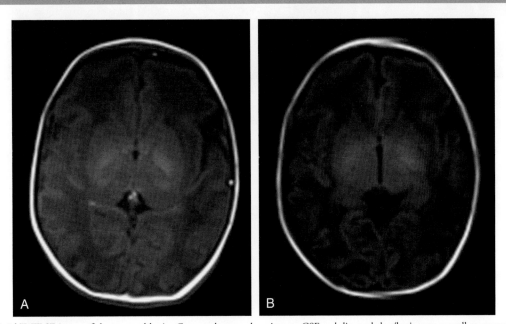

FIGURE 12A. Axial T1W SE image of the neonatal brain. Contrast between hypointense CSF and diencephalon/brainstem, as well as gray-white matter differentiation, are suboptimal.

FIGURE 12B. Axial T1W FLAIR image at the same levels. Robust suppression of CSF signal and improved gray-white differentiation are now evident. Symmetric high T1 signal in the bilateral pallidi is consistent with myelination.

Diagnosis: Newborn myelination.

Discussion
This case was added to illustrate the addition of inversion recovery to T1W sequences to further boost T1 contrast. Initially, inversion recovery was not used with conventional T1W SE sequences due to the excessive lengthening of the TR, which resulted in lengthy imaging times. This was overcome with the development of T1W fast inversion recovery sequences, which basically added the preparatory pulse to a T1W FSE sequence. By adding the 180° inversion pulse (converting thermal equilibrium magnetization from M_0 to $-M_0$), T1 contrast is effectively doubled.

Varying the inversion time can boost the desired contrast within the image, whether it is to improve gray-white differentiation (thus aiding in pediatric myelination staging), or to provide better delineation between tumor and surrounding edema, or to increase conspicuity of lesions bordering CSF and periventricular spaces.[7]

While the use of an FSE sequence allowed for an acceptable imaging time, it is still three to five times longer compared to a T1W SE sequence acquiring the same number of images. Also, the FSE technique causes increased image blur, reducing imaging resolution.[16]

CASES 13 AND 14: COMPANION CASES

Case 13

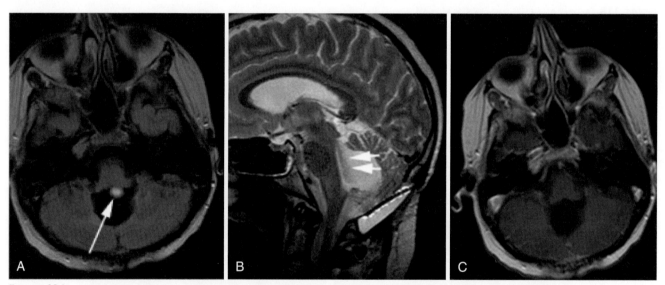

FIGURE 13A. Axial FLAIR image at the level of the clivus. Round hyperintense focus just posterior to the medulla is present *(arrow)*. Patulous fourth ventricle is in keeping with postresection changes in this patient with history of medulloblastoma.

FIGURE 13B. Sagittal T2W FSE image. Bandlike low signal *(double arrows)* within the fourth ventricle is due to flow of CSF protons through the aqueduct of Sylvius.

FIGURE 13C. Postcontrast T1W image at the same level as the FLAIR image. No lesion is detected in the same region as the FLAIR abnormality

Diagnosis: Pseudo-mass from CSF flow artifact on FLAIR.

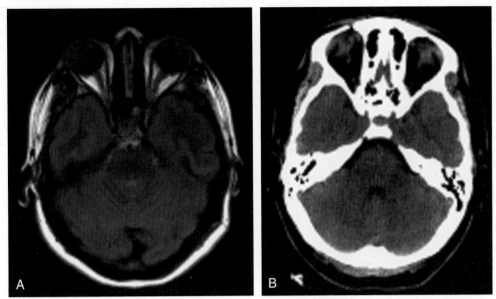

FIGURE 14A. Axial FLAIR image demonstrates high signal in the prepontine cistern and fourth ventricle.

FIGURE 14B. Axial noncontrast brain computed tomography image at the same levels. No evidence of subarachnoid hemorrhage is seen.

Diagnosis: FLAIR CSF flow artifact.

Discussion

We have discussed real pathology causing FLAIR abnormalities, and now we discuss artifacts that can mimic abnormalities. In Case 13, the CSF flow through the cerebral aqueduct has introduced protons that were not subjected to the inverting 180° preparatory pulse, and thus were not suppressed at the CSF null point. The high-signal "nodule" might have raised the possibility of disease recurrence; fortunately, the sagittal T2W sequence provides an explanation for the false FLAIR signal, and the lack of abnormality on the postcontrast T1W image confirms the artifact.

CSF flow artifacts can also give the false impression of subarachnoid disease (Case 14). These artifacts often occur within areas of relative increased CSF flow, including the ventricular foramina and the basilar cisterns (see Fig. 14B). The artifacts are less conspicuous and seen less frequently in regions of reduced CSF flow, such as the cerebral convexities.

Other potential causes of spurious FLAIR signal include delayed excretion of gadolinium into the subarachnoid spaces, which is mainly seen in the setting of renal failure (not much of an issue now given the concern for nephrogenic systemic fibrosis) and sedated patients receiving both propofol and supplemental oxygen.[11]

1. Inversion recovery belongs to the family of preparatory pulse sequences; that is, an RF pulse is delivered prior to the excitation pulse. The tradeoff for using this extra pulse is an increased acquisition time, as the time to inversion (TI) increases the time to repetition (TR)!
2. STIR is a popular technique that relies on the T1 recovery of time of lipid in order to achieve fat suppression.
3. Advantages of STIR over its frequency-selective counterpart are its effectiveness at low field strengths, insensitivity to magnetic field nonuniformities, and increased edema and tumor contrast as a result of additive effects of T1 and T2 weighting (see discussions of Cases 1 through 4).
4. Disadvantages include nonspecific suppression of signal from tissues with similar T1 recovery times as lipids, decreased signal-to-noise ratio, decreased spatial resolution as a result of prolonged acquisition times, and alteration in image contrast (see discussions of Cases 5 and 6).
5. FLAIR is used primarily in neuroimaging to suppress signal from CSF and increase conspicuity of lesions with T2 prolongation. Because of the long T1 relaxation time of CSF, the inversion time in FLAIR is much longer compared STIR.
6. FLAIR is most useful to detect abnormalities within the CSF (blood, proteins, etc.) as well as parenchymal lesions in close proximity to CSF (see discussions of Cases 10 through 12).
7. Frequency-selective saturation and inversion recovery techniques can be combined to achieve more efficient, lipid-specific signal suppression (see discussion of Case 7).
8. Double inversion recovery, which uses two 180° inversion pulses, functions to suppress flowing blood, resulting in "black blood" images in cardiac MRI (see Chapter 10).
9. While inversion recovery is not used in postcontrast T1W sequences for fat suppression, it is the method of choice to null normal myocardium in the delayed-enhancement evaluation of myocardial infarct or fibrosis (see discussion of Case 9).
10. Beware of FLAIR artifacts that mimic CSF abnormalities. Because of CSF flow dynamics, not all CSF protons will be suppressed, resulting in false high signal in cisterns and foramina.

References

1. Delfaut EM, Beltran J, Johnson G, et al: Fat suppression in MR imaging: techniques and pitfalls. *RadioGraphics* 19:373-382, 1999.
2. Lee VS: *Cardiovascular MRI: Physical Principles to Practical Protocols.* Philadelphia, Lippincott, Williams & Wilkins, 2005.
3. Mitchell D, Cohen M: *MRI Principles.* Philadelphia, Elsevier Saunders, 2004.
4. Simonetti O, Finn JP, White RD, et al: "Black blood" T2-weighted inversion recovery MR imaging of the heart. *Radiology* 199:49-57, 1996.
5. Stuckey S, Goh T, Heffernan T, Rowan D: Hyperintensity in the subarachnoid space on FLAIR MRI. *AJR Am J Roentgenol* 189:913-921, 2007.
6. Stemerman D, Krinsky GA, Lee VS, et al: Thoracic aorta: rapid black blood MR imaging with half Fourier rapid acquisition with relaxation enhancement with or without ECG triggering. *Radiology* 213:185-191, 1999.
7. Naganawa S, Satake H, Iwano S, et al: Contrast-enhanced MR imaging of the brain using T1-weighted FLAIR with BLADE compared with a conventional spin-echo sequence. *Eur Radiol* 18:337-342, 2008.
8. Westbrook C, Roth C, Talbot J: *MRI in Practice.* New York, Wiley-Blackwell, 2005.
9. Stradiotti P, Curti A, Castellazi G, Zerbi A: Metal-related artifacts in instrumented spine. Techniques for reducing artifacts in CT and MRI: state of the art. *Eur Spine J* 18:102-108, 2009.
10. Lee MJ, Kim S, Lee SA, et al: Overcoming artifacts from metallic orthopedic implants at high-field-strength MR imaging and multi-detector CT. *RadioGraphics* 27:791-803, 2007.
11. Frigon C, Shaw DWW, Heckbert SR, et al: Supplemental oxygen causes increased signal intensity in subarachnoid cerebrospinal fluid on brain FLAIR MR images obtained in children during general anesthesia. *Radiology* 233:51-55, 2004.
12. Bradley WG: MRI of hemorrhage in the brain. Available at: https://e-edcredits.com/XrayCredits/article.asp?testID=14
13. Noguchi K, Ogawa T, Inugami A, et al: Acute subarachnoid hemorrhage: MR imaging with fluid-attenuated inversion recovery pulse sequences. *Radiology* 196:773-777, 1995.
14. Simonetti OP, Kim RJ, Fieno DS, et al: An improved MR imaging technique for the visualization of myocardial infarction. *Radiology* 218:215-223, 2001.
15. May DA, Pennington DJ: Effect of gadolinium concentration on renal signal intensity: an in vitro study with a saline bag model. *Radiology* 216:232-236, 2000.
16. Rydberg JN, Hammond CA, Iii JH Jr, et al: T1-weighted MR imaging of the brain using a fast inversion recovery pulse sequence. *J Magn Reson Imaging* 6:356-362, 1996.

Chapter 7

Chemical Shift Type 2 Artifact

Scott M. Duncan and Timothy J. Amrhein

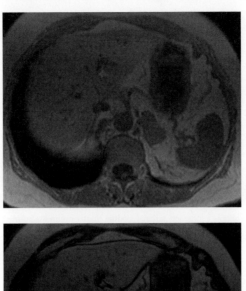

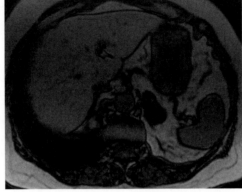

1. Which image is the "in-phase" image and which is the "out-of-phase" image? How can you differentiate the two images?

2. What is the difference between the appearances of the adrenal nodule on the in- and out-of-phase images?

3. Is this lesion benign or malignant?

4. Which series, in or out of phase, is typically acquired first?

5. Why is the subcutaneous fat still bright on the out-of-phase image?

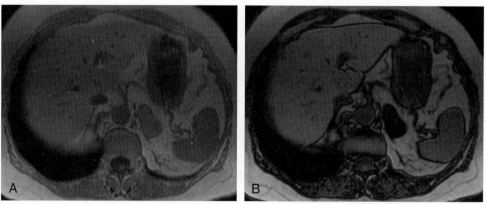

FIGURE 1A. Axial T1-weighted in-phase image. There is a large left adrenal nodule that is isointense to muscle (gray).

FIGURE 1B. Axial T1-weighted out-of-phase image. The left adrenal nodule has lost signal and now appears almost black.

1. The in-phase image is on the left and the out-of-phase on the right. The "India ink" artifact helps to differentiate the two images. The India ink artifact outlines all of the abdominal organs and is only present on out-of-phase images.

2. The nodule appears darker on the out-of-phase image in comparison with the in-phase image because of the presence of fat.

3. This is most likely a benign adrenal lesion because there is fat within the lesion, which is rarely seen with metastatic adrenal nodules.

4. The out-of-phase image is acquired first (see discussion below).

5. Pixels that are almost exclusively fat signal are not suppressed on out-of-phase images. Suppression is seen only in pixels with proportions of both fat and water signal.

Diagnosis: Adrenal adenoma.

Discussion: The signal loss on the out-of-phase image is indicative of fat within the lesion, a finding that is suggestive of an adrenal adenoma. One word of caution: although the signal loss is highly suggestive of an adrenal adenoma, adrenal cortical carcinomas, pheochromocytomas, and clear cell renal cell carcinomas can exhibit these magnetic resonance (MR) characteristics as well.[1] At least 20% signal loss should be identified to ensure the diagnosis of an adenoma.[2] Atypical adrenal nodules warrant consideration of positron emission tomography/computed tomography (PET/CT), adrenal washout CT, or biopsy to confirm the diagnosis.

Physics Discussion

In- and out-of-phase imaging is an essential sequence used in abdominal imaging, especially when evaluating the liver, adrenal glands, and kidneys. This sequence takes advantage of an artifact called "chemical shift" to evaluate for the presence of small proportions of fat. There are two types of chemical shift artifacts. Type 1, or chemical shift misregistration artifact, is present on all sequences to some extent, although it is often imperceptible. Type 1 chemical shift artifact is covered in Chapter 9. Type 2, or chemical shift cancellation artifact, is only present on out of phase sequences and is the focus of this chapter.

Fat and water protons are exposed to slightly different magnetic field strengths as a result of differences in the electromagnetic microenvironments between the two molecules, specifically differences in the electron clouds surrounding the hydrogen nuclei (i.e., protons).[3,4] This results in slightly different Larmor frequencies for protons in these two molecules. Since the protons precess at slightly different frequencies, there are regular intervals when their spins are in phase and out of phase with each other. Adjusting the times to echo (TEs) to times when the nuclei are in and out of phase produces the in- and out-of-phases images.[3] On 1.5T magnetic resonance imaging (MRI) systems, there is an approximately 220-Hz frequency difference between the two molecules. In other words, every 4.4 msec (1 sec/220 Hz) water protons will have done exactly one extrarotation and be back in phase with the fat protons. The signals are in opposite phases (water will have an extra 180° rotation) at 2.2 msec, 6.6 msec, etc. The frequency difference for fat and water is doubled on 3.0T systems, thus the above increments are halved (1 sec/440 Hz).[5]

In- and out-of-phase images are acquired using a T1-weighted gradient-recalled echo sequence. MRI scanners traditionally acquire the out-of-phase images before the in-phase image to eliminate the confounding variable of T2* decay. If the out-of-phase images were acquired after the in-phase images, it would be difficult to determine if the signal loss was from chemical shift artifact or from T2* decay.[6]

The diagnostic utility of in- and out-of-phase imaging is its sensitivity for small amounts of fat within a lesion or organ.[2] Other fat suppression techniques in MR (chemical-selective fat suppression [CSFS] or inversion recovery) and CT can also detect fat within a lesion; however, they are less sensitive for smaller amounts of fat.[7] As in Case 1, identifying lesions with a small component of fat is essential to establishing a diagnosis and to determining its benign or malignant nature. Lesions with small amounts of fat lose signal on out-of-phase images because there is a proportion of both fat and water within an individual pixel. The fat will have a (−) signal value while the

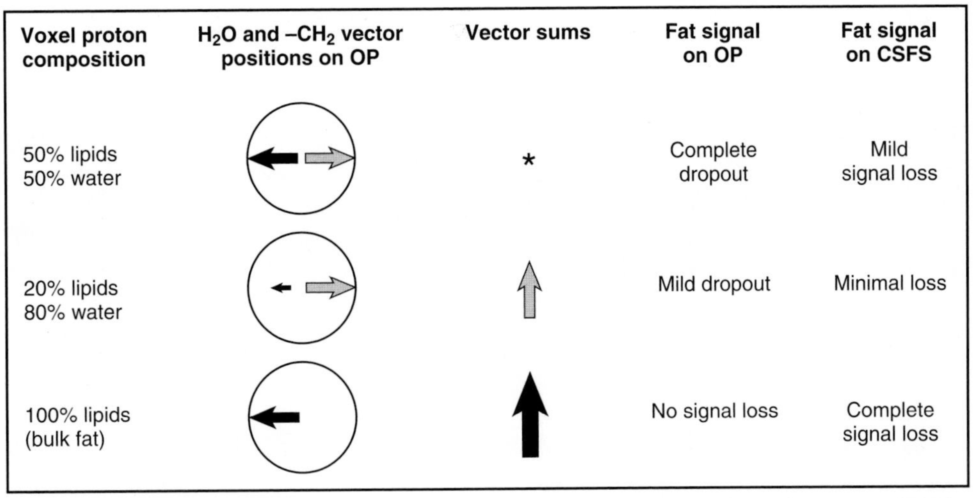
Voxel proton composition
H_2O and $-CH_2$ vector positions on OP
Vector sums
Fat signal on OP
Fat signal on CSFS
50% lipids
50% water
*
Complete dropout
Mild signal loss
20% lipids
80% water
Mild dropout
Minimal loss
100% lipids
(bulk fat)
No signal loss
Complete signal loss

FIGURE 1. Diagram of the appearance of fat on out-of-phase sequence (OP) and 2-point Dixon chemical-selective fat saturation (CSFS) and fat saturation prepulse sequence.

water will have a (+) signal value. When these two signals are summed, a portion of the signal will cancel, resulting in loss of signal within the pixel (the pixel appears darker). To understand why out-of-phase images are more sensitive to fat, compare a T1-weighted fat-saturated sequence with an out-of-phase sequence for a lesion where fat contributes 15% of its signal intensity and water the remaining 85%. In the fat saturation sequence, 85% of the signal will remain in the lesion after the fat saturation prepulse. However, in the out-of-phase image, the 15% fat signal cancels out a portion of the 85% water signal, resulting in only 70% of the original signal. This makes the difference much easier to detect. In summary, out-of-phase sequences magnify the signal loss from fat by a factor of 2, resulting in increased conspicuity of lesions with minimal fat.

If a pixel's signal contribution is 50% from water and 50% from fat, then the two signal contributions will completely cancel each other out and the resultant pixel will have no signal (i.e., be black). The most common location for this to occur is at an interface of fat and water, such as between abdominal organs (containing nearly 100% water signal) and the surrounding mesenteric or retroperitoneal fat. This is the basis for the characteristic India ink artifact identified on out-of-phase images. The India ink artifact is the thin black line that outlines all of the organs in the abdomen. The artifact completely lines the organ on all sides, differentiating it from type 1 chemical shift artifact, which only occurs along the frequency-encoding axis.[3]

Interestingly, areas that are composed solely of fat do not lose intensity on out-of-phase images (look at the appearance of the mesenteric fat in the images in Case 1; note that it retains its high signal intensity) (Fig. 1). This seems counterintuitive. The mesenteric fat and the adrenal nodule both contain fat, so shouldn't they both have suppressed signal? To understand this apparent contradiction, one must remember that MR images are most often magnitude images that make use of only the absolute values to determine signal intensity, and not the vector direction or phase. Therefore, the value in a specific pixel could be positive (water-containing structure) or negative (mesenteric fat), but if they have the same absolute value they will appear similar. Conversely, if a pixel is composed of some combination of fat and water signal, such as an adrenal adenoma, then there will be signal cancellation.

Case 2

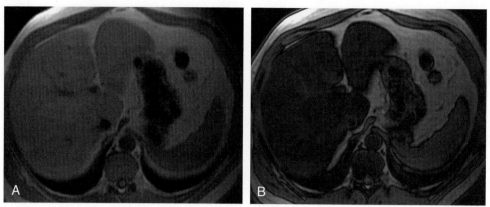

FIGURE 2A. Axial T1-weighted in-phase image. Normal-appearing liver without lesion.

FIGURE 2B. Axial T1-weighted out-of-phase image. Diffuse signal loss throughout the liver.

Diagnosis: Diffuse hepatic steatosis.
Discussion: Signal loss within the liver on the out-of-phase image is diagnostic of hepatic steatosis, which occurs when the liver is incapable of metabolizing triglycerides normally and instead stores them in hepatocytes.[7]

Case 3

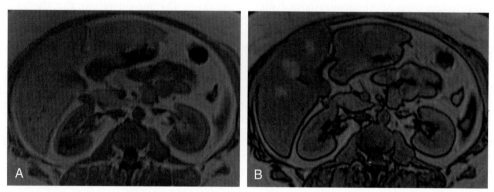

FIGURE 3A. Axial T1-weighted in-phase image. Normal-appearing liver.

FIGURE 3B. Axial T1-weighted out-of-phase image. There is loss of signal throughout most of the liver. There are several hyperintense areas in segments III, IVB, V, and VI of the liver.

Diagnosis: Focal fat sparing.

Physics Discussion
The loss of signal in the liver again signifies hepatic steatosis. The hyperintense "lesions" in the liver are not true lesions, but rather are areas of normal liver that appear bright in comparison with the signal loss in the surrounding liver. One should therefore not mistake these pseudo-lesions for true hepatic masses.[7] Both focal fat infiltration and focal fat sparing demonstrate the same location predilection and are often identified in the region of the gallbladder fossa, adjacent to the teres ligament, anterior to the right portal vein, and in the subcapsular parenchyma.[6]

Case 4

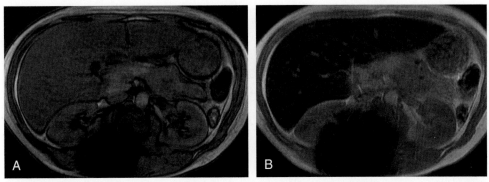

FIGURE 4A. Axial T1-weighted out-of-phase image. There is normal signal intensity of the liver without lesion.

FIGURE 4B. Axial T1-weighted in-phase image. Decreased signal intensity of the liver is seen in comparison with the out-of-phase image. Note the more prominent blooming artifact of the spinal hardware.

Diagnosis: Hemosiderosis.

Case 5

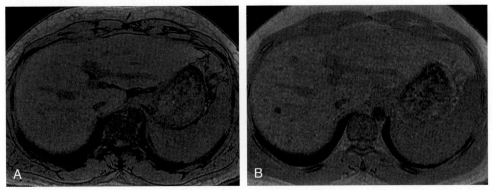

FIGURE 5A. Axial T1-weighted out-of-phase image. Slightly nodular liver without focal lesion.

FIGURE 5B. Axial T1-weighted in-phase image. Multiple tiny foci of black signal are scattered throughout the liver.

Diagnosis: Siderotic nodules in a cirrhotic patient.
Discussion: Approximately one third of patients with cirrhosis will have iron deposition within regenerative and occasionally dysplastic nodules within the liver. These nodules are classified as siderotic nodules. The exact etiology of iron deposition is uncertain.[8]

Case 6

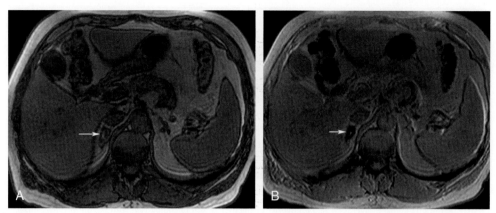

FIGURE 6A. Axial T1-weighted out-of-phase image. A heterogeneous adrenal nodule is seen within the right adrenal gland *(arrow)*.

FIGURE 6B. Axial T1-weighted in-phase image. There is decreased signal intensity of the adrenal nodule *(arrow)* in comparison with the out-of-phase image.

Diagnosis: Adrenal hemorrhage.

Discussion: Appropriate diagnosis of this benign adrenal lesion would prevent unnecessary additional imaging and may even avoid a biopsy attempt.

Physics Discussion

Did you notice the switch? The order of the images in this group of cases was switched. Always look for the India ink artifact to differentiate between the in- and out-of-phase images. Note that the liver and the adrenal nodule get *brighter* on the out-of-phase images. Additionally, the siderotic nodules "drop out" on the in-phase image. This seems counterintuitive, but remember that the out-of-phase images are acquired before the in-phase images, resulting in more T2* decay on the in-phase image.[6] In a normal liver this is often imperceptible. However, when the liver is filled with iron (a diamagnetic substance), there is a resultant increase in the rate of T2* decay, which leads to an in-phase image that has less signal than the out-of-phase image. Similarly, the iron-containing hemosiderin within the adrenal hemorrhage also results in rapid T2* decay and less signal on the in-phase image. Note the increased blooming from the spinal hardware in Case 4 that is more prominent because of the longer TE on the in-phase image.

Case 7

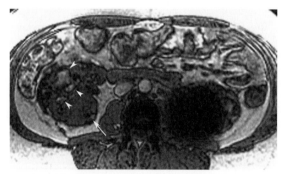

FIGURE 7. Axial T1-weighted out-of-phase image. Several hyperintense lesions are seen within the right kidney *(arrowheads)*. Many of these lesions are intraparenchymal. A slightly exophytic lesion is identified along the posteromedial aspect of the kidney *(arrow)*. The India ink artifact completely surrounds the parenchymal lesions, and separates the exophytic lesion and the renal parenchyma. Note the susceptibility artifact within the left kidney from a surgical clip.

Diagnosis: Angiomyolipoma (AML).

Case 8

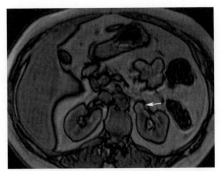

FIGURE 8. Axial T1-weighted out-of-phase image from a different patient. An exophytic lesion is seen arising from the anteromedial aspect of the left kidney *(arrow)*. The India ink artifact extends along the outer margin of the lesion.

Diagnosis: Hemorrhagic cyst.

Physics Discussion

AMLs contain large amounts of fat, which makes them bright on T1-weighted images. Unfortunately, hemorrhagic cysts and hemorrhagic renal cell cancers are also bright on T1. The India ink artifact can help differentiate these lesions.[9] Remember: the artifact always occurs at fat-water interfaces. Thus, when the artifact is identified on all sides of an intraparenchymal lesion, the lesion must contain fat as the renal parenchyma is composed almost entirely of water. An example of this is seen in Case 7, a benign AML. In contradistinction, if the India ink artifact extends along the outer aspect of the lesion, as in Case 8, the fat-water interface is on the outside of the lesion. Since there is surrounding retroperitoneal and mesenteric fat, this implies a predominantly fluid component to the lesion, in this case, a hemorrhagic cyst.

CASE 9

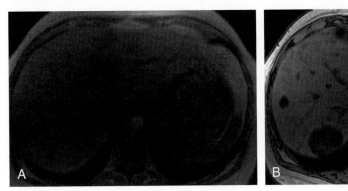

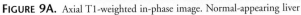

FIGURE 9A. Axial T1-weighted in-phase image. Normal-appearing liver

FIGURE 9B. Axial T1 weighted out-of-phase image. Multiple low-signal masses are seen throughout the liver.

Diagnosis: Hepatic adenomatosis.
Discussion: Hepatic adenomas can be very difficult to detect, as demonstrated by the in-phase image (see Fig. 9A). Some adenomas contain intracytoplasmic fat and will therefore lose signal on the out-of-phase image, becoming quite conspicuous.[10] On the contrast-enhanced sequences (not shown), these masses enhanced, which excluded focal fat deposition as a differential consideration.

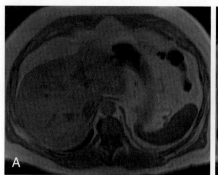 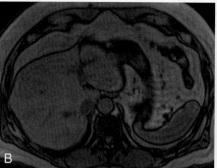 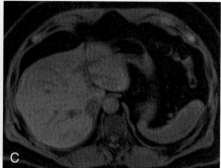

FIGURE 10A. Axial T1-weighted in-phase image. Normal abdomen.

FIGURE 10B. Axial T1 weighted out-of-phase image. Normal abdomen.

FIGURE 10C. "Water-only" image using the 2-point Dixon technique.

Diagnosis: Water-only image for use as a T1-weighted pre-contrast sequence.

Physics Discussion

Initially described by Tom Dixon in 1984, the Dixon technique has had a recent resurgence in popularity with in- and out-of-phase images. The 2-point Dixon technique sums the information from two images to make a third image. By summing in- and out-of-phase images, a "water-only" image is obtained.[11] Remember that the in-phase image is essentially a "water + fat" image and that the out-of-phase image is a "water − fat" image. By adding the two, the fat cancels out, and the resulting image is composed only of water signal:

$$(\text{water} + \text{fat}) + (\text{water} - \text{fat}) = 2 * \text{water and } 0 * \text{fat}$$

Examining the "water-only" image more closely, it does not appear to be the result of adding the in- and out-of-phase magnitude images. For example, look at the subcutaneous fat: the fat is bright on both the in- and out-of-phage images, but it is dark on the "water-only" image. Remember, a pixel displays the absolute value of the signal intensity, not the vector value. However, when the two raw data sets are summed, the vector values are used, resulting in cancellation of the two fat signals.

What is the benefit of a water-only sequence? Essentially, this is a T1-weighted image with signal only from water protons and no signal from fat protons—in other words, a fat-saturated T1-weighted image. This is a third way to generate a fat-saturated image, in addition to a fat saturation pre-pulse and inversion recovery. The sequence does not add additional scanner time (the images are simply generated by a computer using the same equation as above with a small phase adjustment) and may replace the precontrast fat-saturated T1-weighted sequence, decreasing overall scanning time.

"Fat-only" images can also be generated using the 2-point Dixon technique. Instead of adding the two images, the computer subtracts the two images, thereby yielding a "fat-only" image:

$$(\text{water} + \text{fat}) - (\text{water} - \text{fat}) = 0 * \text{water and } 2 * \text{fat}$$

As of yet there is no clear diagnostic utility to the "fat-only" sequence, though it is being investigated.

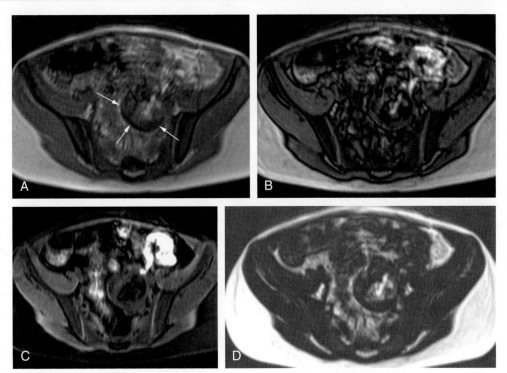

FIGURE 11A. Axial T1-weighted in-phase image demonstrates a left pelvic mass *(white arrows)* with intrinsic high signal intensity internally *(black arrows)*.

FIGURE 11B. Axial T1-weighted out-of-phase image demonstrates persistent high signal intensity centrally. Note the appearance of peripheral low signal about the margins of the mass.

FIGURE 11C. Axial T1-weighted water-only image demonstrates near-complete signal intensity loss of the mass centrally.

FIGURE 11D. Axial T1-weighted fat-only image demonstrates high signal centrally within the mass.

Diagnosis: Ovarian dermoid.

Physics Discussion

When the majority of the protons within a particular voxel are contributed from fat, it will lose signal on the water-only image. This is the finding in Case 11, where the high T1 signal intensity centrally within the pelvic mass lost much of the signal on the water-only image (see Fig. 11C). This confirmed the presence of fat in the mass, a frequent finding in an ovarian dermoid. In contrast, the persistence of the high signal on the out-of-phase image (see Fig. 11B) is due to the predominant fat component with minimal intravoxel phase cancellation. Nonetheless, the identification of the India ink artifact surrounding the margins of the central fat provides indirect evidence of a fat-containing lesion. The fat-only sequence also confirms the presence of fat within the lesion.

Physics

1. There are slight differences between the resonant frequencies of the protons found in fat in comparison with those found in water as a result of differences in their electromagnetic microenvironments.
2. There are regular intervals when fat and water protons are in and out of phase with each other.
3. Setting the TEs to these times results in the in- and out-of-phase images.
4. Type 2 chemical shift artifact, or chemical shift cancellation artifact, is present only on out-of-phase images when there is a proportion of both fat and water signal in a pixel.
5. The (−) value of fat and the (+) value of water in a pixel partially cancel each other out on the out-of-phase image, resulting in signal intensity loss and the lesion appearing darker.
6. The characteristic India ink artifact occurs when a pixel contains 50% water and fat signal. The artifact surrounds the abdominal organs on the out-of-phase sequence.
7. Pixels that contain solely fat do not lose signal because there is no water signal to cancel.

Clinical

1. In- and out-of-phase sequence is essential in abdominal imaging for detecting small proportions of fat.
2. Presence of fat in an adrenal lesion confirms the diagnosis of adrenal adenoma and makes malignancy highly unlikely.
3. Hepatic steatosis results in signal loss within the liver caused by triglycerides within the hepatocytes.
4. In hepatic steatosis, normal areas of liver can appear as hyperintense "lesions" on the out-of-phase sequence because of the signal loss in the surrounding fatty liver.
5. Because the India ink artifact occurs at water-fat interfaces, it can demonstrate the chemical composition of a lesion based on how it outlines a lesion.
6. The liver and spleen can appear brighter on out-of-phase images in the setting of hemosiderosis as a result of increased T2* effects on the in-phase images, which are acquired after the out-of-phase images.
7. The 2-point Dixon technique is used to obtain a "water-only" image, which is actually a fat-saturated T1-weighted sequence.
8. This "water-only" image can be used as the pre-contrast T1-weighted fat-saturated sequence, decreasing scan time.

References

1. Blake MA, Cronin CG, Boland GW: Adrenal imaging. *AJR Am J Roentgenol* 194:1450-1460, 2010.
2. Leyendecker J, Brown J: *Practical Guide to Abdominal and Pelvic MRI.* Philadelphia: Lippincott, Williams & Wilkins, 2004, p 268.
3. Hood MN, Ho VB, Smirniotopoulos JG, Szumowski J: Chemical shift: the artifact and clinical tool revisited. *RadioGraphics* 19:357-371, 1999.
4. Brateman L: Chemical shift imaging: a review. *AJR Am J Roentgenol* 146:971-980, 1986.
5. Merkle EM, Dale BM: Abdominal MRI at 3.0 T: the basics revisited. *AJR Am J Roentgenol* 186:1524-1532, 2006.
6. Merkle EM, Nelson RC: Dual gradient-echo in-phase and opposed-phase hepatic MR imaging: a useful tool for evaluating more than fatty infiltration or fatty sparing. *RadioGraphics* 26:1409-1418, 2006.
7. Earls J, Krinsky G: Abdominal and pelvic applications of opposed-phase MR imaging. *AJR Am J Roentgenol* 169:1071-1077, 1997.
8. Zhang J, Krinsky GA: Iron-containing nodules of cirrhosis. *NMR Biomed* 17:459-464, 2004.
9. Israel GM, Hindman N, Hecht E, Krinsky G: The use of opposed-phase chemical shift MRI in the diagnosis of renal angiomyolipomas. *AJR Am J Roentgenol* 184:1868-1872, 2005.
10. Basaran C, Karcaaltincaba M, Akata D, et al: Fat-containing lesions of the liver: cross-sectional imaging findings with emphasis on MRI. *AJR Am J Roentgenol* 184:1103-1110, 2005.
11. Glover GH: Multipoint Dixon technique for water and fat proton and susceptibility imaging. *J Magn Reson Imaging* 1:521-530, 1991.

Chapter 8

Susceptibility Artifact

Wells I. Mangrum, Elmar M. Merkle, and Allen W. Song

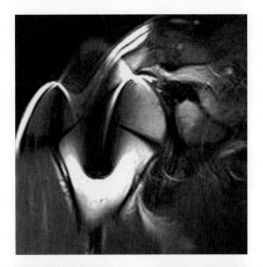

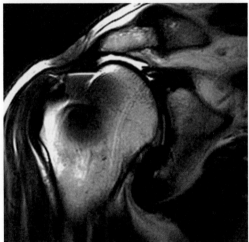

1. What in the shoulder is causing the artifact seen in the images?

2. What is the name of this artifact?

3. What are imaging characteristics of this artifact?

4. Is the artifact more apparent on spin echo or gradient-recalled echo sequences?

5. What would you do to receiver bandwidth and echo train length to reduce the artifact?

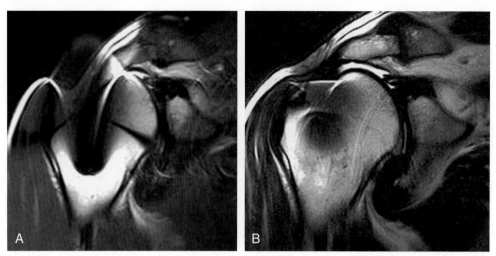

FIGURE 1A. Coronal T2-weighted fast spin echo (FSE) sequence of right shoulder. There is low signal centrally within the humeral head with surrounding high signal. Note that the image distortion is greater in the craniocaudal direction (frequency-encoding direction) than in the medial-lateral (phase-encoding) plane. The artifact limits evaluation of the rotator cuff.

FIGURE 1B. Modified coronal T2-weighted FSE sequence. In an effort to reduce the susceptibility effects, the echo train length was increased from 9 to 23 and the receiver bandwidth was increased from 130 to 435 kHz. Note the significant decrease in susceptibility artifact. The low-signal rotator cuff tendons end abruptly at the level of the acromioclavicular joint. T2 bright signal, consistent with fluid, is seen between the humeral head and acromion.

1. Metal in the proximal humerus causes the artifact.

2. Susceptibility artifact.

3. Susceptibility artifact results in geometric distortion in spin echo imaging and signal loss in gradient-recalled echo imaging.

4. Susceptibility artifacts are less pronounced in spin echo imaging, compared to gradient-recalled echo imaging, due to the 180° refocusing pulse used in spin echo imaging (see discussion below).

5. To reduce susceptibility artifact, one would increase both the receiver bandwidth and the echo train length (see discussion below).

Diagnosis: Torn rotator cuff that is retracted to the level of the acromioclavicular joint with associated fluid in the subacromial/subdeltoid bursa.

Discussion

The magnetic susceptibility of a substance is defined by the effect that the substance has on the local magnetic field. If the material increases the local magnetic field, then the material has a positive magnetic susceptibility; if it decreases the local magnetic field, then it has a negative magnetic susceptibility. Substances that have positive magnetic susceptibilities are considered ferromagnetic or paramagnetic depending on how much they increase the local magnetic field. Iron is a ferromagnetic substance because it significantly increases the local magnetic field. Hemosiderin and deoxyhemoglobin are examples of paramagnetic substances that increase the local magnetic field, but not to the same degree as iron. Diamagnetic materials have a negative magnetic susceptibility and thus decrease the local magnetic field. Free water and most human soft tissue are predominantly diamagnetic. Cortical bone is even more diamagnetic than soft tissue.[1]

Susceptibility artifact occurs when two substances of different magnetic susceptibilities are within close proximity to one another. The substance with the higher magnetic susceptibility will increase the local magnetic field while the adjacent substance with the lower magnetic susceptibility decreases the local magnetic field. The net result is that the local magnetic field is heterogeneous, with high strength next to the paramagnetic/ferromagnetic substance and low strength next to the diamagnetic substance. The susceptibility artifact increases as the difference between the magnetic susceptibilities increases.

Susceptibility artifacts can cause both signal loss and geometric distortion. The signal loss caused by susceptibility artifact is best seen on T2*-weighted sequences (gradient-recalled echo [GRE] sequences). Recall that protons dephase in the transverse plane because of local magnetic field differences (see Chapter 2). When the local magnetic field is highly heterogeneous (such as when metal is in the field), this dephasing can result in significant signal loss. The longer the time to echo (TE), the longer the protons have to dephase and the greater will be the susceptibility-induced signal loss. This effect can be nullified by using the 180° refocusing pulse used in spin echo imaging. The refocusing pulse allows "rephasing" of the protons.

The second manifestation of susceptibility artifact is geometric distortion of the image. Geometric distortion is the dominant manifestation of susceptibility artifact in spin echo imaging. (Geometric distortion also occurs in GRE imaging, but its recognition is often masked by the dominant signal loss from proton dephasing.) In order to understand geometric image distortion, we must first recall that, in the ideal situation, the MRI scanner creates a relatively uniform main

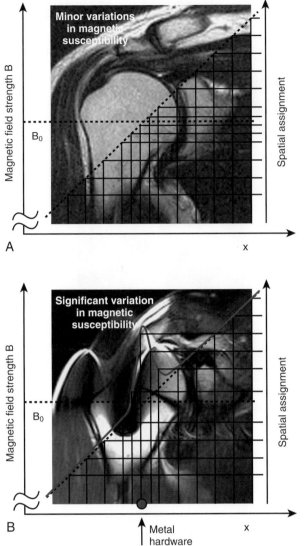

FIGURE 1. Demonstration of susceptibility-induced geometric distortion. **A.** In the normal shoulder, a relatively uniform magnetic gradient is created resulting in a smooth sloping line of the magnetic field. **B.** Metal within a shoulder results in significant distortion of the local magnetic field as demonstrated by the large blip in the otherwise smooth magnetic field. This magnetic field heterogeneity significantly alters the precession frequency of adjacent protons, causing their signal to be interpreted as being in separate parts of the image. As a result, the final image has no signal at the anatomic site of the metal but has high signal adjacent to the anatomic site of the metal, where the signal from the metallic protons is misregistered. *Adapted from Runge VM, Nitz WR, Schmeets SH, et al: The Physics of Clinical MR Taught Through Images. New York: Thieme Medical Publishers, Inc., 2005.*

magnetic field and three sets of linear spatial gradient fields across our body. These fields are required for spatial encoding. Susceptibility effects cause local heterogeneity in these fields, resulting in deviations in the spatial-encoding gradients and distortions in the final image (Fig. 1). The size of the geometric distortion is inversely related to the receiver bandwidth.[2,3] The direction of the geometric distortion is dependent on the imaging sequence. For most conventional imaging, where phase encoding is achieved in separate excitations, the geometric distortion occurs in the frequency-encoding direction. However, in most single-shot acquisitions (e.g., echo-planar imaging [EPI]), the distortion is predominant in the phase-encoding direction as the sampling rate (hence the received bandwidth) is much lower in this direction.

A strategy to reduce susceptibility-induced image distortion is to reduce the length of readout windows for individual spin echoes. This can be achieved by increasing the receiver bandwidth and/or echo train length (this is the strategy used to reduce the geometric distortion in Case 1).[2,3] Alternatively, because geometric distortion occurs in the frequency-encoding direction, one can swap the phase- and frequency-encoding directions and cause the geometric distortion to occur in the orthogonal plane. To uproot the distortion problem altogether, one can measure the magnetic field using a dual-echo sequence, and apply the field correction in the reconstruction process to restore spatial fidelity.

Case 2

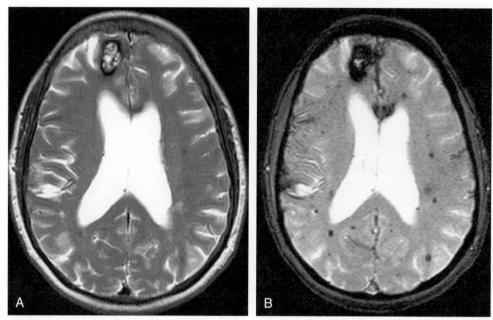

FIGURE 2A. Axial T2-weighted FSE image of the brain. A high-T2-signal lesion with a low-T2-signal rim is identified in the right frontal lobe. The other scattered punctuate foci of low T2 signal in the bilateral cerebral hemispheres are difficult to appreciate.

FIGURE 2B. Axial T2-weighted GRE sequence of the brain. The lesion in the right frontal lobe is again identified. The low-T2-signal rim of the lesion is more pronounced. Additionally, multiple punctuate low-T2-signal foci are distributed diffusely throughout the brain.

Diagnosis: Multiple cavernomas.

Clinical Discussion: The T2 bright lesion with a low-T2-signal rim in the right frontal lobe is characteristic for a cavernoma. Cavernomas chronically bleed and as a result have a characteristic hemosiderin ring. As shown in this case, cavernomas are frequently multiple.[4]

Case 3

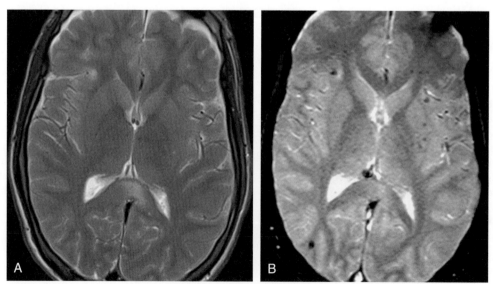

FIGURE 3A. T2-weighted FSE image. Subtle foci of increased signal noted at the gray-white junction of the bilateral frontal lobes and the splenium of the corpus callosum.

FIGURE 3B. T2-weighted GRE image. Multiple low-signal foci are identified in the frontal and parietal lobes bilaterally. These lesions are predominantly centered at the gray-white junction. These lesions are more conspicuous on the GRE sequence.

Diagnosis: Diffuse axonal injury.

Clinical Discussion: The history of trauma and the location of the lesions at the gray-white junction leads one to conclude that these are small foci of hemorrhage in a patient with diffuse axonal injury. Diffuse axonal injury most frequently occurs at the gray-white junction, corpus callosum, basal ganglia, dorsolateral brainstem, and cerebellum.[5]

Case 4

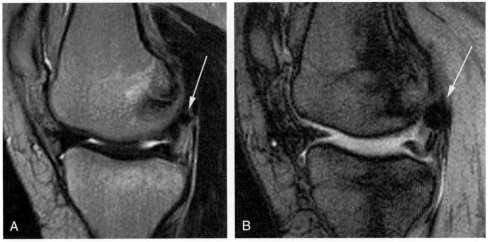

FIGURE 4A. Sagittal T2-weighted FSE image of the knee. A subtle low-T2-signal focus *(arrow)* is identified in the posterior knee joint.

FIGURE 4B. Sagittal T2-weighted GRE image of the knee. The low-T2-signal focus *(arrow)* "blooms" and is much more evident.

Diagnosis: Loose body in the knee joint.

Clinical Discussion: Loose bodies in the knee joint can come from detached cartilage or bone. Free loose bodies within a joint can cause intermittent joint locking and pain.

Physics Discussion

In all three of these cases, the pathology results in susceptibility artifact. In Cases 2 and 3, paramagnetic blood products increase the local magnetic field. In Case 4, the loose body is likely calcified and strongly diamagnetic, again resulting in susceptibility artifact.

The loose body and the blood products are difficult to detect on the spin echo sequences but are readily apparent on the GRE sequences. Spin echo sequences have a 180° refocusing pulse that corrects for the dephasing caused by the magnetic field heterogeneity. Consequently, spin echo sequences are favored when susceptibility effects need to be minimized. Conversely, GRE sequences can be helpful when susceptibility effects need to be enhanced. The dephasing caused by the local changes in the magnetic field is more pronounced with GRE imaging, and results in greater degrees of signal loss. Sometimes this susceptibility-induced signal loss associated with GRE imaging is colloquially referred to as "blooming."

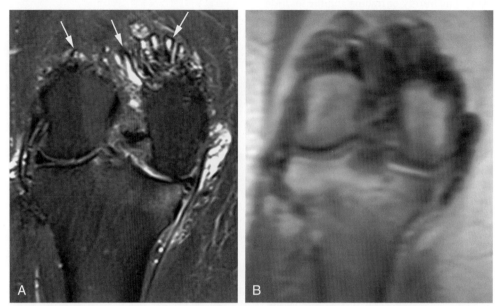

FIGURE 5A. Coronal fat-saturated T2-weighted FSE image of the posterior aspect of the knee joint. Curvilinear low T2 signal intensity is identified within the left knee joint *(white arrows)*.

FIGURE 5B. Coronal GRE localizer sequence. The signal-to-noise ratio is low on this sequence because it was obtained for localizing purposes and not for diagnostic purposes. The low-signal structures within the knee joint "bloom" on this GRE image.

Diagnosis: Pigmented villonodular synovitis (PVNS).

Clinical Discussion: Differential considerations include amyloid arthropathy, hemophilia-related arthropathy, and synovial chrondromatosis. Amyloid arthropathy should not demonstrate the "blooming" artifact seen in PVNS and can be essentially ruled out.[6] Hemophilia can be ruled out by history and by the lack of hemophilia-associated bony abnormalities.[6] Synovial osteochondromatosis will have ossified foreign bodies on plain film; nonossified synovial chrondromatosis is difficult to distinguish from PVNS.

Physics Discussion

As discussed in Case 2, 3, and 4, paramagnetic or diamagnetic substances can cause susceptibility artifact that is more readily detected on GRE sequences. However, GRE images are not always performed. A crude substitute for a routine GRE sequence is the localizer sequence. At our institution, we use a GRE sequence for our localizer sequence. Of course, the resolution of the localizer sequence is poor, but the localizer can confirm the presence or absence of susceptibility artifact, as shown in Case 5.

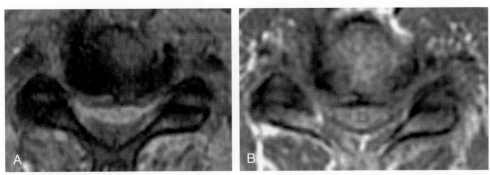

FIGURE 6A. Axial T2-weighted GRE image of the cervical spine shows canal and bilateral neuroforaminal stenosis. Ossification of the posterior longitudinal ligament and ligamentum flavum hypertrophy result in severe canal stenosis. Additionally, uncovertebral and facet degenerative changes result in neuroforaminal stenosis.

FIGURE 6B. Axial T1-weighted FSE image of the cervical spine. The canal stenosis and foraminal stenosis are less pronounced on the FSE image.

Impression: Cervical canal stenosis. Mild bilateral neuroforaminal stenosis.

Physics Discussion
This case shows how susceptibility artifact in GRE imaging can be problematic. Cortical bone and the bone formed by degenerative changes are diamagnetic and cause susceptibility artifact. Consequently, cortical bone and degenerative osteophytosis bloom on GRE imaging, making them appear thicker than they really are. As a result, canal and foraminal stenosis can be overdiagnosed on GRE imaging.

Case 7

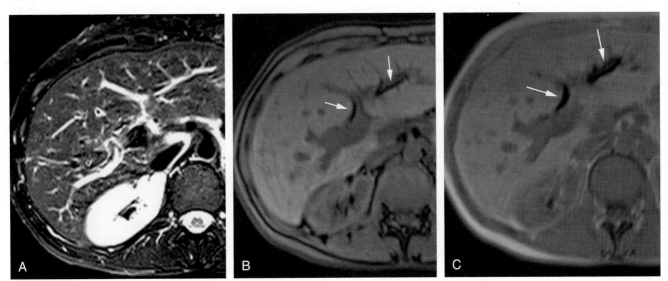

FIGURE 7A. T2-weighted FSE image of the liver. No abnormality is identified.

FIGURE 7B. T1-weighted out-of-phase image of the abdomen (TE = 2.38 msec). A branching low-signal structure is identified centrally within the liver adjacent to the portal veins *(white arrows)*.

FIGURE 7C. T1-weighted in-phase image of the abdomen (TE = 4.76 msec). The branching low-signal structure is more pronounced *(white arrows)*.

Diagnosis: Pneumobilia.
Clinical Discussion: Portal venous gas is another differential consideration for a low-signal branching structure in the liver that is most evident on the longer TE sequence. However, in this case the low-signal branching structures are seen adjacent to the portal veins and not within the veins.

Case 8

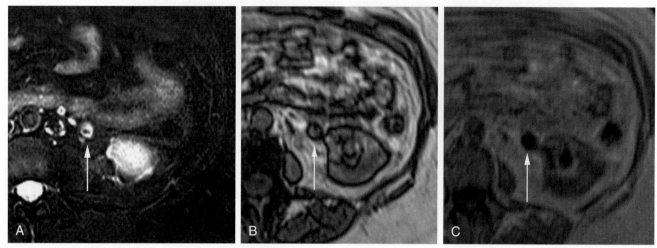

FIGURE 8A. Axial fat-saturated T2-weighted FSE image of the left hemiabdomen. A small filling defect is identified in the left proximal ureter *(arrow)*.

FIGURE 8B. Axial T1-weighted out-of-phase image (TE = 2.38 msec). A low-signal filling defect *(arrow)* is seen within the left ureter.

FIGURE 8C. Axial T1-weighted in-phase image of the abdomen (TE = 4.76 msec). The low-signal filling defect *(arrow)* is more prominent on the in-phase image.

Diagnosis: Left ureteral stone.

Clinical Discussion: The leading differential considerations for a ureteral filling defect include a blood clot, transitional cell carcinoma, and a renal stone. Transitional cell carcinoma would be expected to enhance.[7] A renal stone or a blood clot is a substance that could cause susceptibility artifact. It is rare for transitional cell carcinoma to calcify.

Physics Discussion

Air and liver have widely disparate magnetic susceptibilities and result in susceptibility artifact when adjacent to one another. To best see these effects, one needs to use a GRE sequence such as in- and out-of-phase imaging.[8] As previously described, the lack of a refocusing pulse makes GRE imaging more prone to susceptibility effects.

Comparing the in-phase to out-of-phase imaging also allows one to see the effects of TE on susceptibility artifacts. The in-phase imaging has a longer TE. The longer TE allows the susceptibility-induced dephasing of the protons to have a greater effect. This results in more susceptibility artifact on the in-phase sequence than on the out-of-phase sequence.

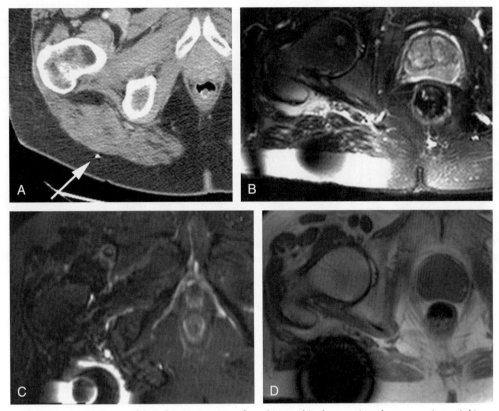

FIGURE 9A. Computed tomography (CT) scan of the pelvis. A tiny piece of metal is noted in the posterior subcutaneous tissues *(white arrow)*.

FIGURE 9B. Axial fat-saturated FSE image of the pelvis. Susceptibility artifact results in signal loss at the site of the metal. The size of the signal loss is much larger than the size of the metal. Chemical-selective fat saturation is insufficient in the immediate surroundings due to metal-induced local alterations of the magnetic field.

FIGURE 9C. Axial short tau inversion recovery (STIR) image of the pelvis. Signal loss is again seen at the site of the metal. The size of the signal loss is roughly equivalent to the signal loss on the FSE image. However, the inversion recovery fat suppression is far superior to that of the FSE chemical-selective fat saturation.

FIGURE 9D. T1-weighted in-phase GRE image of the pelvis. The area of signal loss is much larger than the signal loss seen on the FSE or STIR images.

Diagnosis: The susceptibility effects of metal on different pulse sequences.

Discussion

In this example, the small metal foreign body has a high magnetic susceptibility and results in a significant distortion of the magnetic field despite its small size. The susceptibility effects are enhanced in part because this MRI was performed on a 3T magnet. The higher the magnetic field strength, the greater the susceptibility effects.[1] The greatest signal loss is seen in the in-phase GRE sequence. This is in keeping with the discussions from the previous cases.

Another teaching point from this case is how susceptibility artifact affects fat saturation. As discussed in Chapter 5, homogeneous fat suppression via frequency-selective saturation is dependent on protons within fat having a uniform precession frequency. However, the magnetic field heterogeneity caused by susceptibility effects results in a change of the precession frequency of adjacent fats. Consequently, the fat saturation preparatory pulse may miss the fat that has an altered precession frequency. Inversion recovery imaging, in contrast, is not as affected by local changes in the magnetic field as it depends purely on the T1 relaxation time. Consequently, inversion recovery fat suppression techniques work better in the presence of susceptibility artifacts.

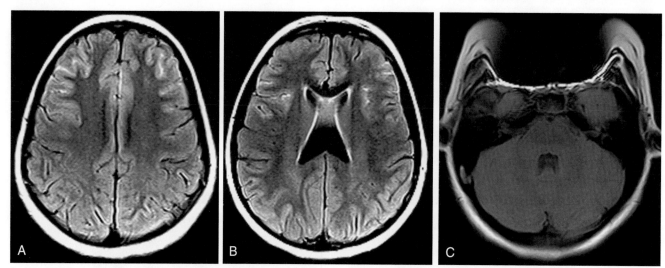

FIGURES 10A AND 10B. Axial fluid-attenuated inversion recovery (FLAIR) images demonstrate increased signal in the region of the leptomeninges of the bilateral frontal lobes.

FIGURE 10C. Axial FLAIR image through the level of the cerebellum. Loss of signal is seen in the anterior half of the face with surrounding hyperintense signal and image distortion.

Diagnosis: Susceptibility artifact from orthodontic braces.

Clinical Discussion: At first appearance, the findings are worrisome for abnormal signal in the leptomeninges possibly from infection, hemorrhage, or neoplasm. However, the more inferior image showing the characteristic signal loss in the region of the mouth (see Fig. 10C) is characteristic for orthodontic hardware.

Physics Discussion

Orthodontic hardware disrupts the local magnetic field. Consequently, the protons in the cerebrospinal fluid (CSF) of the frontal lobes have a magnetic field that is altered by the orthodontic hardware. This alteration in signal is enough to cause incomplete fluid suppression by the fluid-attenuated inversion recovery (FLAIR) sequence, resulting in a pseudo-subarachnoid hemorrhage appearance. Note that the CSF adjacent to the parietal lobes is further away from the orthodontic hardware and experiences normal fluid suppression. This pseudo-subarachnoid hemorrhage is not an uncommon finding in patients with orthodontic braces.

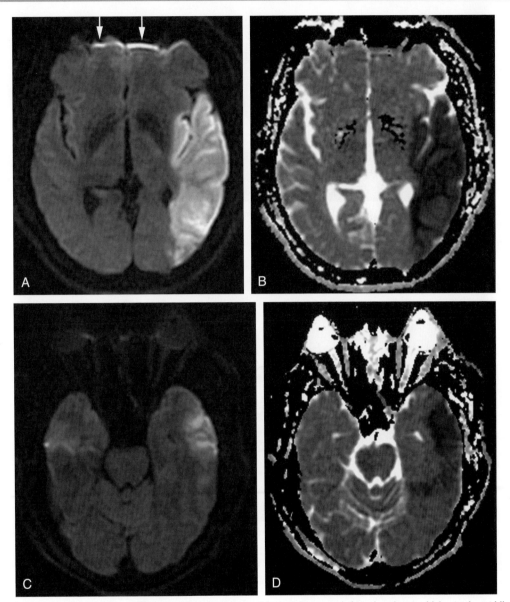

FIGURE 11A. Axial diffusion-weighted image of the brain. High signal is noted in the left temporal, frontal, and parietal lobes in the middle cerebral artery (MCA). An additional thin rim of high signal is seen adjacent to the frontal sinuses bilaterally *(white arrows).*

FIGURE 11B. Apparent diffusion coefficient (ADC) map. Low ADC signal in the left temporal, parietal, and frontal lobes confirms the restricted diffusion in the left MCA distribution. No thin rim of low signal is seen adjacent to the frontal sinuses.

FIGURE 11C. Axial diffusion-weighted image of the brain. High signal is seen in the lateral aspect of the temporal lobe bilaterally, left greater than right.

FIGURE 11D. ADC map. Low ADC values are identified in the lateral left temporal lobe. The right temporal lobe is normal.

Impression: Acute left MCA distribution artifact. High signal adjacent to the frontal sinuses and in the right temporal lobe are normal on the ADC map and due to susceptibility effects.

Physics Discussion

Diffusion images are frequently obtained with echo-planar imaging (EPI). EPI is a GRE sequence that is highly sensitive to susceptibility effects.[1] The differences in magnetic susceptibilities between air in the paranasal sinuses and brain or cortical bone and brain cause susceptibility effects. This is seen as high signal in the brain adjacent to the sinuses on diffusion-weighted images. The ADC maps of these areas will be normal (as shown in this case). Functional MRI is another MRI technique that uses echo-planar imaging and consequently is also highly sensitive to susceptibility effects (see Chapter 17).

Case 12

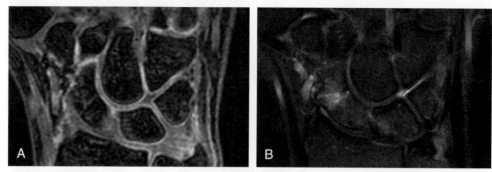

FIGURE 12A. Coronal fat-suppressed T2-weighted GRE image. There is questionable linear distortion of the trabeculae in the waist of the scaphoid. No increased T2 signal is seen in the scaphoid.

FIGURE 12B. Coronal fat-suppressed T2-weighted FSE image. Linear and wedge-shaped increased T2 signal is noted in the waist of the scaphoid.

Diagnosis: Scaphoid waist fracture.

Case 13

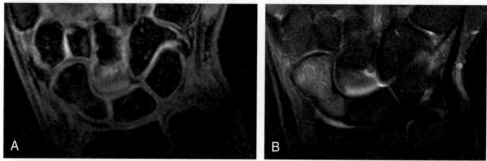

FIGURE 13A. Coronal fat-suppressed T2-weighted GRE image. There is slightly increased T2 signal with associated trabecular distortion in the waist of the scaphoid.

FIGURE 13B. Coronal fat-suppressed T2-weighted FSE image. Linear low T2 signal is noted through the waist of the scaphoid. High T2 signal is noted in the bone marrow of the scaphoid.

Diagnosis: Scaphoid waist fracture with marked surrounding bone marrow edema.

Case 14

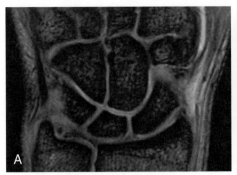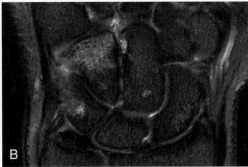

FIGURE 14A. Coronal fat-suppressed T2-weighted GRE image. No abnormality identified.

FIGURE 14B. Coronal fat-suppressed T2-weighted FSE image. Increased T2 signal is noted in the distal half of the hamate and in the distal tip of the triquetrum.

Diagnosis: Contusion of the hamate and triquetrum. A hook of hamate fracture was shown on other images.

Physics Discussion

Trabecular and cortical bone are diamagnetic substances with low magnetic susceptibilities that can result in susceptibility artifact.[9] Case 6 showed an example of how blooming from cortical and degenerative bone can overexaggerate canal stenosis. Cases 12, 13, and 14 show how the susceptibility artifact from cortical and trabecular bone can mask bone marrow edema on GRE imaging. The diamagnetic bone alters the local magnetic field, causing increased dephasing of protons and signal loss. This signal loss hides the signal gain that results from the bone marrow edema. Note that the bone marrow edema is readily apparent on the spin echo sequences because the refocusing pulse "rephases" the dephasing protons.

KEY POINTS

Defining Susceptibility
1. Magnetic susceptibility is defined as the relative ability of a substance to become magnetized when exposed to a magnetic field.
2. Materials can be defined by their magnetic susceptibility to be ferromagnetic, paramagnetic, or diamagnetic.
3. Susceptibility artifact occurs when tissues of widely different magnetic susceptibilities are adjacent to one another, such as metal adjacent to soft tissue.

Methods to Reduce Susceptibility Artifact
1. Spin echo or fast spin echo imaging
2. Long echo train length
3. Shorten TE
4. Increase receiver bandwidth
5. Decrease magnetic field strength (1.5T has less artifact than 3T)

Susceptibility Artifact Can Be Clinically Useful
1. When looking for air: pneumobilia
2. When looking for metal: to detect evidence of surgical changes
3. When looking for blood products: cavernomas, diffuse axonal injury, PVNS
4. When looking for calcification: loose body in the joint, renal stone

Susceptibility Artifact Can Interfere with the Diagnosis
1. Geometric distortion and signal loss from metal hardwire can obscure the image.
2. Susceptibility artifact can create false signal: pseudo-subarachnoid hemorrhage caused by orthodontic braces, signal adjacent to the sinuses in diffusion-weighted sequences.
3. Susceptibility artifact can hide true bone marrow edema: scaphoid fracture, hamate edema.
4. Susceptibility artifact can exaggerate stenosis from degenerative changes.

Sequences Sensitive to Susceptibility Effects
1. GRE sequences in general are highly sensitive to susceptibility artifact.
2. In-phase imaging is more sensitive to susceptibility effects than out-of-phase imaging because of the longer echo time.
3. Echo-planar imaging in diffusion-weighted MRI or functional MRI is sensitive to susceptibility effects.

References

1. Runge VM, Nitz WR, Schmeets SH, et al: *The Physics of Clinical MR Taught Through Images.* New York: Thieme Medical Publishers, Inc., 2005.
2. Harris CA, White LM: Metal artifact reduction in musculoskeletal magnetic resonance imaging. *Orthop Clin North Am* 37:349-359, 2006.
3. Stadler A, Schima W, Ba-Ssalamah A, et al: Artifacts in body MR imaging: their appearance and how to eliminate them. *Eur Radiol* 17:1242-1255, 2007.
4. Maraire JN, Awad IA: Intracranial cavernous malformations: lesion behavior and management strategies. *Neurosurgery* 37:591-605, 1995.
5. Parizel PM, Özsarlak Ö, Van Goethem JW, et al: Imaging findings in diffuse axonal injury after closed head trauma. *Eur Radiol* 8:960-965, 1998.
6. Garner HW, Ortiguera CJ, Nakhleh RE: Pigmented villonodular synovitis. *RadioGraphics* 28:1519-1523, 2008.
7. Leyendecker JR, Barnes CE, Zagoria RJ: MR urography: techniques and clinical applications. *RadioGraphics* 28:23-46, 2008.
8. Merkle EM, Nelson RC: Dual gradient-echo in-phase and opposed-phase hepatic MR imaging: a useful tool for evaluating more than fatty infiltration or fatty sparing. *RadioGraphics* 26:1409-1418, 2006.
9. Majumdar S, Thomasson D, Shimakawa A, Genant HK: Quantitation of the susceptibility difference between trabecular bone and bone marrow: experimental studies. *Magn Reson Med* 22:111-127, 1991.

Chapter 9

Motion, Pulsation, and Other Artifacts

Kimball L. Christianson, Phil B. Hoang, Steve Huang, Mark L. Lessne, Allen W. Song, and Elmar M. Merkle

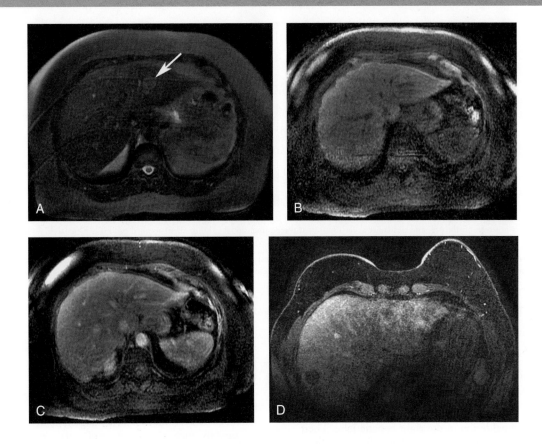

1. What is the differential diagnosis for the bright lesion in the left hepatic lobe in Figure 1A?

2. What is the finding in Figure 1D (different patient)? What other finding in the images suggests the lesion in the right hepatic lobe is artifactual?

3. What is this artifact called and what causes it?

4. Why is the artifact oriented vertically in Figures 1A-C and horizontally in Figure 1D?

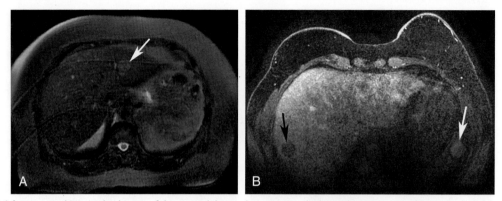

FIGURE 1A. Axial fat-suppressed T2-weighted image of the upper abdomen demonstrates a high signal intensity, round lesion in the left hepatic lobe *(white arrow)*. This lesion is not seen on the pre- and postcontrast fat-suppressed three-dimensional (3D) gradient-recalled echo (GRE) axial T1-weighted (T1W) sequences.

FIGURE 1B. Axial fat-suppressed T1W 3D-GRE sequence from a dedicated breast magnetic resonance (MR) image (different patient) demonstrates a round, low-signal lesion in the right hepatic lobe *(black arrow)* and a round high-signal lesion in the region of the spleen/abdominal wall *(white arrow)*.

1. The differential diagnosis of a subtle, T2 bright lesion in the liver includes hemangioma, metastatic disease, and primary liver tumor. However, given its location, oriented vertically just above the aorta, a pseudo-lesion as a result of pulsation artifact from the aorta is also in the differential.

2. Round low-signal lesion in the right hepatic lobe. There is a subtle high-signal lesion located equidistant to, but left of the aorta along the same horizontal plane as the low-signal lesion in the right hepatic lobe.

3. This artifact is referred to as a "ghosting artifact." Ghosting artifacts appear in abnormal locations as replicas of the moving structure from which they result. They are observed only in the phase-encoding direction and can be the result of any periodic motion such as respiration, arterial pulsation, or cerebrospinal fluid pulsation.

4. Figures 1A through 1C are from an abdominal MR image, and the phase-encoding direction is oriented vertically; therefore, the artifact is also seen along this axis. Figure 1D is from a breast MR image in which the phase-encoding direction is oriented horizontally from right to left.

Part 1: Motion and Pulsation Artifact

Motion is a very common cause of artifacts in magnetic resonance imaging (MRI). Motion artifacts are the result of movement during the data acquisition period. More specifically, when motion is present, tissues excited at a specific location during the radiofrequency (RF) pulse are erroneously mapped to a different location (or often multiple different locations in cases of motion artifacts) during detection. Motion is often divided into two categories: gross body movement and physiologic motion, such as cardiac and respiratory cycles, or blood or cerebrospinal fluid (CSF) flow. In most conventional imaging methods, motion artifact is predominantly manifested in the phase-encoding direction.

The extensive use of spatial gradients complicates and amplifies motion artifacts, as stronger gradients induce larger phase shifts from motion (see *Understanding the Need for Gradients In Image Formation and Its Implication in Motion Artifacts*). While some gradient combinations can compensate for motion (e.g., the flow-compensated gradients; see below for more details), many of the imaging gradient pulses cannot. As such, the inconsistent nature of motion can induce different phase shifts during the image readout period. When viewed from the phase-encoding direction in the final data space, these inconsistencies introduce local deviations that result in ghosting artifacts in the image space as the result of Fourier transformation. For example, a pulsatile effect in one of the data lines (along the frequency-encoding direction) would be viewed as a spike along the phase-encoding direction, which would then result in a streaking line artifact along the phase-encoding direction. More severely, several inconsistent data lines would result in more extensive ghosting artifacts.

In short, motion artifacts are predominantly manifested along the phase-encoding direction. More specifically, random motion results in smearing or blurring in the phase-encoding direction, and periodic motion (cardiac motion and blood vessels) results in ghosting artifacts. Ghosting artifacts appear as replicas of the moving structure at specific intervals along the phase-encoding axis. The motion artifact patterns are dependent on how repeatable the phase shifts were along the phase-encoding direction in k-space. For example, if only one line deviates, then the artifact will be a solid line across the MR image. If it repeats every other line, then the artifact will be a displacement over half the field of view. If all the lines deviate the same way (e.g., after excessive averaging), then there will appear to be no artifact.[11]

Why does flowing blood cause motion artifacts? After application of the dephasing lobe of the slice selection and frequency-encoding gradients, blood moves to a different location and experiences a rephasing gradient of a different strength. The phase shift induced by the dephasing lobe cannot be reversed by a gradient of a different strength, and the phase difference persists as ghost artifacts.[10]

Understanding the Need for Gradients in Image Formation and Its Implication in Motion Artifacts

Why are gradients necessary? If an RF pulse were broadcast without gradients, then every proton along the main magnetic field would be excited. The receiver coil would receive signals from the protons all resonating at the same frequency and with the same phase, making spatial localization and, therefore, a coherent magnetic resonance (MR) image impossible.[9] The three magnetic field gradients required to form an image are the slice selection, frequency-encoding, and phase-encoding gradients. The primary purpose of these gradients is to assign spatial localization to the resultant MR image. For an axial image, the slice selection gradient assigns location in the z direction, the frequency-encoding gradient, or readout gradient, assigns location in the x direction, and the phase-encoding gradient assigns location in the y direction.

The purpose of a slice selection gradient is to expose protons along the z-axis to a different magnetic field, inducing the protons to precess at different frequencies while administering an RF pulse with a very narrow range of frequencies, resulting in excitation of only a thin slice of tissue along the z-axis. Only those protons along the z-axis gradient that have frequencies corresponding to the RF pulse are excited.[9] The range of frequencies transmitted by the RF pulse is referred to as the transmitter bandwidth. The slice thickness can be made thicker or thinner by adjusting the gradient strength or the transmitter bandwidth. Increasing the gradient strength or lowering the transmitter bandwidth results in a thinner slice. Decreasing the gradient strength or increasing the transmitter bandwidth results in a thicker slice.

The frequency-encoding gradient is critically important for spatial localization along the x-axis. Unlike the slice selection gradient, which is applied at the same time as the RF excitation pulse, the frequency-encoding gradient is applied concurrent with echo sampling. The frequency-encoding gradient induces protons along the x-axis at different locations to precess at different frequencies. For example, the protons on the right side of the body will precess a little faster than protons on the left side of the body. With use of the Fourier transform, these differences in frequency can be translated into differences in signal at each spatial location to create the MR image.

The frequency-encoding gradient is also important in the generation of an echo. Over time, proton spins in the presence of a spatial gradient would accumulate phase shifts. The generation of MR signal is dependent on the protons being in phase at just the right time during echo sampling. Gradients' dephasing properties are manipulated in a controlled fashion such that phase coherence can be achieved and an echo generated. This is accomplished by applying a gradient with two lobes that have opposite polarity. The first lobe of the gradient is the dephasing lobe. A second gradient is then applied with opposite polarity and typically twice the duration, called a rephasing lobe. At the midpoint of this rephasing lobe, the sampled protons are most in phase and an echo is generated, referred to as a gradient-recalled echo. If a 180° refocusing pulse is applied prior to the rephasing lobe and after 90° excitation pulse, the generated echo is referred to as a spin echo. Pulse sequences are usually timed so that the gradient-recalled echo and the spin echo occur at the same time. In the case of a spin echo acquisition, the rephasing lobe should be applied with the same polarity (rather than the opposite polarity) as the dephasing lobe because the 180° refocusing pulse results in a complete reversal of phase. The direction of the frequency-encoding gradient is almost always applied along the axis with the widest dimension (e.g., right to left in the abdomen and anterior to posterior in the head).[10]

Finally, a phase-encoding gradient is used for spatial localization along the y-axis. In contrast to the frequency-encoding gradient, the phase-encoding gradient is applied right before the data acquisition (but also after the slice excitation). As such, the protons would have already experienced the gradient and accumulated certain controlled phase shifts. Since the phase-encoding gradient is turned off before the data readout, these phase shifts would remain fixed to ensure the same amount of phase encoding. To complete the coverage for a two-dimensional (2D) image, for example, different phases are assigned with different phase-encoding gradient amplitudes prior to the data acquisition window. A subsequent Fourier transformation can then be used to spatially resolve the image along the phase-encoding direction. It is worth noting that a rephasing gradient (such as that used in slice selection) or a dephasing gradient (such as that used in frequency encoding) is not usually needed for phase encoding. Spatial localization is encoded from differences in phase rather than frequency by applying the phase-encoding gradient after the initial excitation pulse and before echo sampling.[9]

Spatial encoding along the frequency-encoding direction can be performed in its entirety with a single RF excitation pulse. Along the phase-encoding axis, spatial localization usually (save for single-shot imaging techniques, such as echo-planar imaging) requires the application of numerous phase-encoding gradients, each with a different strength, with each new RF excitation. The number of phase-encoding steps required determines the extent of the MR image along the y-axis and, along with the time to repetition (TR), is an important contributor to image acquisition time. Strong phase-encoding gradients create larger differences in phase and allow better discrimination of objects that are close together (better spatial resolution) in the resultant MR image. The down side of a stronger (i.e., steeper) gradient is that protons on one end of the gradient are more out of phase with protons at the other end of the gradient, thereby reducing signal and contrast. Weaker gradients result in better signal and contrast. This principle has important implications in the way k-space is filled. By convention, the center of k-space is the high-contrast region, and the periphery contributes to the fine detail and spatial resolution of the image. It makes sense, then, that the center of k-space is filled first with echoes resulting from the weaker phase-encoding gradients, and the gradient strength increases gradually as k-space is filled from central to peripheral.[9]

Numerous methods can be used to reduce motion artifacts. Increasing the sampling bandwidth (recall the relationship bandwith = 1/time for echo) is a simple method to reduce motion artifact at the expense of the signal-to-noise ratio. While it is true that increasing the gradient strength or the time in which the gradient is applied will increase susceptibility to motion artifact, increasing the strength of the frequency encoding gradient is an exception. The sampling bandwidth increases with increasing (steeper) gradient strength. A steeper gradient means that rephasing of the protons happens more quickly and an echo forms faster, thereby decreasing sampling time.[10]

Another method to reduce motion artifact is called gradient moment nulling. When motion occurs during either the dephasing or rephasing lobe of the gradient, there is incomplete phase cancellation, which leads to a net accumulation of phase referred to as the gradient moment. This phase accumulation can be the result of protons moving with constant-velocity motion (first-order motion), acceleration (second-order motion), or pulsatile or jerk motion (third-order motion). In its simplest form, an applied gradient without motion correction is a unipolar gradient. Application of additional gradient pulses, such as in the form of a bipolar gradient, can rephase the phase shift from both stationary and moving tissues and significantly reduces first-order or constant-velocity motion. Application of more complex gradient pulses can also reduce second- and third-order motion; however, gradient moment nulling works best for first-order motion. Gradient moment nulling requires a longer time to echo (TE); with first-order nulling the increase in TE is negligible, but with second- or third-order nulling, the longer TE can be problematic.[11]

Switching the direction of the frequency- and phase-encoding gradients is a simple way to manipulate motion artifact. Motion artifact is not eliminated with this method, but rather is displaced along another axis. This method can be very helpful in trying to distinguish whether a finding represents true pathology or is due to motion artifact.

Presaturation pulses are another often-utilized method to reduce the effects of motion artifact. This technique is a preferred method if the signal to be nulled is not necessary for image interpretation. Presaturation pulses can be used to null fat if its signal is contributing to the motion artifact. It can also be used to saturate the protons in flowing blood before it enters the volume of tissue being imaged, and is a frequently used technique in time-of-flight (TOF) imaging (see Chapter 11).[10]

Averaging is a motion reduction technique often used to eliminate ghosting artifacts caused by respiratory motion. This method takes advantage of the fact that, on average, normal tissue stays in a relatively constant location with each respiratory cycle while the location of the ghosting artifacts is much more variable with each breath. Averaging is typically accomplished by acquiring more than one signal with each phase-encoding step. The average signal of tissue is much more coherent and contributes more to the overall appearance of the image when compared to the signal produced from the ghosting artifacts.[10]

Respiratory triggering is a method used to decrease respiratory motion artifact. This is accomplished either with a bellows on the upper abdomen that tracks the motion of the respiratory cycle or with a "Navigator" technique, which produces a signal that indicates the position of the diaphragm. Typically the signals are acquired during end expiration with each cycle. Image acquisition takes longer with this technique since signal acquisition is restricted to end expiration. Cardiac gating synchronizes image acquisition with the electrocardiogram, which is very useful in eliminating cardiac motion artifact.

Perhaps the most effective method to reduce respiratory motion is respiratory suspension. Single breath-hold techniques with 2D multislice or three-dimensional (3D) acquisitions can be performed on patients capable of holding their breath. For patients who have difficulty holding their breath, ultrafast imaging techniques can be helpful in producing diagnostic images.[10]

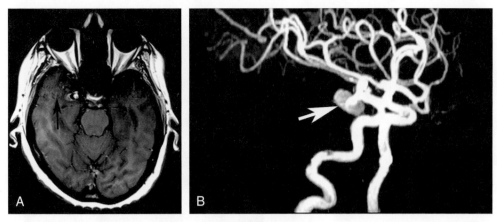

FIGURE 2A. Axial T1W image of the head demonstrates a focal lesion along the medial aspect of the right temporal lobe with central high T1 signal and peripheral low T1 signal. Ghosting artifact is seen on both sides of the lesion extending in the phase-encoding direction *(black arrow)*.

FIGURE 2B. Maximum intensity projection (MIP) image of the circle of Willis from a time-of-flight (TOF) magnetic resonance angiogram (MRA). There is a saccular outpouching seen adjacent to the right supraclinoid internal carotid artery (ICA) *(white arrow)*.

Diagnosis: Right supraclinoid internal carotid artery (ICA) aneurysm.

Discussion

It is extremely important to consider the diagnosis of an aneurysm when developing a differential for an extra-axial parasellar mass. Thrombus within a cerebral aneurysm is composed of blood products of different ages, resulting in the classic appearance of a central flow void with circumferential rings of varying signal intensity extending peripherally. The diagnosis is clinched with recognition of pulsation artifact in the phase-encoding direction, which is due to pulsatile blood flow within the aneurysm. However, lack of artifact does not exclude an aneurysm, since completely thrombosed aneurysms will not produce pulsation artifact. The protons within the moving blood experience a rephasing gradient of a different strength and accumulate phase, which results in the ghosting artifact seen above.

CASES 3 AND 4: COMPANION CASES

Case 3

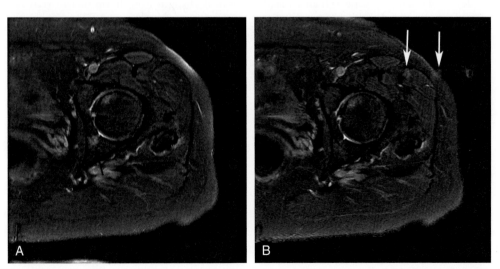

FIGURE 3A. Axial fat-suppressed T2-weighted (T2W) image of the left hip in a patient with breast cancer. Round, high-signal focus is identified in the left posterior acetabulum *(black arrow)*.

FIGURE 3B. Axial fat-suppressed T2W image in the same patient. The frequency- and phase-encoding directions were swapped; the high-signal acetabular focus seen in Figure 3A is no longer identified. Note the vascular pulsation artifact arising from the left femoral artery *(white arrows)*.

Diagnosis: Pseudo-lesion from pulsation artifact.

Case 4

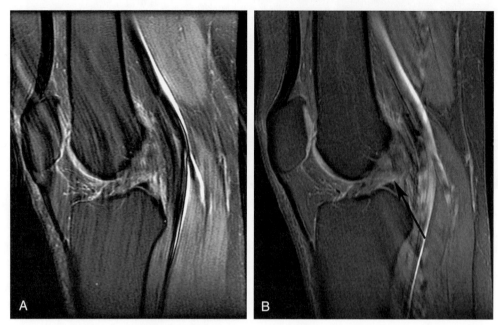

FIGURE 4A. Sagittal fat-suppressed proton density (PD)–weighted image demonstrating extensive ghosting artifact resulting from pulsation of the popliteal artery.

FIGURE 4B. Sagittal fat-suppressed PD-weighted image in the same patient. The frequency- and phase-encoding directions were swapped, resulting in significantly decreased artifact. The anterior cruciate ligament (ACL) tear is now much more easily seen *(black arrow)*.

Diagnosis: Anterior cruciate ligament (ACL) tear obscured by pulsation artifact from the popliteal artery.

Discussion
Vascular pulsation artifact can be a source of confusion if it is mistaken for a true focal lesion, which is evident in Case 3, or obscures a true lesion, illustrated in Case 4. If an artifact is a possibility, a simple way to resolve this is to swap the phase- and frequency-encoding directions. While the artifact is not eliminated, it is shifted into another direction in the image, enabling more accurate evaluation. This is seen in both of the above cases. In Case 3, the phase-encoding direction is shifted from a vertical to a horizontal direction, clearly confirming the lesion to be outside the bone and consistent with a ghosting artifact. In Case 4, the phase-encoding direction is changed from horizontal to vertical, making it much easier to see the obvious ACL tear.

Case 5

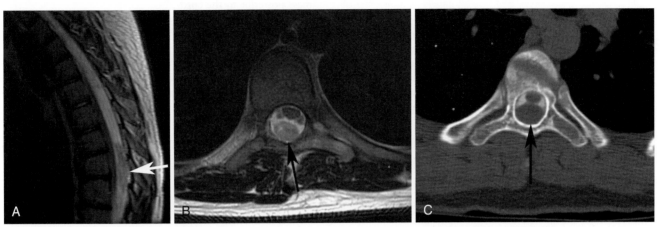

FIGURE 5A. Sagittal T2W image of the thoracic spine demonstrates an ill-defined area of low signal posterior to the cord *(white arrow)*.

FIGURE 5B. Axial T2W image in the same patient. There is an oval intermediate-signal mass posterior to the cord *(black arrow)* corresponding to the lesion on the sagittal image.

FIGURE 5C. Axial computed tomography image from a lumbar myelogram confirms the presence of a low-density oval mass *(black arrow)* posterior to the cord, demonstrating mass effect on the thecal sac and cord.

Diagnosis: Arachnoid cyst.

Case 6

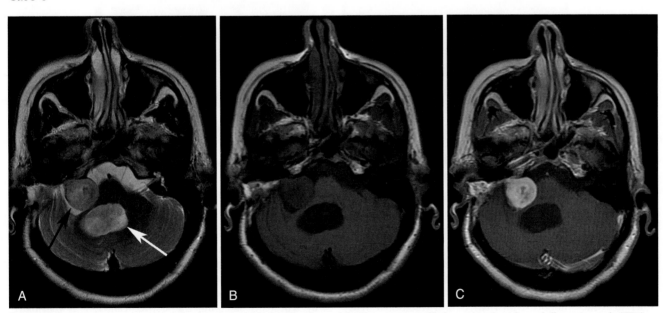

FIGURE 6A. Axial T2W image of the brain though the level of the fourth ventricle. There is a mass *(black arrow)* in the right cerebellopontine angle (CPA) that is heterogeneously high T2 signal. There is a second lesion seen in the expanded fourth ventricle *(white arrow)* that has very similar signal characteristics to the right CPA mass.

FIGURE 6B. Axial noncontrast T1W image in the same patient. The right CPA mass is redemonstrated, but with slightly greater signal than cerebrospinal fluid (CSF). There is homogeneously low signal seen in the fourth ventricle that is isointense to CSF.

FIGURE 6C. Axial postcontrast T1W image shows homogeneous hyperenhancement of the right CPA mass, confirming it as a true pathology. There is no abnormal enhancement seen in the fourth ventricle.

Diagnosis: Acoustic neuroma.

Discussion

CSF pulsation artifact can be a source of confusion when imaging the central nervous system (CNS), potentially resulting in pseudo-lesions or obscuring true pathology. In Case 5, a low-signal area posterior to the spinal cord on both the sagittal and axial T2-weighted (T2W) images looks very similar to CSF pulsation artifact, but an extra-axial mass cannot be excluded particularly given the anterior displacement of the cord. Sometimes the only way to differentiate between the two is to do an additional study. In this patient, a myelogram performed for a separate indication clearly demonstrates a true mass posterior to the cord.

In contrast, Case 6 clearly demonstrates a mass in the right cerebellopontine angle (CPA); however, on the axial T2W image, the fourth ventricle also appears to be expanded with heterogeneous signal intensity within it, similar to the signal of the CPA mass. The axial T1-weighted (T1W) pre- and postcontrast images show persistent dilation of the fourth ventricle, but normal CSF signal with no evidence of enhancement, indicating the heterogeneous signal seen on the T2W image is due to pulsation artifact rather than a true extra-axial mass.

CASE 7

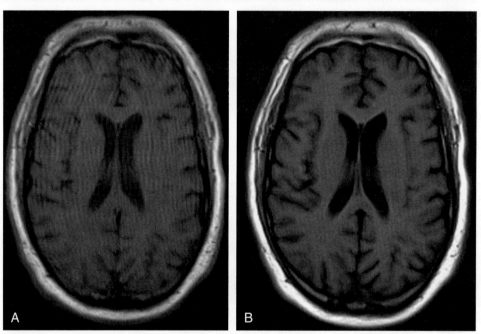

FIGURE 7A. Axial T1W image through the brain is severely degraded by motion artifact.

FIGURE 7B. Axial BLADE sequence with T1 weighting demonstrates significant reduction in the motion artifact.

Discussion

Another simple way of overcoming motion degradation is to use fast imaging sequences. BLADE is a turbo spin echo (TSE) sequence that uses a nonrectilinear sampling of k-space in order to reduce motion sensitivity. As in a traditional TSE sequence, for every TR, one group of parallel lines of k-space is acquired. However, unlike a traditional TSE sequence, each group surrounds the center of k-space, and is rotated relative to the other groups rather than being shifted in the phase-encoding direction relative to the others. This reduces motion sensitivity in two manners: first, motion artifacts get distributed throughout the image, and thus, appear more like an increase in random noise than coherent ghosting; second, by repeatedly sampling the k-space center, it is possible to detect in-plane rigid-body motion and correct for it in the reconstruction. However, because of the redundant sampling of the k-space center, it does take longer to acquire a BLADE image than it does to acquire a traditional TSE image.

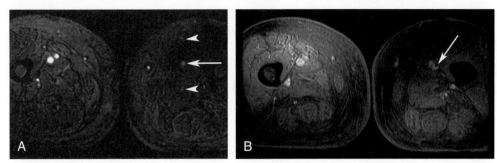

FIGURE 8A. Axial GRE image (bright blood technique) from an MR venography through the upper thighs. There is asymmetric anatomy on the left with only a single vessel seen *(white arrow)*. The *arrowheads* demonstrate ghosting artifacts due to femoral artery pulsation.

FIGURE 8B. Axial postcontrast image from the same study demonstrates a low-signal filling defect *(white arrow)* within the left femoral vein.

Diagnosis: Left femoral vein deep vein thrombosis (DVT).

Discussion

Artifacts are not necessarily bad. For example, in this case the single vessel seen on the axial GRE image in the left thigh could either be a vein or an artery. Sorting this out is very important given the very different clinical implications (occluded artery versus a deep vein thrombosis [DVT]). Recognition of the ghosting artifacts both above and below the vessel confirms the vessel is an artery. In this case, postcontrast images were also performed (Figure 8B) and demonstrate a DVT in the femoral vein. The lack of signal in the left femoral vein in Figure 8A is not diagnostic of DVT as slow flow gives a similar appearance.

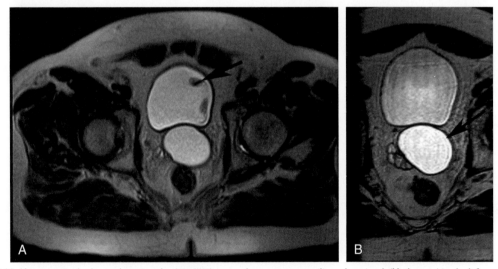

FIGURE 9A. Axial half-Fourier single-shot turbo spin echo (HASTE) image demonstrates curvilinear low signal *(black arrow)* in the left anterior bladder.

FIGURE 9B. Axial SPACE (Sampling Perfection with Application optimized Contrasts using different flip angle Evolutions) image at the same level through the bladder. The curvilinear area of low signal intensity is no longer present. There is a second cystic structure *(black arrow)* posterior to the bladder originating from the seminal vesicle. On other images, it was noted that the left kidney was congenitally absent.

Diagnosis: Flow artifact from a left ureteral jet and Zinner's syndrome.

Discussion

Figure 9A is an axial half-Fourier single-shot turbo spin echo (HASTE) sequence. HASTE is a T2W single-shot, ultrafast imaging technique (acquired in less than half a second) that is very helpful in reducing motion artifact. Single shot means acquiring all of the echoes needed to fill k-space after a single excitation pulse. Also, with the HASTE sequence, a little over 50% of k-space is acquired and the rest is interpolated, which significantly reduces acquisition time. There is no repetition of the excitation (no TR), which eliminates T1 weighting.[10] Although the HASTE sequence is very useful in avoiding the effects of motion, it is still a flow-sensitive sequence, as exemplified by the dark signal of the femoral blood vessels (see Fig. 9A). The turbulent flow from the left ureteral jet in the left anterior bladder creates a curvilinear-appearing signal void. This finding can also be found when there is a large amount of ascites in the abdomen and results from the motion of fluid between excitation and readout. The SPACE sequence (Fig. 9B), in contrast, is a multishot sequence; here, k-space is filled over multiple TRs and the inconstant flow effects of ureteral jets cancel each other out, making the urinary bladder appear homogeneously bright.

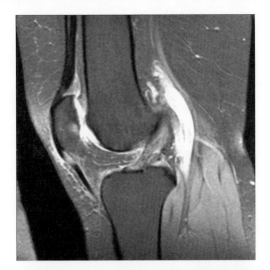

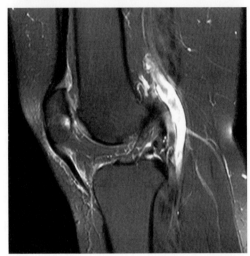

1. The image on the top is proton density (PD) weighted, and the image on the bottom is T2-weighted. What diagnosis might you consider given the signal abnormalities in the proximal patellar tendon on the PD image?

2. What happens to the signal abnormality on the corresponding T2W image? Is this an expected finding?

3. What artifact should be considered when reviewing signal changes in tendons and ligaments?

4. What is the cause of the focal signal abnormality in the proximal patellar tendon on the PD image?

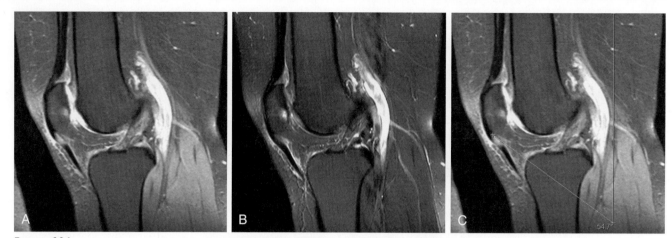

FIGURE 10A. Sagittal PD image of the knee (TE = 17 msec) demonstrates focal high signal intensity of the proximal patellar tendon. Focal subchondral reactive changes are noted in the patella.

FIGURE 10B. Sagittal T2W image (TE = 65 msec) with fat suppression at the same level demonstrates decreased signal intensity in the proximal patellar tendon. The reactive changes of the patella persist.

FIGURE 10C. Sagittal PD image of the knee demonstrates the angle of the proximal patellar tendon oriented at 54.7° to the main magnetic field.

1. In this patient with knee pain, you would consider a diagnosis of patellar tendinosis.

2. The proximal patellar tendon signal abnormality mostly resolves on the T2W image.

3. Magic angle phenomenon.

4. Magic angle phenomenon.

Discussion

The high signal intensity of the proximal patellar tendon in the short echo-time image is due to the magic angle phenomenon. Tissues composed of ordered collagen fibers are normally low signal intensity on all pulse sequences due to the dipolar interactions of the water molecules in contact with the fibers, which leads to a short T2 relaxation time. If the orientation of the fibers is at a certain angle in relation to the main magnetic field, the dipolar interaction approaches zero, leading to a slight *increase* in the T2 relaxation times. While there is a range of angles at which this artifact appears (between 45° and 65°), it is maximal when the tendons are oriented at 54.7° to the main field,[3] producing false high signal on short TE sequences (T1W and PD-weighted). The signal abnormality characteristically resolves on longer TE sequences since the increase in T2 relaxation time is still much shorter compared to the TE, which allows adequate T2 decay to take place.

Part II: Other Artifacts

Many common, clinically relevant artifacts have already been discussed throughout this book, including chemical shift, susceptibility, motion, and contrast-related artifacts. The remaining artifacts discussed in this chapter briefly cover those related to technique, errors in data collection, and magnetic field strength. While many artifacts do not cause significant clinical confusion, they are often a source of poor image quality, which could render an exam nondiagnostic.

Case 11

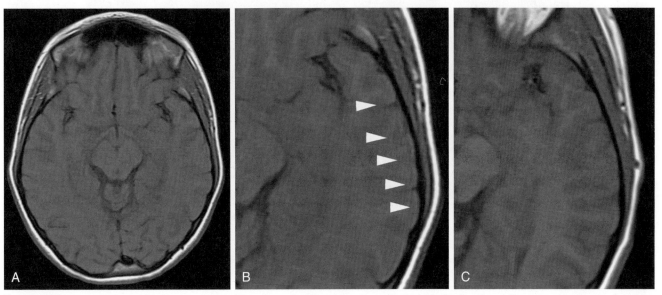

FIGURE 11A. Axial T1W spin echo (SE) image of the brain obtained with a 320 × 192 matrix. Multiple thin hypointense lines traversing the temporal lobes bilaterally are present.

FIGURE 11B. Magnified image of Figure 11A focused over the left temporal lobe better demonstrates these vertical lines *(arrowheads).*

FIGURE 11C. Axial T1W SE image of the same brain acquired with a matrix of 320 × 240. The low-signal lines are no longer seen.

Diagnosis: Gibbs artifact.

Case 12

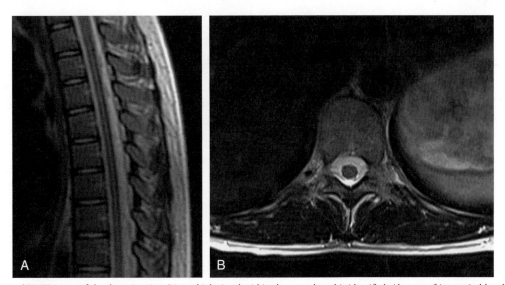

FIGURE 12A. Sagittal T2W image of the thoracic spine. Linear high signal within the central cord is identified. Also note faint vertical bands within the vertebral bodies anteriorly.

FIGURE 12B. Axial T2W image of the midthoracic spine. The spinal cord is normal.

Diagnosis: Gibbs artifact mimicking a cord syrinx.

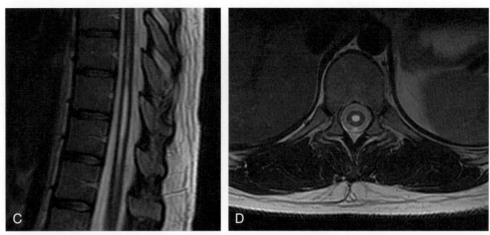

FIGURE 12C. Sagittal T2W image of the thoracic spine, different patient. Linear high signal within the central cord abnormality is present. The signal intensity of the abnormality matches CSF, and the inferior cord appears mildly expanded compared to the upper cord.

FIGURE 12D. Axial T2W image of the midthoracic spine. Cystic high T2 signal abnormality persists in the central spinal cord.

Diagnosis: Cord syrinx.

Case 13

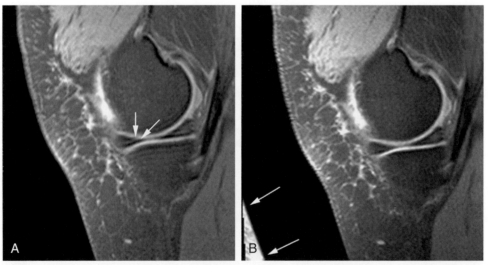

FIGURE 13A. Sagittal PD image of the medial knee. Intrasubstance high signal is seen within the posterior horn consistent with degeneration. Linear signal abnormality extending to the superior articular surface is demonstrated in the anterior horn *(arrows)*, concerning for a tear. Also, multiple periodic curvilinear bands of high and low signal intensity are seen overlying the tibia and femur, which become less conspicuous as they extend farther from the articular surface.

FIGURE 13B. Sagittal PD image at the same level. The linear signal abnormality in the anterior horn, as well as the curvilinear bands overlying the tibia and femur, are no longer seen. Also note wraparound artifact now present in the lower right-hand corner of the image *(arrows)*.

Diagnosis: Gibbs artifact mimicking an anterior horn meniscus tear.

Discussion

The truncation (Gibbs ring) artifact is caused by the limited number of digital samples in k-space and occurs at high-contrast interfaces. Because most examinations undersample in the phase-encoding direction to save time, the highest frequency data are cut off (or truncated); it is these data that represent the sharp-edged interfaces between high-contrast borders.[2] This leads to either an overestimation or underestimation of the signal by the Fourier transform at these boundaries, which is visible as periodic low- or high-signal-intensity lines or bands that "ring" on either side of the interface. This ringing characteristically become less conspicuous the farther from the interface, which differentiates it from the similarly appearing motion artifact.

This artifact is most problematic in spinal cord imaging because of the high-contrast CSF-cord boundary (Case 12). On T1W images, a low-signal band is seen in the cord; the band is correspondingly high signal on T2W images. This pattern raises the possibility of a cord syrinx. However, the axial T2W image of the spinal cord is normal, which verifies the abnormality on the sagittal image as an artifact.

Remedies for truncation include decreasing pixel size, which can be done by either decreasing the field of view (FOV) or increasing the acquisition matrix in the phase-encoding direction. This is illustrated in Case 11, where increasing the matrix from 256×126 to 320×240 during the same study resolved the alternating bands overlying the left temporal lobe.

As mentioned previously, changing the frequency- and phase-encoding directions will not resolve the artifact but could prevent it from affecting the tissue of interest. This is illustrated in Case 13, where the interface between the articular cartilage and menisci results in an artifact mimicking an anterior horn meniscus tear (see Fig. 13A)[8]; by selecting the phase-encoding direction perpendicular to the interface, the effect of the artifact on the menisci was reduced (see Fig. 13B). The change in phase-encoding direction is verified with the identification of the wraparound artifact on the lower left corner of the image.

Of course, the "no free lunch" rule in MRI applies here, since increasing the acquisition matrix results in a longer study and decreased signal to noise ratio (as a result of smaller pixel sizes).

CASE 14

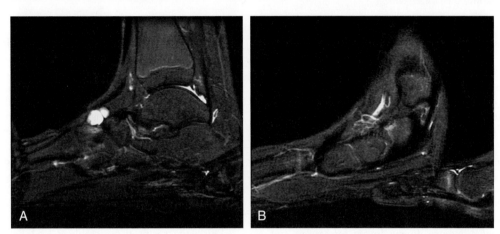

FIGURE 14A. Sagittal T2W image of the foot. Unusual low-signal abnormality is demonstrated in the calcaneus and posterior plantar soft tissues. The septated high-T2-signal cystic lesion dorsal to the midfoot is consistent with a ganglion cyst.

FIGURE 14B. Sagittal T2W image of the more lateral image of the same foot. The patient's toe is located posteriorly in the image.

Diagnosis: Wraparound artifact.

Discussion

This is a typical example of the wraparound artifact, also known as aliasing. It is secondary to the use of a small FOV, with signals arising from tissues outside of the FOV overlapping onto the opposite side of the image. Aliasing is the result of Fourier encoding, as the phases of tissues exhibit cyclic behavior in spatial increments equal to the FOV. In practice, aliasing is primarily an artifact seen in the phase-encoding direction as the frequency-encoding direction is often oversampled (hence widening the FOV). Widening the FOV resolves this artifact, but at the expense of decreased resolution.

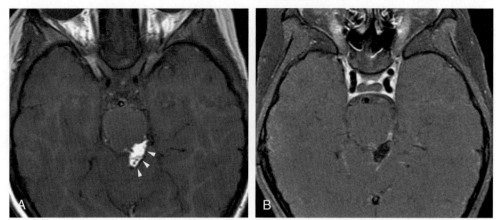

FIGURE 15A. Axial T1W image of the brain. An oval high-signal-intensity lesion is seen compressing the left quadrigeminal plate and adjacent cerebellar vermis; note the thin linear low-signal-intensity border on the posterior margin of the mass *(arrowheads)*.

FIGURE 15B. Axial postcontrast T1W image with fat saturation. There is near-complete signal loss in the quadrigeminal plate mass. The low-signal-intensity posterior margin of the mass is no longer seen.

Diagnosis: Lipoma.

Discussion

The chemical shift misregistration artifact is one of the more commonly seen artifacts in MRI. Signals arising from tissues have both frequency and phase components, which are used in the process of spatial encoding during MR image formation. As noted in previous chapters, protons in fat precess at a different frequency compared to protons in water as a result of differences in molecular environments. Fat and water protons are separated by a chemical shift of 3.5 ppm, which is the equivalent of 224 Hz at 1.5T-strength magnetic field.

This difference in proton frequencies is erroneously interpreted as a *spatial* difference during image formation, and results in a misregistration artifact. The artifact is primarily seen as a linear band of signal abnormality at fat-water interfaces in the body, where the fat-containing voxels are shifted away from their true anatomic positions in the frequency-encoding direction of the image. Note that this misregistration artifact in the frequency-encoding direction, as illustrated in this case, pertains primarily to conventional sequences (spin echo, fast spin echo, and GRE); the misregistration artifact seen in single-shot imaging techniques such as echo-planar imaging occurs in the phase-encoding direction, the details of which are beyond the scope of this discussion.

Case 15 shows this artifact and its potential clinical usefulness. The lipoma compressing the quadrigeminal plate exhibits a thin, low-signal-intensity band along its posterior margin (see Fig. 15A), which occurs in the frequency-encoding direction (note the pulsation artifact arising from the basilar artery, which is seen in the phase-encoding [left-to-right] direction of the image). The presence (and identification) of this artifact suggests its fat-containing properties, and allows for a more definitive diagnosis.

This artifact is most noticeable at 1.5T field strengths, and worsens with increasing field strength as the chemical shift between fat and water protons increases. Technical adjustments to resolve this artifact include decreasing the pixel size (decreasing the FOV) and increasing the receiver bandwidth. Additionally, utilizing fat suppression (see Fig. 15B) to decrease the signal contribution from fat will decrease or eliminate the artifact.

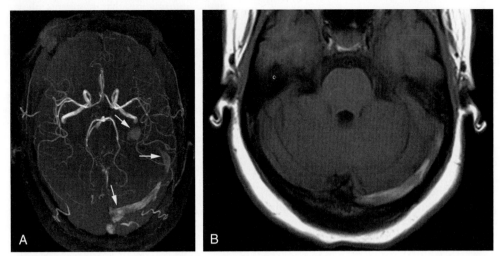

FIGURE 16A. 3D-TOF MIP image of the circle of Willis. The major vessels of the circle of Willis are patent; signal is present in the region of the left transverse sinus and left jugular foramen *(arrows).*

FIGURE 16B. Axial T1W image of the posterior fossa demonstrates bandlike high signal in the left transverse sinus.

Diagnoses: Dural venous thrombosis; T1 contamination artifact.

Discussion

Recall that TOF is a noncontrasted angiographic technique that relies on flow-related enhancement from unsaturated, mobile blood cells. This is commonly used to assess vascular patency (see Chapter 11). Case 16 illustrates an important pitfall that may occur in the interpretation of TOF images, namely T1 contamination artifact.

As the TOF sequence is T1 weighted, tissues with short T1 relaxation times produce signal. This becomes an issue when

subacute hemorrhage or thrombus containing paramagnetic methemoglobin is present.

The 3D-TOF MIP image demonstrates normal signal within the circle of Willis, confirming patency. However, the high signal arising from the left transverse sinus and left jugular foramen represents contamination artifact from subacute thrombus. To avoid this potential pitfall, one should evaluate other sequences (namely the pre- and postcontrast spin echo T1W and fast spin echo T2W sequences) to verify or exclude an abnormality.

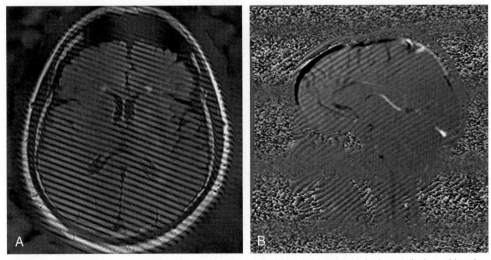

FIGURE 17A. Axial fluid-attenuated inversion recovery (FLAIR) image at the level of the basal ganglia. Multiple periodic lines obliquely traverse the image.

FIGURE 17B. Sagittal phase-contrast CSF flow study in a different patient; similar periodic oblique bands are seen throughout the image, although the orientation of the bands is different than seen in Figure 17A.

Diagnosis: Herringbone artifact.

Discussion

The herringbone, or spike, artifact is caused by a transient corruption during the filling of k-space, most commonly from an electromagnetic spike. The spike is thought to arise from gradients applied at high-duty cycles,[7] which result in a bad data point in k-space. This bad data point is converted into a sinusoidal wave function by the Fourier transform, which is then incorporated into each pixel during image reconstruction. This is manifested as alternating bands propagated across the entire image (see Fig. 17A). The artifact severity increases with the intensity of the electromagnetic spike.

Understanding this artifact requires a basic understanding of the relationship between k-space and the images we interpret. Simply put, each individual data point in k-space contains information that represents all voxels in the MR image. This is what we see with the herringbone artifact; the single abnormal spike in k-space has resulted in an artifact that does not distort just a single pixel, but affects the entire image.

Not only does the presence of a corrupt data point affect the image, but the *location* of the data point in k-space determines its appearance on the image. The lines in the phase-contrast CSF flow image (see Fig. 17B) propagate from right to left in an inferior-to-superior orientation; this is opposite the orientation of the bands seen in Figure 17A. By examining both the angulation and distance between the lines, an estimation of the data spike's location in k-space can be made.[7]

Ways to resolve this artifact include editing (and removing) the bad data point and continuing with subsequent image reconstruction, or simply rescanning the patient if postprocessing capability is limited.

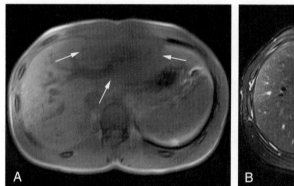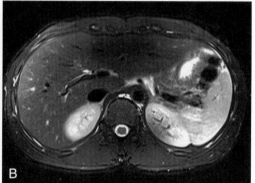

FIGURE 18A. Axial T1W image of the upper abdomen performed on a 3T magnet. Decreased signal intensity of the left hepatic lobe is demonstrated *(arrows)*. Also note the subtle decreased signal of the subcutaneous fat in the anterior midabdominal wall.

FIGURE 18B. Axial T2W image with fat suppression in the upper abdomen at the same examination. Persistent decreased signal intensity of the left hepatic lobe is noted.

Diagnosis: Standing-wave artifact.

Discussion

Inhomogeneous RF excitation of an imaging volume is due to an assortment of dielectric and conductive properties in tissue.[12] At 3T, the RF wavelength measures 234 cm in air; the speed and wavelength of the RF field is shortened to 30 cm within the body as a result of dielectric effects. Coincidentally, 30 cm is also the average field of view for most body imaging examinations. When the RF wavelength approximates the size of the FOV, constructive or destructive interference of the RF field occurs. This leads to local areas of either signal brightening (usually seen in the brain) *or* darkening (shading). This artifact has previously been referred to as the "dielectric resonance" effect, but more recently the terms *standing-wave effects* or *RF interference effects* have been used.[4]

Case 18 is a typical example of this local signal shading. On the T1W image, the decreased signal intensity of the left hepatic lobe may be misdiagnosed as a processes causing local T1 prolongation; however, the corresponding T2W image also shows decreased signal intensity, arguing *against* pathology and *for* artifact. As this exam was performed on a 3T magnet, the characteristic appearance and location of the decreased signal intensity in the left hepatic lobe is the result of destructive RF interference. This artifact tends to occur in thin patients.

A dielectric pad placed between the patient and receiver coil modifies the geometric dimensions of the imaging volume and can decrease RF interference.[1] This artifact is also less severe on 1.5T magnets because the RF wavelength at this field strength is twice that of 3T (468 cm); thus, the RF wavelength in body tissues (60 cm) will be greater than the FOV (30 cm), causing less interference.

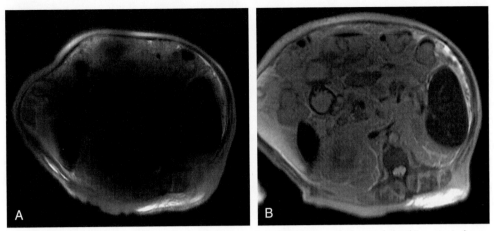

FIGURE 19A. Axial T2W image of the abdomen performed on a 3T magnet. Marked homogeneously decreased signal intensity is demonstrated in the center of the abdomen.

FIGURE 19B. Axial T2W image of the abdomen in the same patient performed 1 day later on a 1.5T magnet. Marked improvement of diagnostic image quality is obtained; a large volume of ascites is evident in the right hemiabdomen. The spleen is enlarged.

Diagnosis: Ascites with conductivity artifact.

Discussion
When a highly conductive medium (ascites, amniotic fluid) is present in the body, a circulating electrical field is formed when under the influence of an external RF field. This in turn produces an electric current; the current acts as its own magnetic field that opposes the main magnetic field. This results in a reduction in the effect of the RF field on the imaging volume and a decrease in signal.

Conductivity artifact, combined with the dielectric effects of the body tissues, produces a significant artifact at 3T,[4] as illustrated in Case 19. The highly conductive ascites promotes signal loss in the central abdomen, rendering the study non-diagnostic. The artifact was immediately recognized and the study subsequently terminated. The exam was completed the next day on a 1.5T magnet, with a marked reduction in the artifact.

Case 19 is an example of an artifact that worsens with increases in magnetic field strength. Other artifacts that are more conspicuous at higher magnetic field strengths include susceptibility, chemical shift, and dielectric effect artifacts.

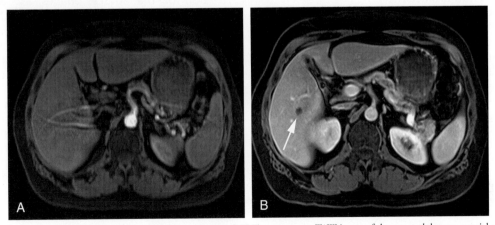

FIGURE 20A. Axial 3D volumetric interpolated breath-hold examination (VIBE) postcontrast T1W image of the upper abdomen, arterial phase. High-signal bands traverse across the center of the image volume. The bands persisted in the remaining images of the sequence (not shown).

FIGURE 20B. Axial postcontrast T1W image, portal venous phase at the same level as Figure 20A. The high-signal bands seen in Figure 20A are no longer apparent. A low-signal lesion in the right hepatic lobe *(white arrow)* is demonstrated; this lesion was not seen on the arterial-phase images.

Diagnosis:
Aliasing artifact in parallel imaging.

Discussion

A GRE T1W, 3D volumetric interpolated breath-hold examination (VIBE) sequence can be used for dynamic contrast-enhanced abdominal imaging. The benefit of 3D acquisitions is superior resolution over 2D sequences due to acquisition of thinner slices.[5] A drawback is that 3D coverage requires a breath hold, which could be challenging for patients. Because of this, parallel imaging (PI) techniques are combined with 3D GRE sequences to shorten examination time.[6]

PI uses signals obtained from multiple phased-array coils, with each coil element acquiring data from a particular region of the body. All PI techniques shorten scan times by intentionally undersampling the k-space (e.g., in the phase-encoding direction). Again, the "no free lunch" rule applies for PI techniques: undersampling k-space leads to a reduction in the FOV. If the anatomy being imaged is *larger* than the FOV, foldover artifacts occur due to aliasing (Case 20). While these artifacts can be mostly removed (i.e., the image can be unfolded) by applying the correct individual coil sensitivity maps, there may still be residual foldover effects resulting from, for example, inaccuracy in the sensitivity maps. In Case 20, the tiny right hepatic lobe lesion was completely obscured by the residual overlapping lines on the arterial-phase image. The lesion is clearly seen on the portal venous-phase image.

KEY POINTS

1. Motion can be divided into two categories, gross body movement and physiologic motion, such as cardiac and respiratory cycles, or blood and CSF flow.
2. In most conventional imaging methods, motion artifact is predominantly manifested in the phase-encoding direction.
3. When motion is present, tissues excited at a specific location during the RF pulse are erroneously mapped to a different location or multiple different locations during detection.
4. Random motion results in smearing or blurring in the phase-encoding direction, and periodic motion (cardiac motion and blood vessels) results in ghosting artifacts.
5. Many techniques such as gradient moment nulling, swapping the direction of the frequency-encoding and phase-encoding gradients, presaturation pulses, averaging, respiratory triggering, and cardiac gating can be used to reduce motion artifacts.
6. The Gibbs ringing, or truncation, artifact is due to the undersampling of k-space and is conspicuous at high-contrast boundaries (CSF-cord, brain-calvarium, cartilage-bone). Decreasing pixel size or increasing the acquisition matrix either improves or eliminates the artifact.
7. While swapping the phase- and frequency-encoding directions does not completely remove the Gibbs ringing artifact, it may prevent the artifact from affecting the tissue in question.
8. The magic angle artifact is seen in tendons and ligaments oriented at certain angles to the main magnetic field. It manifests as artificial high signal on short TE sequences. The artifact is typically not seen on long TE sequences, differentiating it from true pathology.
9. Wraparound artifact represents an error in spatial encoding, as signal from tissues located outside of the FOV are mapped within the FOV, usually on the opposite side. Widening the FOV to include the entire body part resolves this artifact.
10. Chemical shift misregistration results in an error in spatial encoding of fat voxels because of the differences of resonant frequencies between fat and water. This artifact is most evident at fat-water interfaces in the body and is seen in the frequency-encoding direction of the image on conventional sequences.
11. Because TOF sequences are T1 weighted, tissues with high T1 signal (methemoglobin) may appear in the reconstructed MIP image as a T1 contamination artifact, mimicking patent vessels; evaluation of the source images as well as other sequences is necessary to prevent this pitfall.
12. Benefits of imaging at higher magnetic field strengths come at the cost of progressively severe artifacts; examples include artifacts related to dielectric effects, chemical shift, and susceptibility effects.
13. Parallel imaging techniques shorten examination times in 3D GRE volumetric acquisitions by using spatially encoded information obtained in several receiver coils. Because k-space is undersampled, the FOV is reduced and aliasing artifacts result. These artifacts are typically removed by applying the correct individual coil sensitivity maps to unfold the image.

References

1. Cornfeld D, Weinre J: Simple changes to 1.5-T MRI abdomen and pelvis protocols to optimize results at 3 T. *AJR Am J Roentgenol* 190:140-150, 2008.
2. Czervionke L, Czervionke J, et al: Characteristic features of MR truncation artifacts. *AJR Am J Roentgenol* 151:1219-1228, 1988.
3. Erickson SJ, Cox IH, et al: Effect of tendon orientation on MR imaging signal intensity: a manifestation of the "magic angle" phenomenon. *Radiology* 181:389-392, 1991.
4. Merkle EM, Dale BM: Abdominal MRI at 3.0 T: the basics revisited. *AJR Am J Roentgenol* 186:1524-1532, 2006.
5. Rofsky NM, Lee VS, Laub G, et al: Abdominal MR imaging with a volumetric interpolated breath-hold examination. *Radiology* 212:876-884, 1999.
6. Vogt FM, Antoch G, Hunold P, et al: Parallel acquisition techniques for accelerated volumetric interpolated breath-hold examination magnetic resonance imaging of the upper abdomen: assessment of image quality and lesion conspicuity. *J Magn Reson Imaging* 21:376-382, 2005.
7. Zhuo J, Gullapalli RP: MR artifacts, safety, and quality control. *RadioGraphics* 26:275-297, 2006.
8. Turner DA, Rapoport MI, et al: Truncation artifact: a potential pitfall in MR imaging of the menisci of the knee. *Radiology* 179:629-633, 1991.
9. Lee VS: *Cardiovascular MRI: Physical Principles to Practical Protocols.* Philadelphia: Lippincott Williams & Wilkins, 2006.
10. Mitchell DG, Cohen MS: *MRI Principles*, 2nd ed. Philadelphia: Elsevier Saunders, 2004.
11. Brown MA, Semelka RC: *MRI Basic Principles and Applications*, 3rd ed. New York: Wiley-Liss, 2003.
12. Lee VS, Hecht EM, Taouli B, et al: Body and cardiovascular MR imaging at 3.0 T. *Radiology* 244:692-705, 2007.

Chapter 10
Flow-Related Contrast

Scott M. Duncan and Timothy J. Amrhein

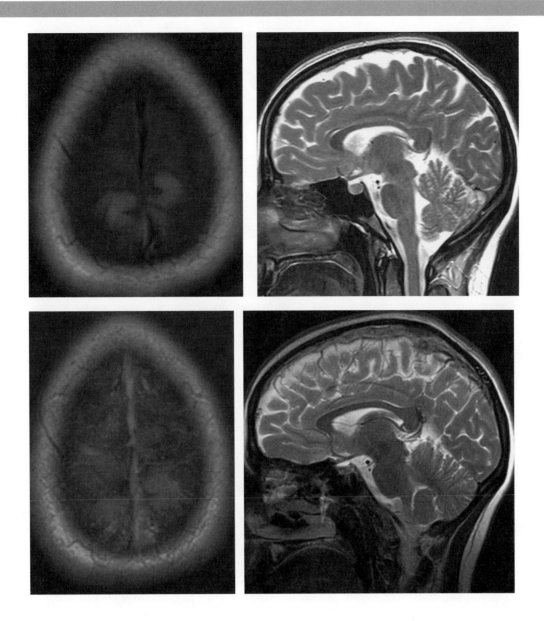

1. Which images are abnormal? Why? What is the diagnosis?

2. Normally, which MRI sequences have flow voids and which exhibit flow-related enhancement?

3. In cardiac imaging, what type of sequence is a "black blood" technique and what sequence is a "white blood" technique?

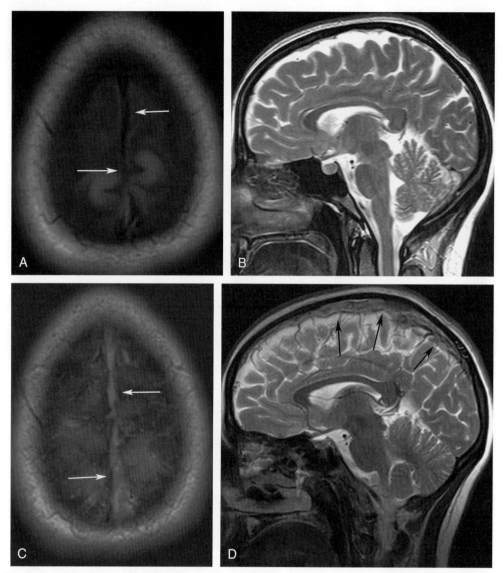

FIGURE 1A. Axial T1-weighted fast spin echo (FSE) image demonstrates a flow void *(arrows)* in a patent superior sagittal sinus.

FIGURE 1B. Sagittal T2-weighted FSE image redemonstrates the thin flow void in the superior sagittal sinus.

FIGURE 1C. Axial T1-weighted FSE image, demonstrates expansion and signal within the superior sagittal sinus and the lack of a flow void *(arrows)*.

FIGURE 1D. Sagittal T2-weighted FSE image redemonstrates the expansion of and signal within the superior sagittal sinus *(arrows)*.

1. The bottom two images (Figs. 1C and 1D) are abnormal because there is signal within the superior sagittal sinus where there should normally be a flow void.

2. Generally speaking, spin echo sequences have flow voids within a vessel. Gradient-recalled echo sequences can have flow-related enhancement resulting in a bright vessel.

3. In cardiac imaging, the "black blood" occurs secondary to a flow void, thus the "black blood" technique is a spin echo sequence. The "bright blood" technique employs a gradient-recalled echo sequence to take advantage of flow-related enhancement.

Diagnosis: Superior sagittal sinus thrombosis.

Physics Discussion

The bright signal within the superior sagittal sinus in Figures 1C and 1D is abnormal as one should expect to identify a flow void in this vascular structure in spin echo imaging. When evaluating a spin echo sequence, always be sure to look for arterial and venous flow voids to exclude an unexpected thrombus.

Vascular Contrast: Flow Voids and Flow-Related Enhancement

Perhaps one of the most confusing topics to understand as a novice to magnetic resonance imaging (MRI) interpretation is the differentiation between flow voids and flow-related enhancement. When should vessels be black and when should they be bright?

The answer is actually quite simple. Spin echo techniques result in flow voids, while gradient-recalled echo techniques result in flow-related enhancement. These are, of course, generalizations and there are exceptions to this rule (we will explore these later). However, in the majority of cases this simple generalization holds true.

Cardiac MRI takes advantage of the distinct flow-related properties of these two magnetic resonance (MR) sequences to image the cardiovascular system. The generic descriptors "black blood" technique and "white blood" technique are the result of flow voids and flow-related enhancement, respectively. In other words, blood is dark in the "black blood" technique primarily as a result of the flow void phenomenon produced by a spin echo sequence. Conversely, blood is bright in the "white blood" technique, based on the flow-related enhancement found in a gradient-recalled echo sequence.

Flow voids and flow-related enhancement are both based on the same "time-of-flight" phenomenon. The basis of this phenomenon is that flowing protons within blood do not experience the same radiofrequency (RF) pulses and magnetization as that of stationary protons. Thus, the signal obtained from flowing protons is different than that from stationary protons.

Let's begin with a discussion of spin echo imaging. Spin echo imaging uses two RF pulses to produce a signal. The first is a 90° pulse that tips the longitudinal magnetization into the transverse plane. Subsequently, a 180° pulse realigns the dephased spins in order to produce an echo. The proton must experience *both* RF pulses to create a signal. For example, if a moving proton is hit with the initial 90° RF pulse and then moves out of the imaging plane before the 180° RF pulse (thereby avoiding the 180° pulse), the dephased protons will not be refocused. This absence of refocusing means that all of the transverse magnetization will remain dephased and no signal will be obtained. Alternatively, if the proton is outside of the imaging slice when the 90° pulse is applied, but then moves into the slice when the 180° pulse is applied, the proton's magnetization will be flipped 180° (reversed or "upside down") in the longitudinal direction. In this scenario, there will be no transverse magnetization to provide a signal (as the initial 90° RF pulse was missed). In both of the provided scenarios, the result is absence of signal, or a flow void.

While we may think of a flow void as a complete loss of signal, there is, in reality, a spectrum ranging from full normal signal to a complete signal void. The amount of signal void is dependent upon the velocity of the proton, the slice thickness, the time to echo (TE), and the course of the vessel. The greater the velocity of the proton, the quicker it will move out of the imaging slice and the less time it has to experience both the 90° and 180° RF pulses. Thinner slices mean that there are shorter required distances to traverse the imaging slice, thus less time to experience both RF pulses (and a greater likelihood of a flow void). Longer TEs mean that there is more time between the 90° and 180° RF pulses (remember that the 90° and 180° pulses are separated by ½ TE). Therefore, there is more time for the moving protons (that have already experienced the initial 90° pulse) to be replaced with "new" protons that have not experienced the first RF pulse prior to signal acquisition. Thus, sequences with long TEs (such as T2 and proton density [PD] images) have the most prominent flow voids. This is an important point to remember. Intraluminal

signal that is concerning for vascular thrombosis, when identified on a T1-weighted sequence (short TE), should be confirmed by comparing to the corresponding T2 or PD sequences as these are less sensitive to slow flow and more specific to the diagnosis of thrombosis.

Finally, the course of the vessel also has implications for the presence or absence of a flow void. The time-of-flight phenomenon only applies to flow that is perpendicular to the imaging plane. When vessels take a course that is oblique or parallel to the imaging plane, the protons stay within the imaging slice for an extended period of time, increasing the probability that they both experience RF pulses and produce signal. Thus, if a vessel courses obliquely or parallel to the imaging plane, an intravascular signal may be seen despite normal flow within the vessel.

Blood velocity within the arterial system is usually great enough to result in a complete intraluminal signal void regardless of the obliquity of the vessel (examples include the petrous internal carotid artery and the middle cerebral artery). Conversely, the relatively reduced venous velocity may not result in a complete signal void despite patency, especially if the vessel takes an oblique course. As a result, if intraluminal signal is identified within a vein on a spin echo sequence, the possibility of a thrombus should be raised, but should be confirmed with a more flow-sensitive sequence (such as phase contrast).

In gradient-recalled imaging, the time-of-flight phenomenon has the opposite effect of that seen in spin echo sequences. Recall that in gradient-recalled echo sequences there is only one RF pulse, with phase refocusing dependent upon the application of a gradient. Additionally, the times to repetition (TRs) in gradient sequences are very short and are repeated multiple times. Thus, the proton's longitudinal magnitude does not fully recover before the next RF pulse is applied. After several TRs are applied, the amount of longitudinal magnetization recovered reaches equilibrium with the amount of magnetization that is tipped into the transverse plane. This is called "saturation." A flowing proton that is entering a slice has not experienced the multiple previous RF pulses and will produce more signal than the adjacent partially saturated nonmobile protons. This is the basis of "flow-related enhancement" (Fig. 1).[1]

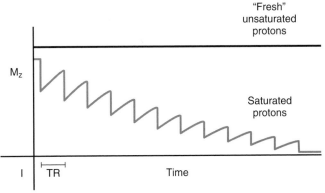

FIGURE 1. Comparison of magnetization of stagnant and moving protons after multiple RF pulses. The moving, unsaturated protons always have maximal signal. However, the stagnant protons are repeatedly hit with RF pulses. The curve shows how the signal progressively decreases after multiple RF pulses. Eventually, a steady state is reached where the longitudinal magnetization recovered is equal to the magnitude of magnetization flipped into the transverse plane by the next RF pulse (saturation). *(Adapted from Lee VS: Cardiovascular MRI: Physical Principles to Practical Protocols. Philadelphia: Lippincott Williams & Wilkins, 2006, p 22.)*

Since flow-related enhancement is also a time-of-flight phenomenon, the same variables that determine the flow voids in spin echo imaging (i.e., the velocity, slice thickness, etc.) also affect the flow-related enhancement in gradient-recalled echo imaging. For example, increased time between RF pulses also results in increased time of flight effect in gradient-recalled echo imaging. However, the difference is that the end result is increased flow-related enhancement in gradient-recalled echo imaging rather than the increased flow voids seen in spin echo imaging. Another difference is that, since gradient-recalled echo sequences make use of only one RF pulse and no refocusing 180° "echo" pulse, the relative time between RF pulses is represented by the TR rather than the TE. The longer the TR in a gradient-recalled echo sequence, the more pronounced the enhancement of flowing protons.

Gradient-recalled echo images are often acquired via excitation of a three-dimensional (3D) "slab" of tissue, rather than excitation of multiple contiguous two-dimensional (2D) slices. With 3D acquisition, a proton must traverse the entire volume of excited tissue to escape the multiple repeated RF pulses, which means it must travel much further than with the contiguous single-slice 2D acquisition technique. This fact results in an effect termed the "entry slice phenomenon." As flowing protons course antegrade through a vessel, they become more and more saturated by the RF excitation pulses sent into the 3D tissue slab. This results in progressive loss of signal within the downstream aspect of the vessel. The images therefore demonstrate bright signal within the vessel at the beginning of the tissue slab, progressive loss of intraluminal vascular signal over the course of the tissue slab, and the least amount of intraluminal signal at the end of the slab. The entry slice phenomenon is dependent upon the direction of flow within the vessel. For example, in the abdominal aorta there is brighter signal superiorly (since the flow courses superior to inferior), while the phenomenon results in brighter signal at the inferior aspect of the inferior vena cava (flow from inferior to superior). The flow-related enhancement will extend further into the imaged volume with higher velocities, with longer TRs, and with contiguous slices/slabs that are acquired countercurrent to flow.

Gradient Moment Nulling

The time-of-flight phenomenon is the major determinant of vessel contrast in MRI. However, there are several additional factors that attenuate signal within flowing blood, thereby resulting in an accentuation of flow voids in spin echo sequences and a decrease in flow-related enhancement in gradient-recalled echo sequences.

The application of a gradient results in dephasing of protons secondary to exposure to slightly different magnetic field strengths, which results in slightly different precession frequencies. This dephasing leads to signal cancellation and an overall decrease in signal. In order to correct for this signal loss, a bipolar gradient (two equal gradients with opposite polarity) can be applied, which will realign the dephased spins. Bipolar gradients work well for stationary protons, but are less successful in the case of mobile protons (such as in flowing blood). Flowing protons change their positions between the application of the two lobes of the bipolar gradient (i.e., the dephasing and rephasing lobes) and therefore do not experience equal and opposite gradients. This difference results in the accumulation of a net phase shift for the mobile protons. The amount of phase shift is dependent on the velocity of the mobile protons (a principle employed in phase-contrast imaging). According to the principle of laminar flow, velocities are not uniform throughout a vessel, with faster flow centrally and slower flow near the vessel wall. Therefore, intravascular protons will accumulate different amounts of phase and, when summed together, will result in signal cancellation and decreased or absent signal within the vessel.

While this signal loss is tolerable for simple anatomic imaging applications, if the goal is an evaluation of the vasculature, the imaging quality can be improved via utilization of a correction technique called a flow compensation gradient or gradient moment nulling. A flow-compensated gradient is a second bipolar gradient that is a mirror image of the first gradient (i.e., the lobes are applied in the opposite order, negative then positive) When diagramed, it appears as a trilobed gradient since the negative lobes are applied back to back (Fig. 2). This technique causes mobile protons to acquire a phase shift

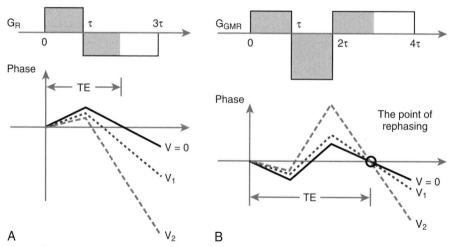

FIGURE 2. Gradient moment nulling. *Black arrow* represents protons with no flow. *Dashed lines* represent protons with constant velocity. (A) There is no flow compensation. The stationary protons do not have a net phase shift at TE but the flowing protons do. (B) The application of gradient moment nulling (a trilobed gradient) results in net 0 phase shift for all protons regardless of their velocity. Note: this only accounts for protons with constant velocity.

that is equal and opposite to that acquired during the first bipolar gradient, which results in no net phase shift. Unfortunately, this compensation technique is only successful for flowing protons with a constant velocity. Higher order flow, such as pulsatility and jerk, can be compensated by larger, more complex gradient schemes, though these are rarely used.[2] Additionally, areas of turbulence cannot be compensated for and always result in decreased signal. The tradeoff for the application of gradient moment nulling is that of additional scan time

as the TE or TR must be lengthened to allow time for the second bipolar gradient to be inserted into the sequence.

An additional way to compensate for flow-related dephasing is by shortening the TE or TR, which reduces the time that protons have to dephase before the signal is acquired. Cardiac imaging employs short TEs and TRs to help compensate for higher order flow without using more complex and time-consuming gradients.

CASE 2

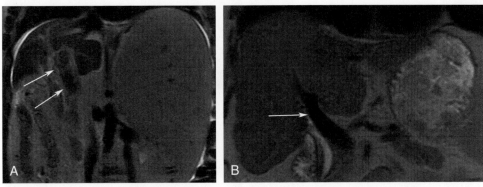

FIGURE 2A. Coronal T2-weighted half-Fourier single-shot turbo spin echo (HASTE) image of the abdomen demonstrating an expanded portal vein containing heterogeneous signal *(white arrows)*. Note the small liver and the markedly enlarged spleen.

FIGURE 2B. Coronal T2-weighted HASTE image of the abdomen in a normal patient demonstrating the normal size and expected flow void of a patent portal vein.

Diagnosis: Portal vein thrombosis.

Discussion: The portal vein contains heterogeneous signal, is expanded, and lacks a normal flow void, findings that are consistent with portal vein thrombosis. Additionally, there are signs of portal hypertension, including marked splenomegaly.

CASES 3 AND 4: COMPANION CASES

Case 3

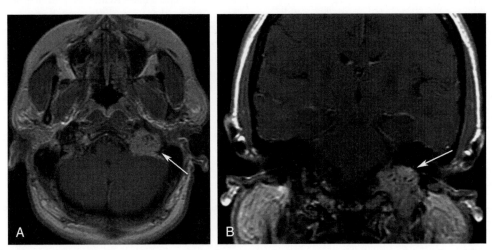

FIGURE 3A. Axial postcontrast T1-weighted image demonstrates an enhancing mass in the region of the left jugular foramen *(arrow)* that contains speckled areas of internal low signal.

FIGURE 3B. Coronal postcontrast T1-weighted image redemonstrates the left jugular foramen mass *(arrow)*. The speckled low-signal areas represent flow voids.

Diagnosis: Glomus jugulare.

Discussion: The glomus tumors (paragangliomas) have a typical "salt and pepper" appearance, which can be identified on either T2-weighted or postcontrast T1-weighted images.[3] The "salt" or white portion of the tumor is secondary to the marked enhancement (representing hypervascularity) of the lesion on postcontrast T1 images as well to as the high water content resulting in T2 hyperintensity. The "pepper" or black portions of the lesion are a result of prominent internal flow voids.

Case 4

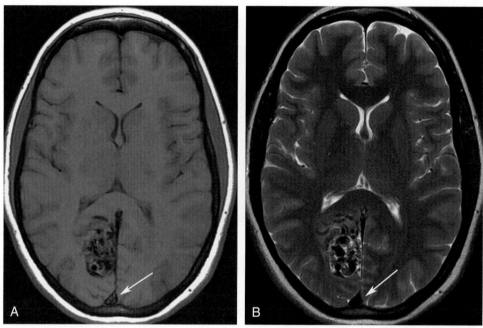

FIGURE 4A. Axial T1-weighted spin echo (SE) image of the brain (TE = 15 msec) demonstrates a heterogeneous mass in the right occipital lobe in this pediatric patient. Multiple serpentine flow voids are identified. Note the incomplete flow void within the superior sagittal sinus *(arrow)*.

FIGURE 4B. Axial T2-weighted SE image of the brain (TE = 116 msec) redemonstrates a heterogeneous mass in the right occipital lobe. Note that the flow voids are more prominent than those identified on the T1-weighted image. Additionally, note that there is now a complete flow void within the superior sagittal sinus *(arrow)*.

Diagnosis: Arteriovenous malformation (AVM).

Physics Discussion

Identification of flow voids within a lesion can be useful for its characterization, providing clear evidence of hypervascularity and thereby narrowing the differential diagnostic possibilities. In Case 4, one notes that the flow voids (including those within the superior sagittal sinus) are more prominent on the T2-weighted image in comparison with the T1-weighted image. This occurs as a direct result of the longer TE (116 msec versus 15 msec on the T1-weighted image), which allows more time for the protons to leave the imaging plane and "escape" the 180° echo pulse. Remember, to acquire signal in a spin echo image, the proton must experience both the initial 90° excitation pulse and the 180° refocusing pulse. Furthermore, susceptibility artifacts will be more prominent with longer TEs as there is more time for T2* effects to degrade acquired signal. Sequences with longer TEs (usually T2) are therefore the most sensitive for the evaluation of flow voids and for determining vessel patency.

Case 5

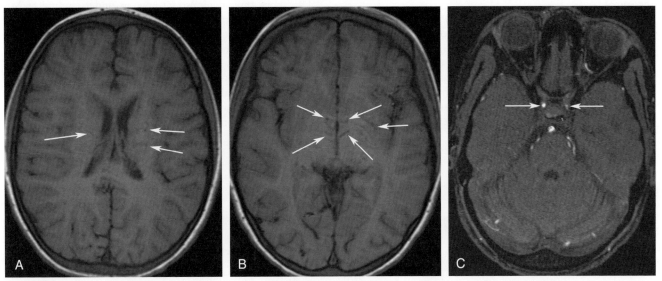

FIGURE 5A. Axial T1-weighted image at the level of the corona radiata. Multiple curvilinear low-signal structures are visualized within the periventricular white matter consistent with flow voids *(arrows)*.

FIGURE 5B. Axial T1-weighted image at the level of the thalamus and basal ganglia redemonstrating the flow voids *(arrows)*.

FIGURE 5C. Axial time-of-flight image at the level of the supraclinoid internal carotid arteries (ICAs) demonstrating narrowing of the ICAs, left greater than right *(arrows)*.

Diagnosis: Moyamoya disease.

Discussion: The term *moyamoya* is Japanese for "puff of smoke," a name derived from the characteristic appearance of this disease on a conventional angiogram. There are multiple etiologies of the disease ranging from idiopathic (most prominent in the Japanese population) to sickle cell disease, the causative basis in this patient. The unifying feature is intimal hyperplasia and narrowing of the distal carotid arteries, which results in increased collateral flow within the lenticulo-striate vasculature.[4]

Case 6

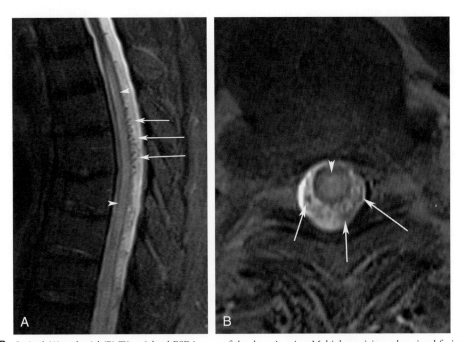

FIGURES 6A AND 6B. Sagittal (A) and axial (B) T2-weighted FSE images of the thoracic spine. Multiple serpiginous low-signal foci are identified dorsal to the cord consistent with flow voids *(arrows)*. Note the edema (T2 hyperintensity) and expansion of the cord *(arrowhead)*.

Diagnosis: Dural arteriovenous (AV) fistula with ischemia of the spinal cord.

Discussion: Dural AV fistulas most commonly affect elderly men and are classically found in the thoracolumbar spine. The AV fistula is located inside the dura mater, close to the spinal nerve root where the arterial blood from a radiculomeningeal artery enters a radicular vein. The increase in spinal venous pressure leads to decreased drainage of normal spinal veins. Increased pressure within the venous system results in flow voids that may exhibit a serpiginous pattern or may manifest as black "dots" studding the spinal cord.[5]

Physics Discussion

The above cases demonstrate how an understanding of MR vascular physics principles can be used to identify pathology and elucidate diagnoses. Flow voids in unexpected locations can signify the presence of collateralization secondary to arterial occlusive disease or can provide the telltale sign of an abnormal vascular pathway, as in the case of the dural AV fistula. One should always include an evaluation for normal and abnormal flow voids in an MR search pattern. Flow voids will be more pronounced on sequences with longer TEs (T2 and PD).

CASE 7

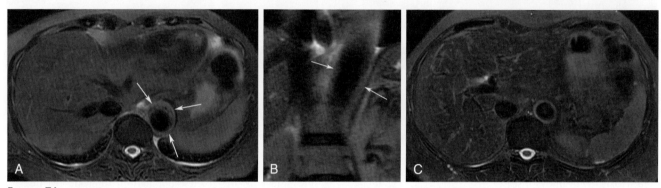

FIGURE 7A. Axial T2-weighted HASTE image of the abdomen. Diffuse thickening of the aortic wall is seen *(arrows)*.

FIGURE 7B. Coronal T2-weighted HASTE image of the abdomen providing an additional view of the smooth thickening of the aortic wall *(arrows)*.

FIGURE 7C. Axial T2-weighted HASTE image of the abdomen 6 months after the initial images, which demonstrates a normal thin aortic wall. The patient underwent interval treatment with steroids.

Diagnosis: Aortitis.

Discussion: The circumferential diffuse smooth-wall thickening of the aorta is concerning for an aortitis. Based on clinical symptomatology and the imaging findings, the patient was treated with steroids. A subsequent MRI (see Fig. 7C) exhibited complete resolution of the aortic wall thickening.

Physics Discussion: Flow voids, in addition to providing information about the presence or absence of intraluminal blood flow, also augment the contrast between the lumen and the vessel wall, allowing for excellent evaluation of some forms of vessel pathology.[1] In this case, the flow void results in improved conspicuity of the diffuse thickening of and heterogeneous signal within the aortic wall, aiding in the diagnosis of aortitis.

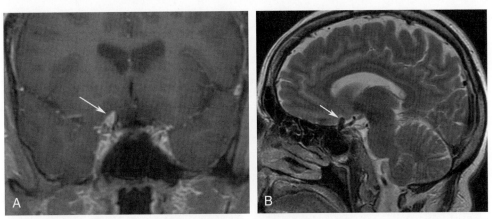

FIGURE 8A. Coronal postcontrast T1-weighted image of the brain. A small enhancing mass is seen adjacent to the right cavernous sinus *(arrow)*.

FIGURE 8B. Sagittal T2-weighted SE image of the brain. There is a vascular flow void that extends superiorly *(arrow)* and corresponds to the mass seen on the coronal T1-weighted image.

Diagnosis: Supraclinoid ICA aneurysm.

Physics Discussion: There is a wide differential diagnosis for the enhancing mass identified on the coronal postcontrast T1-weighted image, which includes a meningioma and a nerve sheath tumor, as well as an aneurysm. However, recognizing the presence of a corresponding flow void on the T2-weighted image allows the diagnosis of an aneurysm to be made. The identification of flow voids in the suprasellar region can be especially helpful in diagnosing aneurysms in this region of complex anatomy.

CASES 9 AND 10: COMPANION CASES

Case 9

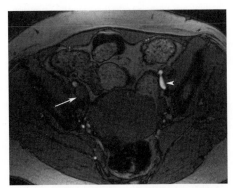

FIGURE 9. Axial T1-weighted gradient-recalled echo (GRE) image of the pelvis demonstrates a filling defect within and expansion of the right external iliac vein *(arrow)*. Compare to the normal left external iliac vein *(arrowhead)*.

Diagnosis: Right external iliac vein thrombus.

Case 10

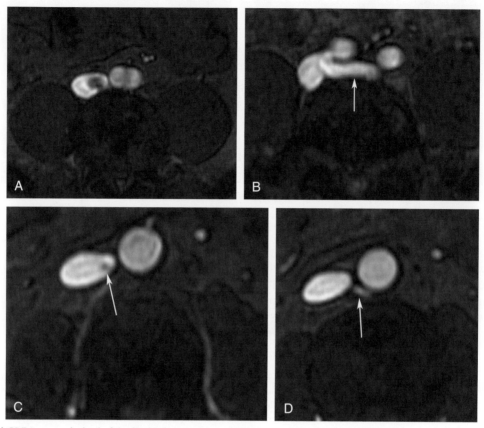

FIGURE 10A. Axial GRE image at the level of the distal inferior vena cava (IVC) demonstrating an apparent filling defect.

FIGURE 10B. Axial GRE image caudal to the first image. Transverse course of the left common iliac vein *(arrow)* emptying into the IVC.

FIGURE 10C. Axial GRE image more superiorly at the level of the midabdomen. An additional smaller filling defect is identified within the IVC *(arrow)*.

FIGURE 10D. Axial GRE image just caudal to the prior image, which demonstrates a transversely oriented lumbar vein emptying into the IVC *(arrow)*.

Diagnosis: Inflow artifacts mimicking thrombi within the IVC.

Physics Discussion

Ultrasound of the bilateral lower extremities is an integral part in the evaluation of deep vein thrombosis (DVT), but is limited by its inability to visualize the more central venous structures. MRI has therefore become an important adjunct imaging modality, providing information about the patency of the deep veins within the pelvis and abdomen. MR venography (MRV) has been proven to be more accurate than traditional contrast venography for diagnosing pelvic thrombus.[6] The inherent flow-related enhancement characteristic of gradient sequences results in a hyperintense appearance to the lumen of patent vessels. A filling defect with associated expansion of the vessel diameter, as seen in Case 9, therefore raises the suspicion for a thrombus. However, pitfalls with this technique include slow flow and flow coursing perpendicular to the imaging slice, both of which can mimic a venous thrombus. This commonly occurs in areas of inflow to the IVC, as in this case at the left iliac vein and at the level of a draining lumbar vein. To increase the specificity of the MRV, a T2-weighted fat-suppressed turbo

spin echo sequence is added to assess for edema within the adjacent soft tissues, an expected finding in an acute DVT. Phase-contrast images may also be obtained to further increase specificity and confidence of interpretation.[7]

Case 10 provides two examples of the lack of sensitivity to in-plane flow on gradient images in a single patient.[8] Evaluated separately, both of these filling defects could represent thrombi. However, the images immediately inferior demonstrate the transverse course of the causative draining vein. This transverse (rather than inferior-to-superior) course increases the time that the intraluminal protons remain within the imaging slice, which, coupled with the relatively slow flow/transit time of venous blood, results in saturation of the protons by the multiple RF pulses sent into the imaging slice. The saturated protons are therefore unable to contribute signal during image acquisition, leading to low signal and apparent filling defects. Common locations for this to occur include the distal IVC at the confluence of the iliac veins, and at the level of the bilateral renal veins. If persistent concern for thrombus remains, phase-contrast images or contrast-enhanced T1-weighted MRV images can be obtained to add specificity.

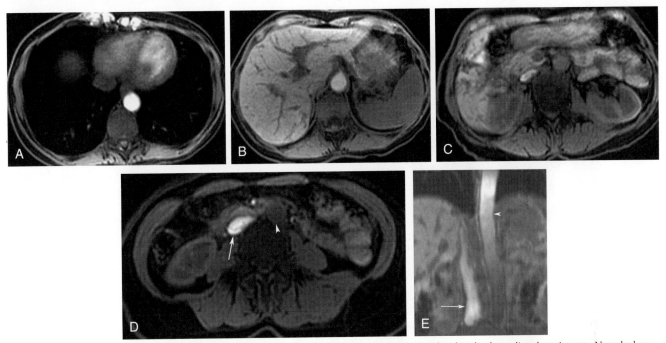

FIGURE 11A. Axial water-only 2-point Dixon GRE image of the lower chest demonstrates bright signal within the descending thoracic aorta. Note the low signal within the IVC.

FIGURE 11B. Axial water-only 2-point Dixon GRE image several centimeters inferior to the first image (at the level of the liver), which demonstrates a slightly less bright aorta. The IVC is isointense to the hepatic parenchyma.

FIGURE 11C. Axial water-only 2-point Dixon GRE image even more inferiorly (at the level of the kidneys). There is intermediate signal within the aorta. The IVC is now brighter than the aorta.

FIGURE 11D. Water-only 2-point Dixon GRE image at the level of the pelvis (most inferior image), which demonstrates a dark aorta *(arrowhead)* and a very bright IVC *(arrow)*.

FIGURE 11E. Coronal reformation based on an axially acquired 3D in-phase GRE imaging dataset. The aorta becomes progressively darker from superior to inferior *(arrowhead)*, while the IVC becomes progressively brighter from superior to inferior *(arrow)*.

Diagnosis: Normal entry phenomenon on a gradient sequence.

Physics Discussion

Gradient-recalled echo images are typically acquired via repeated saturation of a 3D slab of tissue. This results in progressive increased saturation of protons within the imaged tissue slab and a concomitant decrease in acquired signal. The axial images reformatted from the acquired 3D dataset exhibit high signal within the superior aorta because the aorta is receiving "fresh" or unsaturated protons from above the imaged tissue slab.[9] These protons are naïve to the saturation pulses and therefore have their full longitudinal magnetization available to provide signal to the image. The axial images acquired from more inferior in the imaged tissue slab include signal derived from intraluminal protons that have been exposed to more and more of the excitation pulses and are therefore more saturated. This results in less longitudinal magnetization available to produce signal and accounts for the progressively decreased signal intensity within the inferior aorta. The protons within the most inferior aspect of the aorta are completely saturated and appear dark. The opposite effect is occurring within the IVC: the most inferior image has the brightest signal as the IVC receives "fresh" or unsaturated protons from below the imaging slab. By the same principle, the superior aspect of the IVC is dark. This is a striking example of entry phenomenon on a gradient sequence, which is dependent upon the direction of flow.

Case 12

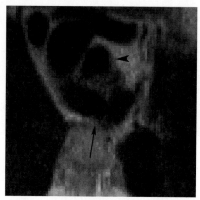

FIGURE 12. Axial HASTE image at the level of the aortic arch, which demonstrates a right aortic arch with an aberrant left subclavian artery *(arrow)* coursing posterior to the trachea *(arrowhead)* and esophagus.

Diagnosis: Right-sided aortic arch with an aberrant left subclavian artery.

Discussion: There are two types of right-sided aortic arches, a mirror-image aortic arch and a right-sided aortic arch with an aberrant left subclavian artery. Two important differences between these two entities should be noted. First, the right-sided aortic arch with a mirror-image branching pattern is almost always (> 95% incidence) associated with other cardiac anomalies, most commonly tetralogy of Fallot or a truncus arteriosus. A right-sided aortic arch with an aberrant left subclavian artery is only rarely (5% to 10% incidence) associated with other cardiac anomalies. Furthermore, the right-sided aortic arch with an aberrant left subclavian artery results in a vascular ring that is completed by the ductus arteriosus on the left side of the mediastinum. This complete vascular ring can lead to dysphagia and wheezing.[10]

Case 13

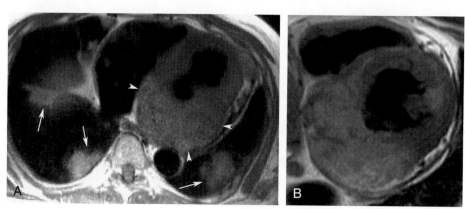

FIGURE 13A. Axial HASTE image at the level of the left atrium and ventricle. A soft tissue mass involves most of the left atrium *(arrowheads)*. Note the multiple bilateral pulmonary nodules *(arrows)*.

FIGURE 13B. Oblique FSE image at the level of the left atrium and ventricle redemonstrating the left atrial mass. Note the improved spatial resolution in comparison with the HASTE image.

Diagnosis: Renal cell carcinoma (RCC) metastatic to the heart and lungs.

Discussion: In this case, black blood images (spin echo–based sequences) are used to identify and characterize a left atrial mass. The black blood technique provides improved delineation of the mass and great vessels. Differential diagnostic considerations for an infiltrating mass in the myocardium include primary malignancies such as angiosarcomas, liposarcomas, and rhabdomyosarcomas as well as metastatic disease.

Physics Discussion

Cases 12 and 13 are two examples of the cardiac "black blood" technique. In Case 12, the black blood technique adeptly demonstrates the vascular anatomy of the mediastinum. In Case 13, it is used to better evaluate the vessel walls and myocardium.[1] As was previously described, black blood images are spin echo–based sequences that take advantage of flow voids to null signal within vascular structures. While standard fast

spin echo (FSE) techniques are occasionally employed in order to obtain high-resolution images, their lengthy acquisition times preclude routine use in areas of high motion.

Most cardiac imaging is performed using a half-Fourier single-shot turbo spin echo, or HASTE, sequence (also called single-shot fast spin echo [SSFSE]). As the name implies, this sequence involves a single 90° RF pulse in combination with a long echo train length (usually > 70) in order to fill k-space. As an additional time-saving measure, only a little more than half of k-space is filled (e.g., 56%) and the remainder is interpolated via the inherent symmetry of k-space. These two properties allow for very rapid imaging. Acquisition of a single image takes less than half a second.[1] As a result, an entire image series through the thorax can be acquired in a single breath hold. While this technique provides increased speed and reduced motion artifact, it also results in a diminished signal-to-noise ratio (because only slightly more than half of k-space is sampled), diminished contrast-to-noise ratio, and decreased spatial resolution. This decreased spatial resolution is shown in Case 13. Note the increased conspicuity and clarity of the pulmonary nodules on the FSE image. Additionally, on the HASTE image the intracardiac mass appears relatively indistinct, while on the FSE sequence there is improved differentiation between the normal intermediate-signal myocardium and the hyperintense metastatic lesion as a result of an improved contrast-to-noise ratio. Because of this improved resolution and enhanced discrimination, a second lesion along the anterolateral wall of the left ventricle can be identified.

Black blood cardiac images are acquired during diastole in an effort to reduce motion artifact. However, during diastole there is reduced blood flow (particularly within the cardiac chambers), resulting in diminished or nonexistent flow voids. To compensate, a double inversion recovery technique is added that completely nulls the signal from flowing blood. An initial inversion recovery pulse is applied to the entire slab of tissue,

which inverts all spins. Subsequently, a second inversion recovery pulse is applied only to the slice being imaged. With this technique, all stationary protons within the imaging slice have experienced two 180° inversion pulses (for a total of 360°) and have reverted back to their normal longitudinal magnetization. They are thereby available to produce signal during the excitation pulse and image acquisition. However, flowing protons (i.e., those within the blood pool) are not located within the imaging slice during the second inversion pulse and therefore do not revert back to their normal longitudinal magnetization. Rather, they move into the imaging slice immediately prior to the excitation pulse and image acquisition. As a final measure, the time to inversion (TI) is set to the null point of blood, further reducing the signal acquired from flowing blood. This combination of techniques provides excellent "black blood" images.[1] For further discussion of the double inversion recovery technique, please see Chapter 6.

CASE 14

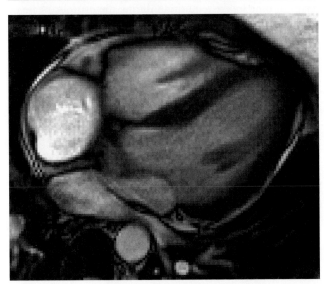

FIGURE 14. Balanced steady-state free precession 4-chamber view of the heart demonstrating a thin septum within the left atrium.

Diagnosis: Cor triatriatum.

Discussion: Cor triatriatum represents an abnormal septum within the left atrium that causes partitioning of the atrium into two chambers.[11] This often results in an obstruction leading to pulmonary venous hypertension and pulmonary edema. More severe forms can cause identifiable heart failure on a neonatal chest radiograph.

Physics Discussion

White or bright blood imaging is one of the workhorses of cardiac MRI. It is used in the evaluation of the cardiac lumen, evaluation of cardiac valves, evaluation for cardiac defects, and most commonly, evaluation of cardiac function. In other words, it provides the physiologic information compared to the anatomic information of the black blood technique, though it is also good at delineating some anatomy. Bright blood sequences are usually electrocardiography (ECG) gated and displayed in cine form.[1] Unfortunately, that can make it

difficult to illustrate them in book format. Functional information, particularly wall motion abnormalities, is much better appreciated and more obvious in the cine form.

As was mentioned previously, the white blood technique takes advantage of flow-related enhancement with gradient images in much the same way as black blood technique takes advantage of flow voids in spin echo technique. Similar to the black blood technique, the white blood technique adds a few wrinkles to ensure there is adequate signal intensity from the blood beyond relying on flow-related enhancement.

The gradients used in cardiac MRI are very fast with TRs that are shorter than T2* times. The result is that there is residual transverse magnetization that has not decayed when the next RF pulse arrives. This residual magnetization can affect the signal of the next acquisition.

There are two ways to address the residual magnetization. The first is by spoiling or crushing the residual magnetization using a gradient. The spoiler gradient takes advantage of one of the recurring themes in MRI, that exposing protons to a magnetic gradient will result in rapid dephasing. With gradient imaging, the spins are dephased and then rephased using a bipolar gradient. The signal acquisition (TE) occurs when the rephasing gradient lobe equals the dephasing gradient lobe. The spoiler gradient works by leaving the rephasing gradient on after the TE, which rapidly dephases the spins again and destroys (a.k.a. spoils or crushes) the residual transverse magnetization. The spoiled gradient technique is used in time-of-flight imaging.

About 10 years ago, cardiac imaging used spoiler gradients in the white blood technique. The white blood results from flow-related enhancement, as described earlier. That method worked well except for two problems. First, since it relies on flow-related enhancement, there is a built-in delay to allow "fresh" spins to enter the slice. Second, the extra spoiler gradient results in longer acquisition times and longer TRs.

Over the last 5 to 10 years, there have been technologic advances in gradient manufacturing that allow them to be switched and adjusted very rapidly. With these new advances, new and better imaging sequences could be used. Out of this arose the "steady-state" sequences. In steady-state imaging, the residual transverse magnetization is used to obtain more signal in subsequent excitations. The initial RF pulse tilts the magnetization vector partially into the transverse plane. The subsequent RF pulses knock the magnetization vector back and forth across the z-axis. The appearance is similar to a metronome, used in music. The result is that both the transverse and longitudinal magnetization enter a steady state, not just the longitudinal magnetization, as in spoiled gradient imaging.

There are several advantages to the steady-state technique over the spoiled gradient technique. First, since it uses the residual transverse magnetization instead of wasting it, there is increased signal-to-noise ratio. Secondly, since the transverse magnetization is added back to the longitudinal magnetization, the steady state is reached quicker, in as little as a single TR. Thirdly, the TRs are extremely short (< 5 msec), allowing for very rapid imaging. For, example a typical 4-chamber white blood cine sequence with ECG gating can be performed in less than 20 seconds—in other words, a single breath hold for most patients.

Another benefit of the steady-state sequence is that the images have both T1 and T2 weighting. In other words, molecules with long T2 and short T1 times will have bright signal (both water and fat). Since blood has a long T2 and short T1

time, it is bright on steady-state images. Thus, the bright signal in steady-state white blood images is mostly attributable to inherent T1 and T2 signal from the blood, not flow-related enhancement. Therefore, the TR does not have to be lengthened to wait for "fresh" spins to enter the slice, and there will not be lack of signal because of slow flow.

Flow-related enhancement does contribute some signal in the steady-state sequence; however, the majority of the signal is due to inherent bright signal of the blood. Since multiple powerful gradients are being used and both residual transverse and longitudinal magnetization is being reused, there is increased sensitivity to artifacts from field inhomogeneities and susceptibility.[1]

Most sequences in cardiac MRI, including both the white and black blood images, are ECG gated. Gating of white blood images allows for the evaluation of dynamic cardiac function and physiology throughout the cardiac cycle. Examples include motion of the myocardium and valve leaflets. The images are typically reviewed in cine form. Gating in black blood images serves to time image acquisition during the diastolic phase of the cardiac cycle, thereby limiting cardiac motion artifact. ECG gating has many similarities to gating in nuclear cardiology. However, the detailed technique of ECG gating is beyond the scope of this book.

CASES 15, 16, AND 17: COMPANION CASES

Case 15

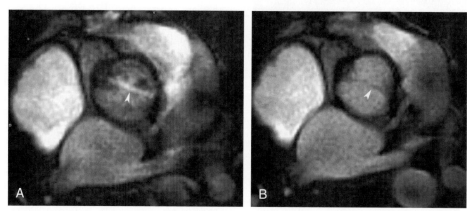

FIGURE 15A. Steady-state free precession image focused over the aortic valve during systole demonstrating a linear jet of flow *(arrowhead)* consistent with a bicuspid aortic valve.

FIGURE 15B. Steady-state free precession image focused over the aortic valve during diastole confirming the presence of only two aortic valve leaflets *(arrowhead).*

Diagnosis: Bicuspid aortic valve with aortic stenosis and aortic regurgitation.
Discussion: The bicuspid aortic valve is a common congenital cardiac anomaly with an incidence in the general population of 0.9% to 2.0%. Bicuspid aortic valves are present in 54% of adult patients with aortic stenosis.[12] Aortic stenosis results in turbulent flow with increased velocities across the valve manifesting as linear heterogeneous signal within the proximal aorta during systole on MR images.

Case 16

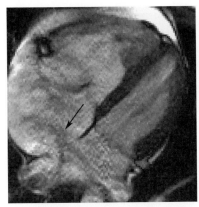

FIGURE 16. Steady-state free precession 4-chamber image demonstrates a large atrial septal defect with a turbulent jet of flow across the defect *(arrow)*. Note the enlarged right atrium and ventricle secondary to volume overload from the left-to-right shunt.

Diagnosis: Ostium secundum atrial septal defect.
Discussion: The excellent contrast between the white blood and dark septum clearly demonstrates the communication between the right and left atrium and the absence of an intact septum. Additionally, the darker turbulent flow extending into the right atrium provides added conspicuity. Identifying secondary signs such as an enlarged right atrium and right ventricle is also important.

Case 17

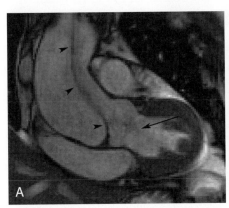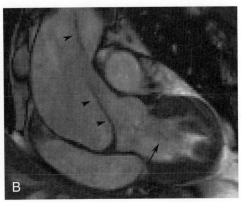

FIGURES 17A AND 17B. Steady-state free precession images centered over the left ventricular outflow tract (LVOT). Note the dilated ascending aorta extending into the aortic root as well as a dissection flap within the ascending aorta *(arrowheads)*. A jet of dark signal representing turbulent flow extends retrograde from the aortic valve into the left ventricle consistent with aortic regurgitation *(arrows)*.

Diagnosis: Marfan syndrome with annuloaortic ectasia, a dissection of the ascending aorta, and resultant aortic regurgitation.
Discussion: In contradistinction to ascending aortic aneurysms from atherosclerotic disease, aneurysms secondary to Marfan syndrome result in dilation of the aortic root, termed *annuloaortic ectasia*. A defect in the gene that encodes for the glycoprotein fibrillin results in a weakened vascular interstitium and can lead to dissections, as seen in Case 17.[13] Aortic insufficiency is a common complication in these patients, occurring secondary to the annuloaortic ectasia as well as to dissections of the ascending aorta.

Physics Discussion
White blood images are excellent for evaluation of the cardiac valves. The hyperintense signal from the blood pool provides superb contrast with the low-signal cardiac valves. Furthermore, turbulent jets of flow from stenotic or regurgitant valves manifest as conspicuous areas of dark signal on the white blood pool background. Remember, turbulent blood flow results in protons of varying velocities, which therefore acquire differing amounts of phase shift in the setting of a gradient.

This phase shift results in cancellation of signal and results in the characteristic dark signal or flow void. Flow-compensated gradients are unable to correct for this dephasing as it is random. Areas of turbulent flow with resultant signal loss are identified in the right atrium adjacent to the ostium secundum atrial septal defect in Case 16 (see Fig. 16) and within the left ventricle secondary to regurgitant flow in Case 17 (see Fig. 17B).

On occasion it can be difficult to determine whether a jet of turbulent flow is secondary to valve regurgitation versus valve stenosis. Intuitively, the direction that the jet is oriented should help one make this determination. In order to identify the direction of the turbulence, one must first locate the position of the valve, which may require several reviews of the cine. Another way to help locate the valve and determine the direction of turbulence is to examine the contour of the jet. Turbulent jets start out from a small point and extend outward from the point in a fan-shaped configuration. Thus, the narrower portion of the jet represents the valvular side of the jet and the broad fan-shaped end represents the direction of turbulent flow. Using these two techniques, it should be relatively easy to determine the origin of the turbulent flow.

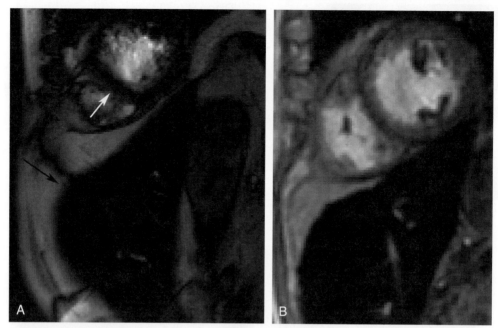

FIGURE 18A. Steady-state free precession short-axis image of the heart and upper abdomen. The myocardium *(white arrow)* exhibits very dark signal secondary to susceptibility artifact from iron deposition. Additionally, note the black signal within the liver *(black arrow)*.

FIGURE 18B. Spoiled gradient short-axis image of the heart and upper abdomen demonstrates myocardium with intermediate gray signal. Redemonstrated is black signal within the liver.

Diagnosis: Hemochromatosis affecting the myocardium and resulting in severe susceptibility artifact.

Physics Discussion

Over the past several years, steady-state imaging has become the primary sequence employed in white blood imaging, replacing the spoiled gradient sequence. Faster scanning times and an improved signal-to-noise ratio have spurred this transition. However, steady-state images are very sensitive to susceptibility artifacts.[1] In this case, hemochromatosis resulted in diffuse iron deposition within the myocardium, causing significant susceptibility artifact and making evaluation of the myocardium impossible. An astute MR technologist recognized this problem and attempted a spoiled gradient image, which successfully decreased the degree of susceptibility artifact. However, note that there remains considerable susceptibility artifact within the liver parenchyma, even on the spoiled gradient images. This is because the iron concentration within the liver is much higher than that within the myocardium.

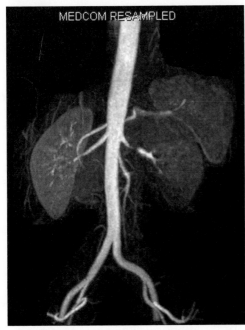

FIGURE 19. Maximum intensity projection (MIP) image of a contrast-enhanced magnetic resonance angiography (CE-MRA) of the abdomen. Focal severe stenosis of the left renal artery with post-stenotic dilation. Note asymmetric enhancement of the left kidney as compared to the right renal artery.

Diagnosis: Atherosclerotic narrowing of the left renal artery.

Physics Discussion

In one respect, contrast-enhanced magnetic resonance angiography (CE-MRA) is similar in principle to its ionizing counterpart, contrast-enhanced computed tomographic angiography (CE-CTA), in that an intravascular contrast agent is injected intravenously, with images obtained during peak vascular enhancement. However, the method of vascular enhancement is dissimilar; while CE-CTA depends on increasing the density of vessels with the use of iodinated contrast agents, CE-MRA depends on T1 shortening of blood cells by the use of paramagnetic gadolinium chelates. In other words, during CE-CTA the iodine molecules are depicted, while during CE-MRA the effect of the gadolinium molecules on the surrounding molecules (e.g., blood) is depicted!

Because vessel enhancement is brief, ultrafast, 3D spoiled gradient echo sequences are used to acquire images during peak vascular enhancement. Volumetric 3D acquisitions enable thin-slice acquisitions, which allow multiplanar reconstruction and creation of high-resolution maximum intensity projection (MIP) images. K-space filling is centric, which maximizes signals primarily containing information about tissue contrast.

Case 19 illustrates the benefit of CE-MRA; the MIP image clearly shows the severe stenosis and post-stenotic dilation of the left renal artery. Another benefit of this examination was the ability to depict the asymmetric enhancement of the kidneys resulting from the stenosis.

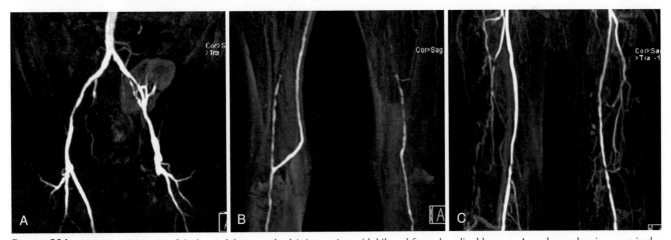

FIGURE 20A. CE-MRA MIP image of the lower abdomen and pelvis in a patient with bilateral femoral-popliteal bypasses. A renal transplant is present in the left hemipelvis. Moderate stenosis of the mid-left external iliac artery is present, with the anastomosis of the left renal transplant artery patent. The proximal extent of a right femoral-popliteal bypass is patent. A left femoral-popliteal bypass is occluded at its origin.

FIGURE 20B. CE-MRA MIP image of the thigh. The distal right femoral-popliteal bypass is patent. The left femoral-popliteal bypass is occluded.

FIGURE 20C. CE-MRA of the lower extremity. Significant trivessel disease bilaterally with single-vessel runoff to the feet.

Diagnosis: Multifocal peripheral vascular disease.

Physics Discussion

The main difference in CE-MRA of the extremities is the difference in image acquisition. The lower extremities are divided into stations (similar to traditional angiography), which are imaged individually at extremely fast acquisition times. A single intravenous bolus of gadolinium chelate is injected, and the MRI table moves distally as it "chases" the contrast bolus from the proximal station (thighs) to the distal station (legs, ankle).

Physics

1. Spin echo sequences result in flow voids.
2. Gradient-recalled echo sequences exhibit flow-related enhancement.
3. Flow voids and flow-related enhancement are both based on the same "time-of-flight" phenomenon.
4. The time-of-flight phenomenon is based on the fact that flowing protons within blood do not experience the same RF pulses as that of stationary protons.
5. The amount of flow void is not binary. Rather, there is a spectrum ranging from full normal signal to a complete signal void.
6. Sequences with long TEs (such as T2 and PD images) have the most prominent flow voids.
7. Vessels taking an oblique course to the imaging plane result in an increase in the amount of time that protons stay within the imaging slice and thereby increase the probability that they experience both RF pulses (and result in a signal).
8. In gradient-recalled echo sequences, a proton's longitudinal magnitude does not fully recover before the next RF pulse is applied. Multiple repeated TRs in gradient-recalled echo images result in the achievement of an equilibrium between the amount of longitudinal magnetization recovered and the amount of magnetization that is tipped into the transverse plane. This is called "saturation" and results in decreased signal based on the proton's inherent T1 and T2* properties.
9. Flowing protons moving into a slice are unsaturated and have full signal. This is the basis of "flow-related enhancement."
10. With 3D acquisition, a proton must traverse the entire volume of excited tissue to escape the multiple repeated RF pulses. The result is an effect termed the *entry slice phenomenon.*
11. Entry slice phenomenon results in progressive loss of signal within the downstream aspect of the vessel. It is dependent on direction of blood flow.
12. Bipolar gradients are unable to correct phase shift in moving protons, which results in further signal loss.
13. Flow-compensated gradients are a second "mirror-image" bipolar gradient that can account for phase shifts in flowing protons.
14. Most "black blood" cardiac imaging is performed using a half-Fourier single-shot fast spin echo, or HASTE, sequence (also called single-shot fast spin echo [SSFSE]). These sequences involve a single 90° RF pulse in combination with a long echo train length (usually > 70) in order to fill k-space.
15. Black blood cardiac images are acquired during diastole to reduce motion artifact.
16. Decreased blood flow during diastole is countered by application of a double inversion recovery technique that completely nulls the signal from flowing blood.
17. Steady-state images are very sensitive to susceptibility artifacts.
18. Spoiled gradient images provide decreased magnetic susceptibility, but take longer to acquire.
19. In CE-MRA, the lower extremities are imaged in stations and the gadolinium bolus is "chased" down the extremities.

Clinical

1. One should always include an evaluation of the vasculature for flow voids on spin echo–based sequences.
2. Venous thrombosis will manifest as intrinsic signal with the vessel on spin echo images.
3. Confirmation of flow voids identified on short TE sequences (i.e., T1-weighted images) should be done by evaluating long TE sequences (T2 and PD).
4. Identifying abnormally positioned or unexpected flow voids can be exceedingly helpful in establishing a diagnosis.
5. T2-weighted images are usually included in evaluating for DVT to look for soft tissue edema, a finding expected in acute thrombosis.
6. The relative lack of sensitivity to in-plane flow on gradient images can result in "in-flow" phenomena in areas where the vasculature courses parallel to the imaging plane. Common areas where in-flow artifacts are seen include the distal IVC at the confluence of the iliac veins, and at the level of the bilateral renal veins.
7. In cardiac imaging, a "white blood" technique is a gradient-recalled echo–based sequence and a "black blood" technique is a spin echo–based sequence.
8. Standard cardiac imaging sequences include HASTE and SSFSE.
9. On white blood cardiac images, look for linear areas of dark signal that represent areas of increased velocity and turbulent flow. These can be seen in valvular stenosis, valvular regurgitation, and septal defects.

References

1. Lee VS: *Cardiovascular MRI: Physical Principles to Practical Protocols.* Philadelphia: Lippincott Williams & Wilkins, 2006.
2. Miyazaki M, Lee VS: Nonenhanced MR angiography. *Radiology* 248:20-43, 2008.
3. Edelman RR: *Clinical Magnetic Resonance Imaging*, 3rd ed. Philadelphia: Saunders Elsevier, 2006.
4. Hasuo K, Mihara F, Matsushima T: MRI and MR angiography in moyamoya disease. *J Magn Reson Imaging* 8:762-766, 1998.
5. Krings T Geibprasert S: Spinal dural arteriovenous fistulas. *AJNR Am J Neuroradiol* 30:639-648, 2009.
6. Orbell JH, Smith A, Burnand KG, Waltham M: Imaging of deep vein thrombosis. *Br J Surg* 95:137-146, 2008.
7. Spritzer CE, Norcock JJ Jr, Sostman HD, Coleman RE: Detection of deep venous thrombosis by magnetic resonance imaging. *Chest* 104:54-60, 1993.
8. Glockner JF, Lee CU: Magnetic resonance venography. *Appl Radiol Online* 39(6), 2010.
9. Bradley WG Jr: Carmen Lecture. Flow phenomena in MR imaging. *AJR Am J Roentgenol* 150:983-994, 1988.
10. Brant WE, Helms CA: *Fundamentals of Diagnostic Radiology.* Philadelphia: Lippincott Williams & Wilkins, 2007.
11. Krasemann Z, Scheld H-H, Tjan T, Krasemann T: Cor triatriatum. *Herz* 32:506-510, 2007.
12. Yener PN, Oktar GL, Erer D, Yardimci MM, Yener A: Bicuspid aortic valve. *Ann Thorac Cardiovasc Surg* 8:260-267, 2002.
13. Judge DP, Dietz HC: Marfan's syndrome. *Lancet* 366:1965-1976, 2005.

Chapter 11

Time-of-Flight Imaging

Scott M. Duncan and Timothy J. Amrhein

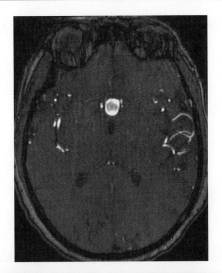

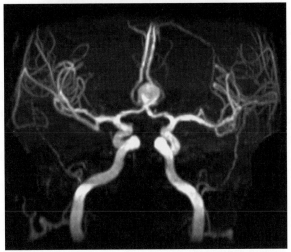

1. Does time-of-flight (TOF) imaging use gadolinium-based contrast agents?

2. Why do the arteries have signal but not the veins?

3. What else can be bright on TOF besides flowing protons?

4. What parts of the body are usually imaged with TOF as opposed to contrasted angiography, and why?

5. In how many dimensions can TOF detect flow?

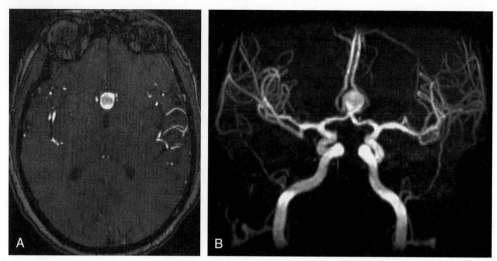

FIGURE 1A. Axial time-of-flight (TOF) image. A large high-signal lesion is seen anterior to the third ventricle consistent with an anterior communicating artery aneurysm.

FIGURE 1B. Maximum intensity projection (MIP) TOF image of the anterior circulation. Redemonstration of the anterior communicating artery aneurysm.

1. Time-of-flight imaging does not use gadolinium-based contrast agents.

2. The signal from veins is eliminated by applying a saturation band above the desired imaging plane to saturate signal in the veins.

3. TOF has some T1 weighting, so tissues with short T1 times, such as fat, can be bright, similar to inflowing blood.

4. The most common anatomic locations for using TOF are in the circle of Willis and the feet. These areas are susceptible to venous contamination with contrasted angiography, and at the same time, have inflowing spins perpendicular to the axial imaging plane. Venous contamination can be prevented with TOF by applying a saturation band to remove venous signal.

5. TOF imaging can detect flow in just one dimension, in the plane perpendicular to the imaging plane.

Diagnosis: Saccular anterior communicating artery aneurysm.

Discussion: Time-of-flight (TOF) imaging is an angiographic technique that does not require gadolinium to obtain contrast within the vasculature. With the increased awareness of nephrogenic systemic fibrosis (NSF), this technique has become much more commonly employed when contrast angiography is contraindicated. Even when contrasted angiography can be used, TOF is often used in evaluating the circle of Willis vasculature. In Case 1, the aneurysm is well visualized on the maximum intensity projection (MIP); note that venous flow-related contrast has been eliminated.

Physics Discussion

Much of the physics of TOF angiography is similar to what was discussed in Chapter 10; however, it will also be reviewed in this chapter in order to keep the discussion coherent. TOF angiography is a gradient sequence that optimizes certain parameters to produce bright signal within the vessel while suppressing the nonmobile background tissue. The suppression of background tissues is achieved via signal saturation. The bright signal within the vessel is a result of flow-related enhancement.

The suppression of background signal through saturation is performed by applying multiple radiofrequency (RF) pulses in succession to the slice of interest. In TOF imaging, the time to repetition (TR) is so short that protons' longitudinal magnetization does not completely recover before the next RF pulse. This results in less magnetization available to flip back into the transverse plane with subsequent RF pulses. After several repeated RF pulses, the proton reaches a steady state in which the amount of longitudinal magnetization recovered is equal to the amount flipped into the transverse plane by the next RF pulse.[1] This is called "saturation" or "magnetization equilibrium." (For a more detailed description of this phenomenon, please refer to Chapter 10, with special attention to Figure 1 in that chapter.) Saturation is not an "all-or-nothing" phenomenon, but rather a spectrum. There are multiple variables that affect the degree of saturation, including the flip angle and the TR.

Saturation occurs in nonmoving protons. However, a flowing proton that is moving perpendicular to the imaging plane will not have been exposed to the multiple previous RF pulses and will therefore have all of its longitudinal magnetization available when it moves into the imaging plane (i.e., not be saturated) (Fig. 1). Therefore, it will have high signal in comparison with the adjacent saturated stagnant spins. This property is known as flow-related enhancement, and is a time of flight phenomenon; thus time of flight angiography. There are several variables that affect the amount of flow-related enhancement moving spins will have, including TR, slice thickness, velocity, and direction.[2]

The TR and the flip angle are two important parameters that affect the degree of signal saturation and flow-related enhancement. Shortening the TR results in less time for longitudinal magnetization recovery and less magnetization left

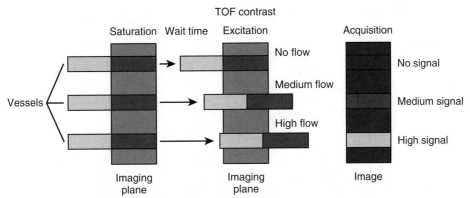

FIGURE 1. Signal intensity is based on the rate of flow within a vessel. The protons within the imaging plane are saturated. Depending on the velocity of flow within a vessel (i.e., high, medium, or none), a certain amount of new, unsaturated protons will enter the imaging plane. When the image is acquired, vessels with high flow will have bright signal because many new, unsaturated protons have entered the imaging plane. Vessels with little or no flow will appear dark, as few new unsaturated protons have entered the field.

for the next pulse. The end result of a short TR is improved signal saturation. Shorter TRs are also beneficial because they mean shorter imaging times and less potential for motion artifact. But shortening the TR does have a drawback. Shorter TRs may not allow enough time for the flowing saturated spins to exit the slice and new unsaturated spins to enter the slice. Thus, shorter TRs can reduce flow-related enhancement. One way to improve flow-related enhancement while maintaining a short TR is to obtain thinner imaging slices. Thinner slices mean shorter distances that the moving protons need to traverse to exit the image slice, which allows the protons *within* the vessel to be refreshed more quickly. The net result is improved flow-related enhancement. The use of thinner slices comes at the cost of longer imaging time (because more image slices need to be obtained per centimeter of tissue). However, this increased time is offset by the fact that the thinner slices allow for shorter TRs. A typical TR for TOF is 25 to 50 msec with a slice thickness of less than 1 mm.

The flip angle of the excitation pulse is another parameter that affects the saturation of stagnant spins. Increasing the flip angle means that more longitudinal magnetization is tipped into the transverse plane, which, for a constant TR, results in less longitudinal magnetization available for the next RF pulse. Therefore, the higher the flip angle, the more magnetization that that does not return to the longitudinal plane, resulting in increased saturation (less signal). The larger the flip angle, the less residual longitudinal magnetization available for the next RF pulse, and the greater the resultant saturation of stationary protons. For TOF imaging, most flip angles range from 45° to 60°. Finally, it should be noted that short TRs and large flip angles in gradient-recalled echo sequences promote T1 weighting (see Chapter 1). Thus, high signal on TOF can be secondary to things other than flow, including fat or subacute blood products.

There are several factors that decrease flow-related enhancement. *Flow-related dephasing,* as was discussed in Chapter 10, is one such factor. Recall that this can be compensated for by using gradient moment nulling or short times to echo (TEs). Typical TEs for TOF angiography are in the magnitude of less than 10 msec. Using short TEs minimizes the need for complex, time-consuming, higher order flow compensation gradients.[2] Remember, gradient moment nulling only compensates for first-order flow (constant velocity). The major drawback is

increased imaging time that is required to insert extra gradients.

Flow velocity is not uniform throughout the lumen of the vessel. For example, the normal laminar flow within a vessel results in higher velocities in the center of the vessel and lower velocities at the periphery. Additionally, there are also microscopic variations in velocity within a vessel due to turbulence and other factors. These small variations in velocity result in dephasing of spins within a single voxel, called intravoxel dephasing. Protons that are within the same voxel and are out of phase with each other will have some of their signal canceled, resulting in decreased signal. Smaller voxel sizes are used to minimize the amount of dephasing, which has the added benefit of improved spatial resolution. However, like everything else in magnetic resonance imaging (MRI), this comes at a cost in the form of longer acquisition times and decreased signal-to-noise ratio.

Another limitation to TOF is that it only detects flow in a single plane, perpendicular to the imaged slice. This makes sense because, if a proton is moving in the plane of the slice, it will experience all the repetitive RF pulses applied to that slice and be saturated like stagnant spins. Therefore, the imaging plane should be oriented perpendicular to the direction of flow. Most vasculature is oriented vertically, making the axial plane the best for TOF. By extension, tortuous vessels or vessels than run in a transverse or oblique plane, such as the subclavian or renal arteries and veins, are not well evaluated by the TOF technique.

There are a few more limitations to TOF that need to be noted when protocoling or evaluating a study. First, TOF often overestimates the degree of stenosis compared to computed tomography (CT) and conventional angiography. This happens because of intravoxel dephasing of the inflowing blood experiencing magnetic field inhomogeneities. The dephasing of spins leads to less signal within the vessel and an apparent increased stenosis. Turbulent flow also leads to rapid dephasing that cannot be corrected. Thus, areas where there is turbulent flow, such as in regions of stenosis, will have less signal and appear more narrow than they really are.[3] Additionally, in general MRI has less spatial resolution compared to CT and conventional angiography.

The major disadvantage of TOF compared with contrast-enhanced magnetic resonance angiography (MRA) is acquisition time. Gadolinium-enhanced MRA takes only 10 to 15 seconds, whereas TOF often takes 4 or more minutes to acquire, which means significantly longer scan times and increased susceptibility to motion. For this reason, TOF is usually only used to image a small volume of tissue (usually < 10 cm), though if necessary it can be used to image larger areas.

TOF is usually acquired in the reverse order that flow is being detected. For example, in the brain, imaging would commence at the vertex. This ensures that inflowing spins have not been saturated from imaging of the previous slice. If slices were acquired along the direction of flow, the incoming protons would be saturated by the RF pulses that were applied to the preceding slices.

TOF images can be acquired using a two-dimensional (2D) or three-dimensional (3D) technique. There are several advantages of the 3D technique; however, it is not appropriate to use in all scenarios. The 3D technique has better signal-to-noise ratio, and is better for evaluating tortuous vessels.[2] However, it can only be used in vessels with high velocities. This makes intuitive sense because a whole slab of tissue is excited for 3D imaging, which means that the proton has to transverse the entire slab instead of a single slice in order to be refreshed. If the slab is too thick, there will be bright signal in the vessels of the first slices with progressive decrease in signal toward the end of the volume, similar to the entry phenomenon discussed in Chapter 10. To avoid this problem, the flip angles are usually smaller, in the range of 20° to 35° for 3D-TOF. (Remember, smaller flip angles result in more residual longitudinal magnetization and less saturation of both stagnant and flowing protons.) 3D technique is usually used when evaluating the circle of Willis, the aorta, and the proximal lower extremities. 2D technique is usually used in the peripheral arteries of the feet, and when imaging veins, because of the slower flow.

The multiple overlapping thin-slab angiography (MOTSA) technique combines 2D and 3D techniques to take advantage of the best features of both. It consists of several thinner 3D slabs that are overlapped to provide high resolution and high signal-to-noise ratio, while still maintaining high signal within the vessel because the slabs are thinner. This technique is commonly used for the circle of Willis.

One of the major advantages of TOF is the ability to null unwanted flow-related enhancement signal coming from the opposite direction. This is why it is often used in the head and the feet even when contrast angiography is available. Think back to experiences you have had reading CT angiograms (CTAs) of the circle of Willis or a CT lower extremity runoff. In each of these cases the MIP and even the raw axial data can be difficult to interpret because there is so much venous contamination that it is difficult to differentiate artery from vein. TOF eliminates the unwanted venous contamination by sending in a saturation pulse peripheral to the imaging slice to saturate any signal from venous flow coming into the slice. For example, when imaging the circle of Willis, a venous saturation band will be applied near the vertex. To image only the veins, the saturation ban is reversed and placed central to the imaging slice to eliminate arterial contamination.

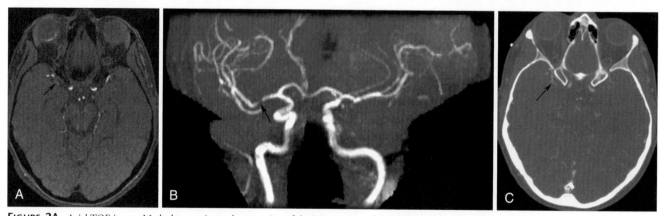

FIGURE 2A. Axial TOF image. Marked narrowing and attenuation of the M1 segment of the right middle cerebral artery (MCA) is seen *(arrow)*.

FIGURE 2B. MIP TOF image of the anterior circulation. MIP shows near occlusion of the right MCA *(arrow)*.

FIGURE 2C. Axial computed tomographic angiography (CTA) image. There is only minimal narrowing of the right MCA *(arrow)*.

Diagnosis: Stenosis of the right middle cerebral artery (MCA) overestimated by MRI.

Physics Discussion

The case is a great example of TOF overestimating stenosis because of dephasing, transverse course of the artery, and turbulent flow. On the magnetic resonance (MR) image, the vessel looks severely attenuated and stenotic, but on the computed tomographic angiography (CTA) image it is almost normal. Notice that, on the MIP image, the artery looks nearly occluded. MIP images exaggerate stenosis because faint vascular enhancement cannot be distinguished from the background by the computer algorithm and is thus suppressed from the image.[3] Beware of determining stenosis using MIP images; always revert back to the raw data for measurements. This is true for both CTA and MRA.

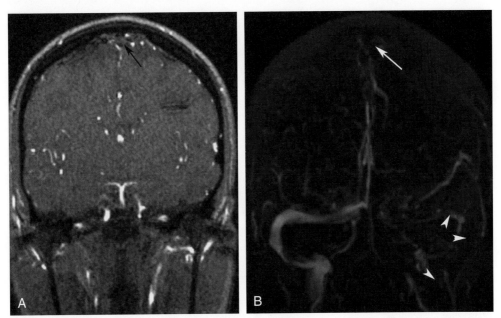

FIGURE 3A. Coronal TOF image. There is absence of flow within the superior sagittal sinus *(arrow)*. Note flow within the basilar artery.

FIGURE 3B. MIP TOF image. There is absence of flow within the superior sagittal sinus *(arrow)*. Also note absence of flow within the left transverse and sigmoid sinuses, along with the left jugular vein *(arrowheads)*.

Diagnosis: Venous sinus thrombosis involving the superior sagittal sinus, as well as the left transverse and sigmoid sinuses and jugular veins.

Discussion: Patients with venous sinus thrombosis often present with nonspecific symptoms. Thus, thrombosis is occasionally noticed or suggested on MR exams that were performed for other reasons. Unfortunately, spin echo techniques are not accurate enough for proper evaluation of the dural sinuses.[4] The TOF sequence is much more sensitive and specific for the detection of thrombosis,[4] and should be added to an MR exam anytime there is a question of dural sinus thrombosis.

Physics Discussion

Venous flow is best imaged by lengthening the TR, and decreasing the flip angles to allow time for the slow-flowing venous sinuses to demonstrate flow-related enhancement. The longer TR and smaller flip angle mean less suppression of background tissue. Notice the background tissues have a brighter signal than other TOF images.

This is one of the few times when coronal slices are used instead of axial slices. This maximizes evaluation of the superior sagittal sinus, which runs in the anterior-posterior (AP) plane; in addition, the transverse and sigmoid sinuses have a posterior-to-anterior (PA) direction of flow. Coronal slices are oriented perpendicular to the AP/PA direction, making them ideal to produce flow-related enhancement. Institutions have different protocols, and some prefer to use the axial plane to evaluate the dural venous sinuses because an arterial saturation band can be used.

Were you surprised to see arterial flow in this image? You shouldn't be. Venous sinus flow is both in the AP (superior sagittal sinus) and in the PA (transverse and sigmoid sinus) direction; thus, if a saturation band were applied, the flow in one direction would be nulled. Additionally, the arteries predominantly flow from inferior to superior and have just a small component in the AP or PA direction; thus, minimal flow would be suppressed if a saturation band were applied.

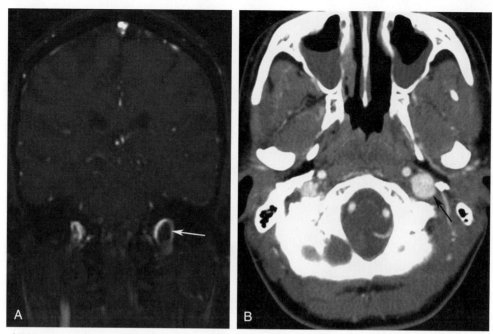

FIGURE 4A. Coronal TOF image. An apparent filling defect is seen within the left jugular vein *(arrow)*.

FIGURE 4B. Axial computed tomographic venography (CTV) image. Widely patent left jugular vein *(arrow)*.

Diagnosis: Apparent thrombus within the left jugular vein, shown to be an artifact (flow defect) on computed tomographic venography (CTV).

Physics Discussion: This case nicely demonstrates one of the pitfalls of TOF, the lack of sensitivity to slow flow, especially when the flow is primarily directed in the plane of the image.[5] The flow of the left jugular vein is primarily superior to inferior and relatively slow. Thus, the protons within the jugular vein were not able to be refreshed by incoming flow and the signal was saturated by the repeated RF pulses. The potential for a false-positive result was realized by the radiologists, and the more sensitive CTV was ordered, which shows that the jugular vein is widely patent.

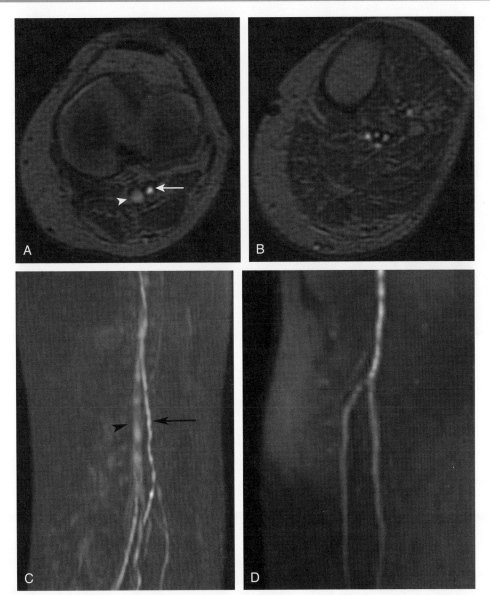

FIGURE 5A. TOF image at the level of the popliteal fossa. Both arterial *(arrow)* and venous *(arrowhead)* signal are identified.

FIGURE 5B. TOF image at the midcalf. Multiple high-signal vessels are seen; it is difficult to separate the arteries and veins.

FIGURE 5C. MIP TOF image of the proximal calf. More superiorly, it is relatively easy to separate the popliteal artery *(arrow)* from the popliteal vein *(arrowhead)*. However, distally, the separation is very difficult.

FIGURE 5D. MIP TOF image with venous suppression.

Diagnosis: Lack of venous suppression during an MRA runoff.

Physics Discussion: What is artery and what is vein? It is quite difficult to differentiate when the venous saturation band is not applied. The mistake helps illustrate how beneficial venous saturation in TOF can be in regions that have significant venous contamination during contrast angiography (head and feet).[6] Note that more superiorly, when only a few vessels are present, the artery can be distinguished from the vein by its smaller size and its brightness (resulting from higher velocity). More inferiorly, when multiple vessels are involved and the flow is slower, all bets are off.

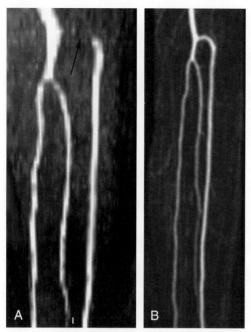

FIGURE 6A. MIP TOF image. There is apparent complete occlusion of the proximal anterior tibial artery *(arrow)*.

FIGURE 6B. MIP from contrast-enhanced MRA. The proximal anterior tibial artery is widely patent and normal in appearance.

Diagnosis: Transverse flow within the anterior tibial artery simulating stenosis.

Discussion: There is an apparent complete occlusion of the proximal anterior tibial artery on the TOF image; however, more distally the arteries appear very normal. This should raise a red flag that the "stenosis" may be artifactual. In this case contrast was given and time-resolved images were obtained. The MIP demonstrates a normal-appearing, widely patent proximal anterior tibial artery.

Physics Discussion
Because of the transverse orientation of the proximal anterior tibial artery, the blood is moving in the axial plane, and the flowing saturated protons are not refreshed by unsaturated new spins; thus, signal from the vessel was lost, resulting in an apparent stenosis.[3] This can also occasionally occur in the transversely oriented petrous portion of the internal carotid artery, as well as in the renal arteries.[6]

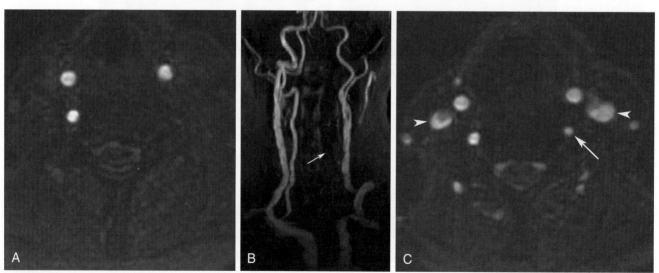

FIGURE 7A. Axial TOF image. There is absence of signal within the left vertebral artery.

FIGURE 7B. MIP TOF image. There is complete absence of signal within the left vertebral artery from its origin to the basilar artery *(arrow)*.

FIGURE 7C. Axial TOF image without saturation band applied. Flow within the left vertebral artery is seen *(arrow)*. Note the venous flow in the jugular veins *(arrowheads)* and other neck veins.

Diagnosis: Subclavian steal.

Physics Discussion

On the initial TOF images (see Figs. 7A and 7B), there is complete lack of signal within the left vertebral artery along its entire course. Without thinking about how the images were acquired, it would be easy to assume there is complete occlusion of the vertebral artery. Remember, a saturation band is applied to saturate venous flow, which will also saturate any arterial flow flowing superior to inferior. That makes subclavian steal with reversal of flow within the vertebral artery a differential possibility.[7] In this case the TOF sequence was repeated without the saturation band, which shows the flow within the vertebral artery (see Fig. 7C) confirming the diagnosis of subclavian steal. Notice that the left vertebral artery is not as bright as the right vertebral artery because of the slower flow. The image acquisition from superior to inferior likely also suppressed some of the signal within the artery.

On a side note, did you recognize that the cerebrospinal fluid (CSF) is bright? That is not signal from water (remember, TOF is T1, not T2, weighted, and water is T1 dark); instead, it is signal from flow within the CSF space.

CASE 8

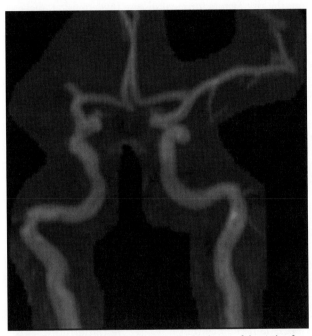

FIGURE 8. MIP TOF image of the anterior circulation of the circle of Willis. Abrupt cutoff of the proximal right MCA is seen.

Diagnosis: Acute right MCA stroke.

Discussion: As mentioned previously, TOF is used for the circle of Willis because of the ability to suppress venous contamination.[8] The MIP nicely demonstrates the abrupt occlusion of the right MCA without the overlying venous structures.

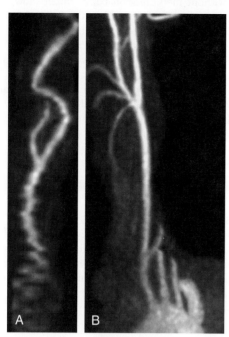

FIGURE 9A. MIP TOF of the right carotid artery. There is a significant motion artifact at the origin of the carotid limiting evaluation. The patient could not receive contrast due to acute renal failure.

FIGURE 9B. MIP contrast-enhanced MRA of the right carotid artery in a different patient. There is no motion artifact. The aortic arch and proximal great vessels are easily evaluated and normal. Note some venous contamination.

Diagnosis: Significant respiratory motion artifact on TOF imaging limiting evaluation.

Physics Discussion

The juxtaposition of these two MIP images demonstrates the major drawback to TOF angiography; its significantly longer imaging time and, by extension, increased susceptibility to motion. In the TOF image, the proximal carotid is completely blurred and it is impossible even to discern the aortic arch. Clearly, this is not an ideal angiographic technique for imaging over large areas or in close proximity to the chest. However, in the age of NSF, more and more patients are not able to receive gadolinium contrast because of poor renal function. In addition, the risk factors for renal disease (hypertension, diabetes, smoking, obesity) are the same as for vasculopathy. The result is that a significant portion of the patients being evaluated for vascular disease cannot receive CT or MRI contrast. Thus, in the past few years there has been a significant increase in non-contrast MRA using TOF. Despite its limitations, it is often the only option in patients with severe renal dysfunction.

Note that, as you move further away from the chest on the MIP TOF image, the respiratory motion artifact decreases so that the image distal to the bifurcation is of high quality, which is why it can be used successful when evaluating the circle of Willis.

KEY POINTS

Physics

1. TOF is a noncontrast angiographic technique that is becoming more popular as a result of increased awareness of NSF.
2. TOF is a gradient sequence that suppresses background signal and enhances flow-related contrast to produce angiographic images.
   a. Stagnant, background tissue is saturated by using short TRs and large flip angles.
   b. Flow-related enhancement is improved by using short TEs, thin slices, and small voxels.
3. One major advantage of TOF is the ability to eliminate flow coming from the opposite direction. This allows for suppression of unwanted venous flow in the head and feet. As a result, TOF is the MR sequence of choice in these areas even when contrast angiography is available.
4. Limitations to TOF include its overestimation of stenosis and its long acquisition time, making it more susceptible to motion.
5. Images can be acquired using a 2D or 3D technique. The 3D technique has better spatial resolution and signal-to-noise ratio, and is better for evaluating tortuous vessels. However, it takes longer and is not good for evaluating large volumes.
   a. The MOTSA technique combines the 2D and 3D technique to take advantage of the good qualities of each technique.
6. TOF can only detect flow in one dimension; thus, it is usually acquired in the axial plane. For this reason it is suboptimal at evaluating tortuous vessels, obliquely oriented vessels, or vessels that course parallel to the imaging plane.

Clinical

1. MIP TOF images will overestimate stenoses; always refer back to source images to determine the degree of stenosis.
2. Dural sinus thrombosis is well evaluated with TOF. The images can be obtained in either the coronal or axial plane.
3. The proximal portion of the anterior tibial artery often shows minimal signal because of its transverse orientation. Be wary of diagnosing stenosis or occlusion in this region if the other vessels appear normal.
4. In subclavian steal, the affected vertebral artery will appear completely occluded because of the saturation band that nulls reversed flow. To differentiate between subclavian steal and complete occlusion, repeat the TOF sequence without the saturation band.

References

1. Edelman R, Hesselink J, Zlatkin M: *Clinical Magnetic Resonance Imaging* (Vol 1). Philadelphia: Saunders, 1996.
2. Lee V: *Cardiovascular MRI: Physical Principles to Practical Protocols*. Philadelphia: Lippincott Williams & Wilkins, 2006, p 402.
3. Kaufman J, McCarter D, Geller SC, Waltman AC: Two-dimensional time-of-flight MR angiography of the lower extremities: artifacts and pitfalls. *AJR Am J Roentgenol* 171:129-135, 1998.
4. Vogl T, Bergman C, Villringer A, et al: Dural sinus thrombosis: value of venous MR angiography for diagnosis and follow-up. *AJR Am J Roentgenol* 162:1191-1198, 1994.
5. Ayanzen RH, Bird CR, Keller PJ, et al: Cerebral MR venography: normal anatomy and potential diagnostic pitfalls. *AJNR Am J Neuroradiol* 21:74-78, 2000.
6. Miyazaki M, Lee VS: Nonenhanced MR angiography. *Radiology* 248:20-43, 2008.
7. Huston J, Ehman RL: Comparison of time-of-flight and phase-contrast MR neuroangiographic techniques. *RadioGraphics* 13:5-19, 1993.
8. Yang JJ, Hill MD, Morrish WF, et al: Comparison of pre- and postcontrast 3D time-of-flight MR angiography for the evaluation of distal intracranial branch occlusions in acute ischemic stroke. *AJNR Am J Neuroradiol* 23:557-567, 2002.

Chapter 12

Time-Resolved Contrast-Enhanced Magnetic Resonance Angiography

Kimball L. Christianson, Allen W. Song, Elmar M. Merkle, and Charles Y. Kim

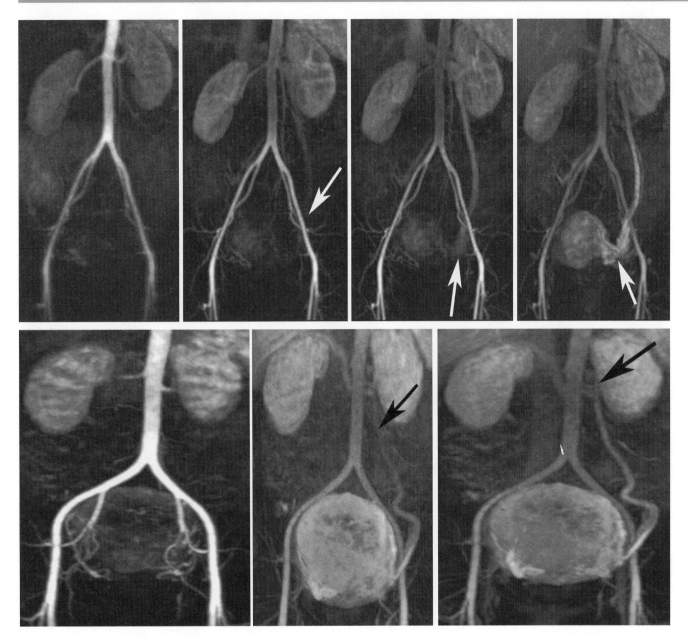

1. What magnetic resonance imaging technique is being used here?

2. What is the diagnosis in the top row of images? What is the diagnosis in the bottom row of images (different patient)?

3. How is this technique useful in interpreting the pathology in these two cases?

4. What does time-resolved imaging mean?

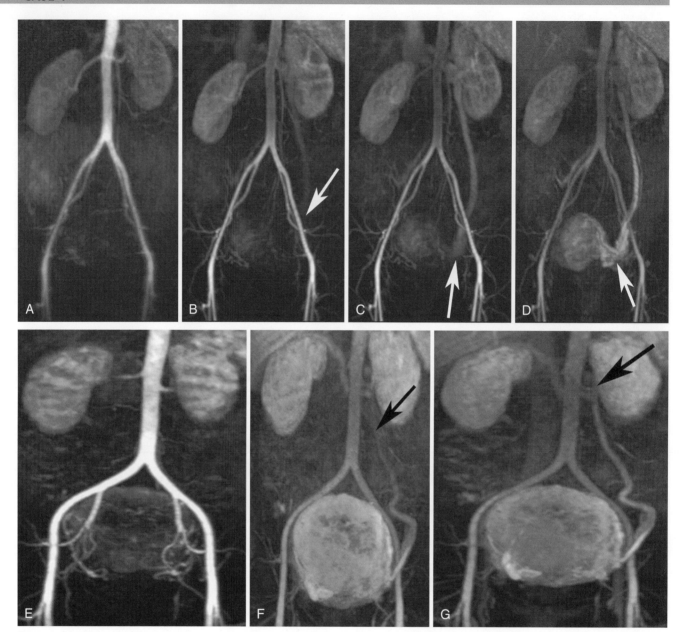

FIGURES 1A THROUGH 1D. Time-resolved magnetic resonance angiography (MRA) with interleaved stochastic technique (TWIST) sequence. A through D sequentially show how the contrast flows in a retrograde fashion in the left gonadal vein. The leading edge of the bolus is annotated with *white arrows* in B, C, and D.

FIGURES 1E THROUGH 1G. Time-resolved MRA TWIST sequence. These images also demonstrate a leading edge (also annotated with *black arrows* in F and G) demonstrating flow in the opposite and correct direction toward the left renal vein.

1. Time-resolved contrast-enhanced MRA.

2. The top row of images demonstrates a dilated left gonadal vein with retrograde flow of contrast in the left ovarian vein, which can be seen with pelvic congestion syndrome. The bottom row of images demonstrates a dilated left gonadal vein with normal direction of blood flow towards the left renal vein.

3. The direction of flow is crucial to making the diagnosis in this case. Static imaging would demonstrate a dilated left gonadal vein in both cases; however, time-resolved

imaging with its high temporal resolution allows visualization of the direction the blood is flowing.

4. Time-resolved imaging is the rapid sequential acquisition of images so that the blood flow dynamics (or any other nonstatic property) can be visualized in a real-time manner. When performing time-resolved imaging, there is usually a localized area of interest. A three-dimensional volumetric slab of the area of interest is imaged numerous times during a contrast bolus with very fast acquisitions and very high temporal resolution, with some sacrifice of spatial resolution.

Discussion: Time-resolved magnetic resonance angiography (MRA) can be a helpful tool in making the diagnosis of pelvic congestion syndrome (PCS). PCS is a cause of chronic pelvic pain currently thought to be due to incompetent valves within the ovarian veins that result in reflux of blood and symptoms of congestion and a feeling of fullness in the pelvis. Static imaging, such as computed tomography (CT) and conventional MRA, is limited in evaluation of PCS, as stated in Answer 3 above. The gold standard in diagnosing PCS is angiography. However, time-resolved MRA is a very good alternative because it is noninvasive and does not require ionizing radiation. Endovascular therapy of PCS can be performed by embolization of the ovarian veins using coils or sclerosant.1

Physics Discussion

Many of the modalities that are used in radiology, including plain films, CT, and much of magnetic resonance imaging (MRI), involve static imaging. Although static images with high resolution are obviously vital to making many diagnoses, sometimes temporal resolution is needed in order to accurately make a diagnosis. Modalities such as ultrasound and fluoroscopy have a high temporal resolution, allowing dynamic imaging to be performed. With the development of time-resolved techniques, MRI now has the capability to perform dynamic imaging. Time-resolved MRA applies very fast imaging techniques that enable multiple acquisitions during a single contrast bolus, thereby offering information on the dynamics of contrast enhancement and actual blood flow dynamics. This is made possible by techniques that have a very rapid image acquistion while still maintaining sufficient spatial resolution. Time-resolved sequences typically employ three-dimensional (3D) sequences that take about 2 to 5 seconds per acquisition.2 Some examples of the use of time-resolved techniques include arteriovenous malformations, peripheral vascular disease, thoracic veins, and differentiating between the true and false lumen in aortic dissection.

Time-resolved MRA offers several advantages over static contrast-enhanced MRA, computed tomographic angiography, and conventional angiography. MRA affords a noninvasive examination without use of ionizing radiation. Time-resolved MRA demonstrates the direction of blood flow, which is helpful to detect abnormal retrograde flow or reflux and is especially helpful for evaluating collateral vessels. The limitations of time-resolved MRA include general MRI contraindications—pacemaker, metallic implants, claustrophobia—as well as limited spatial resolution and nephrogenic systemic fibrosis in patients with renal insufficiency.

In order to understand the concepts behind time-resolved MRA, it is important to understand the concept of k-space. K-space is where the raw signal resides; the echoes (i.e., magnetic resonance [MR] signals) received by the receiver coils of the magnet are mapped out as spatial frequencies in the k-space. As such, the k-space units are in inverse distance, and the k-space map and MR image (units in distance) are mutually convertible by the Fourier transformation. The coordinates of k-space are referred to as kx and ky in two dimensions and kx, ky, and kz in three dimensions. The center of k-space contributes more to the majority of signal intensity of the MR image and the peripheral k-space contributes to the fine spatial details. This concept is very important in understanding time-resolved imaging. The filling of k-space can be done in many

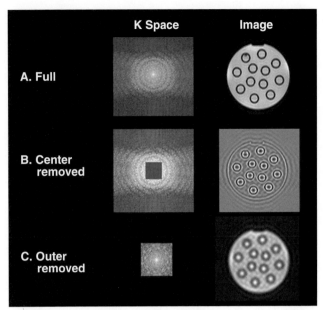

FIGURE 1. Effects of removing k-space from specific regions. (A) None of k-space has been removed and the image has good contrast and resolution. (B) The center of k-space has been removed and the edges and detail of the objects are seen, but there is very little contrast. (C) The periphery of k-space has been removed and there is good contrast but the edges appear blurry and lack the fine detail. *(Reprinted with permission from Jacobs MA, Ibrahim TS, Ouwerkerk R: MR imaging: brief overview and emerging applications. RadioGraphics 27:1213-1229, 2007, Figure 8.)*

different ways, which are controlled by the so-called trajectories. Linear k-space trajectories fill k-space one line at a time corresponding to each echo. This linear filling of k-space can be done from one edge of k-space to the next, which is a sequential linear trajectory. Alternatively, the central lines of k-space can be filled first with the more peripheral lines filled subsequently. This is known as linear centric k-space filling (Fig. 1).

Inherent in understanding how to decrease acquisition times is having a fundamental understanding of the factors that influence acquisition time:

Acquisition time = TR × Number of phase-encoding steps ×

Number of acquisitions / Echo train length

All of these components can be manipulated to decrease acquisition times; however, this chapter focuses primarily on methods that decrease the number of phase-encoding steps and undersample the k-space with unique k-space trajectories.

One of the strategies used to decrease the number of phase-encoding steps and therefore decrease acquisitions time is called partial Fourier k-space acquisition. This is accomplished by filling only a part of k-space, and then by either determining the remainder of k-space from the information already obtained (since the complex k-space data has conjugate symmetry) or simply performing zero filling of k-space. For example, the central portion of k-space can be quickly obtained if the periphery of k-space is filled in with zeroes, thus dramatically reducing the number of phase-encoding steps. Also, because all of k-space is filled (central actual data and periphery zeroes), the desired matrix size is still acquired and the spatial resolution interpolated.2

Other methods of k-space filling have been developed that enable faster imaging techniques such as time-resolved imaging. Most of these techniques are faster because they preferentially fill the center of k-space over the periphery, which is termed undersampling. One of these approaches to filling k-space is keyhole imaging. This technique typically starts by filling the full extent of k-space in the first acquisition. On later acquisitions of k-space, only the central portion of k-space is filled and the peripheral parts of k-space are copied from the prior acquisition. This technique increases the temporal resolution significantly in the later acquisitions because it not only samples the center of k-space but also maintains spatial resolution in the latter acquisitions by copying lines of the peripheral k-space from the initial k-space acquisition. This technique can also be modified by sampling several lines of the periphery of k-space at different time points along with the central portion of k-space, rather than just copying them from the initial acquisition. This improves the spatial resolution of the data acquired from the periphery of k-space along the different time points.[2,3]

View sharing is another technique employed primarily in cardiac cine imaging to increase temporal resolution while maintaining the acquisition time. In cardiac cine imaging, numerous frames or images of the cardiac cycle are obtained with every heartbeat. The filling of k-space with this technique is referred to as segmented because only a portion of k-space is filled in every frame during one heartbeat. With the next heartbeat, another few lines of k-space are filled in every frame,

and so on until all the k-spaces are filled over numerous heartbeats. View sharing significantly increases the number of frames acquired with each heartbeat and, therefore, increases temporal resolution. This is accomplished by acquiring a limited number of lines of k-space from every other frame and copying the remainder of the needed k-space lines from the completed frames acquired before and after.[2]

Parallel imaging using multiple receiver coils is another powerful technique that reduces the number of phase-encoding steps, thereby reducing image acquisition time. A distinct advantage of parallel imaging is that it does not sacrifice spatial resolution, because the distinct spatial sensitivity profiles of individual coils at different spatial locations can be effectively used to recover the missing spatial information. Moreover, parallel imaging can be employed in concert with the above techniques to perform time-resolved imaging.[2]

Two different techniques for parallel imaging are commonly used: sensitivity encoding (SENSE) and simultaneous acquisition of spatial harmonics (SMASH). Undersampling k-space by decreasing the number of phase-encoding steps results in a phenomenon known as wraparound artifact or aliasing. Essentially this occurs when the field of view is smaller than the body part being imaged. With wraparound artifact, part of the image on one side is folded over to the other side. With SENSE, this wraparound artifact is eliminated during image processing in the image space. This is accomplished by being able to distinguish the difference in signals contributing to the true image and those signals contributing to the aliased portion

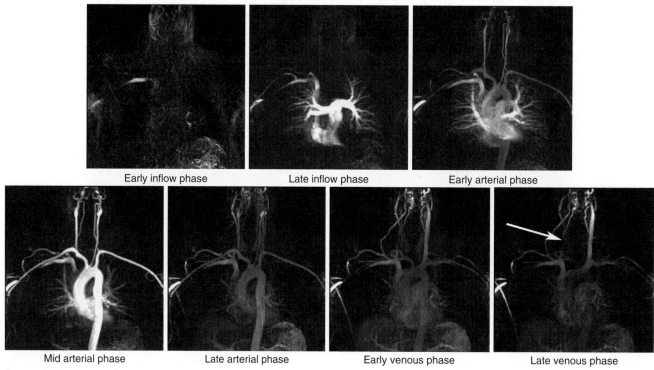

Early inflow phase   Late inflow phase   Early arterial phase

Mid arterial phase   Late arterial phase   Early venous phase   Late venous phase

FIGURE 2. Seven images from a time-resolved MRA of the chest in a patient with a right internal jugular vein stenosis *(white arrow, late venous phase image).* After contrast administration, numerous rapid acquisitions are taken in the coronal plane at very short (2- to 5-second) intervals. In the inflow-phase images, the gadolinium bolus is initially observed traveling through the right subclavian vein, into the superior vena cava and right heart and out to the pulmonary arteries. Next come the arterial-phase images, which become very important later in the study in differentiating arteries from veins as some of the contrast in the arteries often remains throughout the entirety of the study. The venous-phase images demonstrate very good opacification of the central veins. *(Reprinted with permission from Kim CY, Mirza RA, Bryant JA, et al: Central veins of the chest: evaluation with time-resolved MR angiography. Radiology 247:558-566, 2008.)*

of the image, based on the known spatial sensitivity profile of individual coils at different locations. Once the correct signals are distinguished and calculated, each voxel can be reassigned its appropriate signal intensity, whether it be within the aliased portion of the image or within the true image. Then the image can be reconstructed with a full field of view without any aliasing. Similarly to SENSE, SMASH takes advantage of differing sensitivity profiles of individual receiver coils to restore the image, but all operations are carried out in the k-space domain.[2]

The most commonly used sequences currently applied in contrast-enhanced MRA are as follows:

- Time-resolved angiography with interleaved stochastic technique (**TWIST**)—Siemens
- Time-resolved imaging of contrast kinetics (**TRICKS**)— GE Healthcare
- Time-resolved angiography using keyhole (**TRAK**)— Philips Healthcare

All of these sequences use various combinations of the techniques described above to decrease acquisition times and increase temporal resolution while maintaining adequate spatial resolution (Fig. 2).

CASE 2

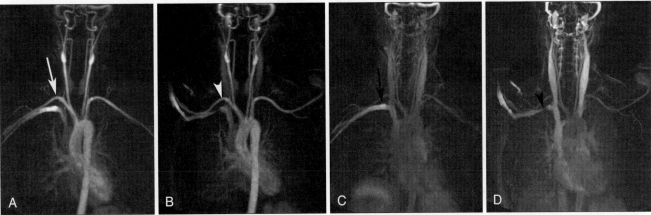

FIGURE 2A AND 2B. Time-resolved MRA images in the arterial phase with the arms down (A) and the arms up (B). The right subclavian artery retains its normal caliber with the arms down (*white arrow,* A) and up (*white arrowhead,* B).

FIGURES 2C AND 2D. Images taken during the venous phase with arms both down (C) and up (D). In D, the *black arrowhead* demonstrates narrowing of the right subclavian vein that occurs when the patient's arms are up versus the nromal-appearing caliber when the arms are down (*black arrow,* C).

Diagnosis: Thoracic outlet syndrome.

Discussion: *Thoracic outlet syndrome* is a term that describes abnormal compression of either the brachial plexus, subclavian artery, or subclavian vein as they travel in the space between the clavicle and the first rib. Compression can be due to both bony and soft tissue etiologies. The symptoms depend on which part of the neurovascular bundle is affected. Clinically, symptoms can sometimes be elicited or exacerbated with elevation of the arms. Time-resolved MRA can be very helpful in determining whether the symptoms are due to compression of the artery or the vein. In this case there is marked narrowing of the right subclavian vein when the arms are elevated. If thrombus forms within the vein, this is referred to as effort thrombosis or Paget-Schroetter syndrome.

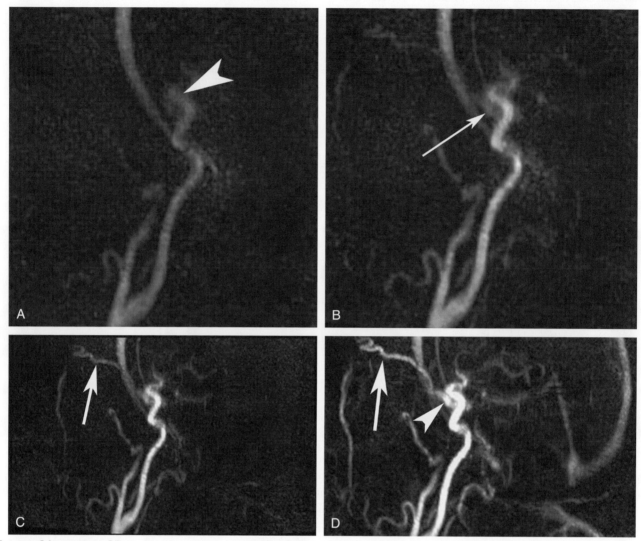

FIGURES 3A THROUGH 3D. Sequential sagittal time-resolved MRA of the internal carotid artery distribution. (A) Early arterial phase image. The *white arrowhead* in A is the cavernous portion of the internal carotid artery. (B) Slightly later time-point with almost immediate ipsilateral filling of the cavernous sinus *(white arrow)*. (C) Late arterial phase image shows retrograde filling of the superior ophthalmic vein *(white arrow)*. (D) Early venous phase image demonstrates increased prominence of the cavernous sinus *(white arrowhead)* and superior ophthalmic vein *(white arrow)*.

Diagnosis: Carotid-cavernous (CC) fistula.

Discussion: These images portray how time-resolved imaging can be extremely helpful in making the diagnosis of a CC fistula. The high temporal resolution particularly throughout the arterial phase allows very good visualization of the early-filling cavernous sinus, which clinches the diagnosis. CC fistulas are most commonly due to trauma but can also be due to ruptured aneurysms and atherosclerotic disease. The patient often presents with proptosis, chemosis, and an orbital bruit from venous congestion. Findings on static MR and CT images include asymmetrical enlargement of the superior ophthalmic vein, proptosis, and extraocular muscle enlargement.

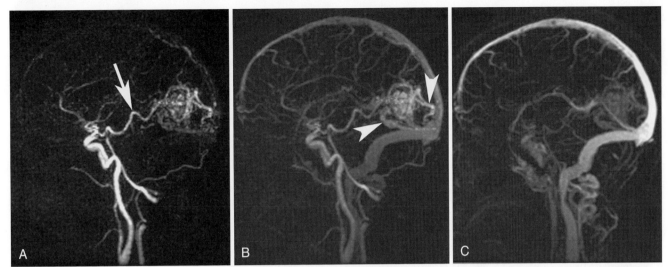

FIGURES 4A THROUGH 4C. Sagittal time-resolved MRA image of the brain. (A) Early arterial-phase image shows immediate enhancement of a tangle of vessels in the occipital region of the brain. The *white arrow* denotes an enlarged posterior cerebral artery feeding the tangle of vessels. (B) Early venous phase demonstrates venous drainage from this vascular abnormality via superficial cortical and tentorial branches that drain into the distal superior sagittal sinus and proximal right transverse sinus *(white arrowheads)*. (C) Mid-venous phase image demonstrates some degree of washout from the vascular abnormality.

Diagnosis: Arteriovenous malformation (AVM).

Discussion: A cerebral AVM is a direct shunt between one or more large feeding arteries and one or more draining veins with an intervening vascular nidus. These lesions are developmental in origin. There is approximately a 1.5% to 3% overall yearly risk of hemorrhage of AVMs, including a risk of death with the first bleed of approximately 10%.[5] The Spetzler-Martin criteria are most commonly used to grade these lesions from 1 to 6. The lesions are graded on size (1 to 3 cm, 3 to 6 cm, > 6 cm), venous drainage (either deep or superficial), and whether they involve eloquent cortex or not. The higher the number, the more difficult they are to resect. Conventional high-resolution MRA is somewhat limited in evaluation of these lesions because it can be difficult to sort out arteries from veins. Contrast-enhanced time-resolved MRA is especially helpful in diagnosing and characterizing AVMs, because the high temporal resolution of this technique enables the differentiation between AVMs and venous malformations based on the timing of the enhancement of the abnormal vessels. Furthermore, this technique helps to distinguish the arterial supply and draining veins.

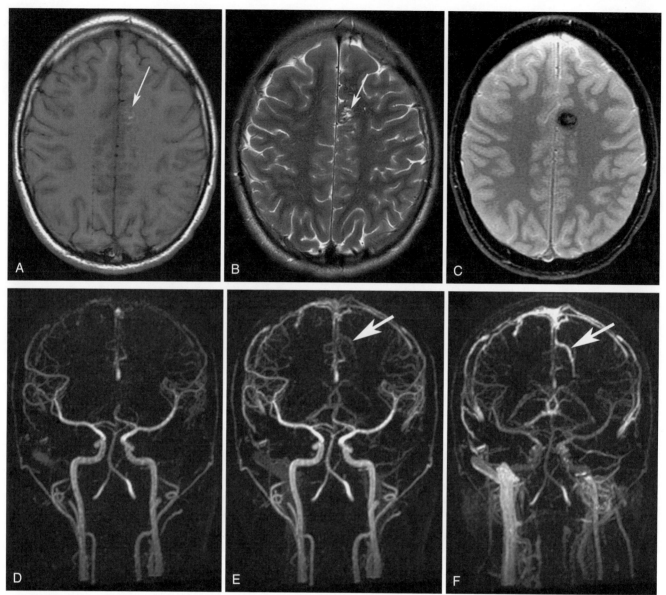

FIGURES 5A THROUGH 5C. Axial T1-weighted (A), T2-weighted (B), and gradient-recalled echo (GRE) (C) sequences that demonstrate a lesion in the left medial frontal lobe with increased signal centrally on the T1- *(white arrow)* and T2-weighted images. On the T2-weighted image there is a subtle low-signal rim *(white arrow)* surrounding the lesion. This low-signal rim blooms on the GRE sequence.

FIGURES 5D THROUGH 5F. Coronal time-resolved MRA images in the early arterial phase (D), late arterial phase (E), and early venous phase (F). The contrast-filled structure in E *(white arrow)* becomes more apparent on the venous-phase image *(white arrow, F)*. There is no large artery feeding this structure, and it appears to be draining toward the dural surface.

Diagnosis: Cavernous hemangioma (Figs. 5A through 5C); developmental venous anomaly (DVA) (Figs. 5D through 5F).
Discussion: The noncontrast images (see Figs. 5A through 5C) demonstrate the classic findings of a cavernous hemangioma as described above. The increased signal within the lesion on the T1- and T2-weighted images is due to methemaglobin. The low peripheral T2 signal surrounding the lesion that becomes even darker on the gradient-recalled echo image is a result of susceptibility artifact from hemosiderin deposition. Developmental venous anomalies are often associated with cavernous hemangiomas. Dynamic imaging in this case is helpful in establishing the diagnosis of a DVA and excluding an AVM (see Figs. 5D through 5F). DVAs represent abnormal venous drainage of normal brain, which is likely due to a congenital insult. It is important to distinguish a DVA from an AVM because DVAs are incidental findings and their removal can result in a venous infarct.

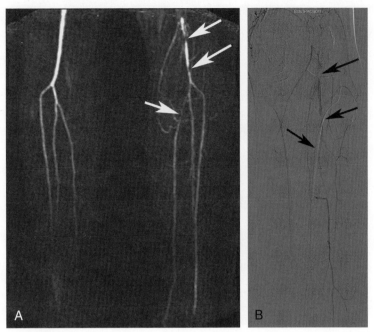

FIGURES 6A AND 6B. (A) Time-resolved MRA in the arterial phase of both lower extremities. (B) Subtracted angiographic image of the left leg in the same patient. The *arrows* in both images denote stenosis of the popliteal artery, tibioperoneal trunk, and anterior tibial artery.

Diagnosis: Peripheral vascular disease involving the left lower extremity.

Discussion: In conventional high-resolution MRA of the lower extremities, the images are obtained in three stations starting proximally and moving distally. The table is moved between each station to cover the entire runoff region. Although this works well for the first two stations (the distal aorta and iliac vessels and the arteries in the thigh), it can be very difficult to time the bolus correctly in the distal legs, and venous contamination can be very problematic. With proximal and distal arterial stenoses and occlusions, the timing of the arterial-phase enhancement can vary dramatically between the lower legs, which further complicates image acquisition timing for static MRA. Time-resolved MRA can be very helpful in this scenario. Because with time-resolved MRA, numerous image acquisitions are obtained at very short intervals, similar to conventional angiography, it is much more reliable in obtaining a diagnostic arterial phase of both lower legs, particularly in the setting of asymmetric arterial flow with severe peripheral vascular disease.

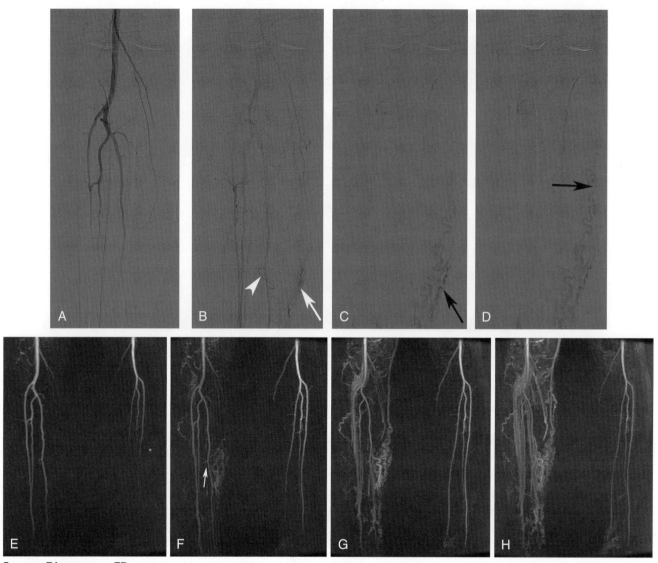

FIGURES 7A THROUGH 7D. Digitally subtracted images from an arteriogram. (B) A late arterial-phase image that shows early filling of a tangle of vessels in the left calf *(white arrow)* and a dominant feeding artery off of the posterior tibial artery *(white arrowhead)*. (C and D) Images showing progressive filling of the dilated venous channels *(black arrows)*.

FIGURES 7E THROUGH 7H. Time-resolved MRA images. (E) Image demonstrating earlier filling of the right distal arteries than the left. (F) A *white arrow* denotes the same feeding artery as seen on the arteriogram, with filling of a tangle of vessels in the medial calf. (G and H) Images demonstrating progressive enhancement of extensive venous structures, making it more and more difficult to distinguish vein from artery.

Diagnosis: Arteriovenous malformation.

Discussion: This case and Case 6 both demonstrate how time-resolved MRA is very comparable with an angiogram in diagnosing certain conditions without the radiation and the invasiveness of angiography. It is clear both on the angiogram and the time-resolved MRA that dynamic imaging is very helpful not only in making the diagnosis but in identifying the feeding arteries to the lesion for treatment planning.

KEY POINTS

1. Although static images with high resolution are obviously vital to making many diagnoses, temporal resolution is sometimes helpful or necessary to accurately make certain vascular diagnoses.

2. Modalities such as ultrasound and fluoroscopy have a high temporal resolution and allow dynamic imaging to be performed. With the development of time-resolved techniques, MRI now has the capability to perform dynamic imaging.

3. Time-resolved MRA involves exciting a 3D volumetric slab of the area of interest that is imaged numerous times during a contrast bolus with very fast acquisitions and very high temporal resolution, with some sacrifice of spatial resolution.

4. Some examples of the use of time-resolved techniques include AVMs, peripheral vascular disease, deep vein thrombosis, thoracic outlet syndrome, CC fistulas, and PCS.

5. Decreasing acquistion times in order to perform time-resolved imaging is primarily achieved by decreasing the number of phase-encoding steps through k-space undersampling as well as parallel imaging.

6. Some examples of time-resolved imaging sequences are TWIST, TRICKS, and TRAK.

References

1. Kim CY, Miller MJ Jr, Merkle EM: Time-resolved MR angiography as a useful sequence for assessment of ovarian vein reflux. *AJR Am J Roentgenol* 193:W458-W463, 2009.

2. Lee VS: *Cardiovascular MRI: Physical Principles to Practical Protocols*. Philadelphia: Lippincott Williams & Wilkins, 2006.

3. Edelman RR, Hesselink JR, Zlatkin MB, Crues JV III: *Clinical Magnetic Resonance Imaging*, 3rd ed. Philadelphia: Saunders Elsevier, 2006.

4. Kim CY, Mirza RA, Bryant JA, et al: Central veins of the chest: evaluation with time-resolved MR angiography. *Radiology* 247:558-566, 2008.

5. Hadizadeh DR, von Falkenhausen M, Gieseke J, et al: Cerebral arteriovenous malformation: Spetzler-Martin classification at subsecond-temporal-resolution four-dimensional MR angiography compared with that at DSA. *Radiology* 246:205-213, 2008.

Chapter 13
Phase Contrast
Scott M. Duncan and Timothy J. Amrhein

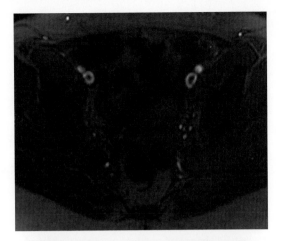

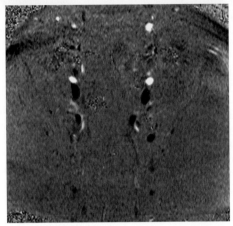

1. What are possible etiologies for the low signal intensity within the bilateral external iliac veins? Are there bilateral deep vein thromboses (DVTs)? If not, why are there filling defects on the gradient-recalled echo (GRE) image?

2. What is the most sensitive magnetic resonance (MR) sequence for detecting slowly flowing blood?

3. Why do the arteries and veins have opposite signal intensities on the phase-contrast image (i.e., the arteries appear hyperintense or white and the veins appear hypointense or black)?

4. Which two types of information can you obtain with a phase-contrast sequence?

5. In which plane is flow being detected on this phase-contrast image, perpendicular or parallel to the image?

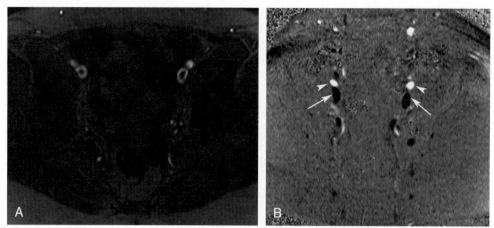

FIGURE 1A. Axial T1-weighted gradient-recalled echo (GRE) image. Filling defects are seen in the bilateral external iliac veins.

FIGURE 1B. Axial phase-contrast image. There is hyperintense signal in bilateral external iliac arteries *(arrowheads)*. Hypointense signal is seen in the bilateral external iliac veins *(arrows)*.

1. The low signal intensity centrally within the bilateral external iliac veins may represent thrombus or flow artifacts on the GRE image. However, the phase contrast image confirms that there is no DVT and this represents flow artifacts. There are two reasons for the filling defects on the GRE images. First, there is a component of flow-related dephasing. Second, the flow in the veins is too slow to result in flow-related enhancement.

2. Phase contrast is the most sensitive MR sequence for detecting slowly flowing blood.

3. The labeling of flow direction is arbitrary. Hyperintense (white) signal signifies flow in one direction and hypointense (black) signal signifies flow in the opposite direction. In this case, the hyperintense signal represents craniocaudal flow and hypointense signal represent caudocranial flow.

4. One can generate two images from a phase-contrast sequence, a phase-contrast image and a magnitude image.

5. Through-plane flow, or flow that is perpendicular to the imaging plane, is detected on the phase contrast image.

Diagnosis: Patent vasculature without deep vein thrombosis (DVT).

Discussion: The central areas of low signal within the iliac veins on the gradient-recalled echo (GRE) image are concerning for bilateral venous thrombosis. However, this finding could also be secondary to slow-flowing blood. A phase-contrast image through the concerning level was obtained for further clarification. On the phase-contrast image, there is hypointense signal within the bilateral external iliac veins confirming flow within the vessel and excluding a thrombus.

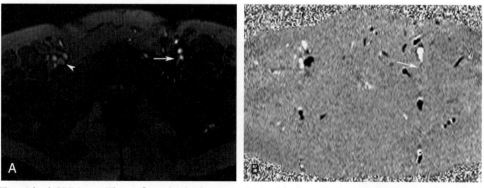

FIGURE 2A. Axial T1-weighted GRE image. There is flow-related enhancement in the right femoral vein *(arrowhead)*, and no flow-related enhancement in the left femoral vein *(arrow)*.

FIGURE 2B. Axial phase-contrast image. Hypointense, black signal is seen at the confluence of the right superficial and deep femoral veins. Only gray signal is seen on the left *(arrow)*. Hyperintense, white signal is seen in the bilateral femoral arteries laterally.

Diagnosis: DVT in the left femoral vein.

Discussion: In this case, the phase-contrast image supports the findings on the GRE image and confirms a left femoral vein DVT. Given phase contrast's increased sensitivity to slow flow, the absence of signal within the left femoral vein means the diagnosis of a DVT can be made with more confidence.[1,2]

Physics Discussion

Phase contrast is an additional noncontrast magnetic resonance (MR) angiographic technique. The information from phase contrast can be utilized in two separate ways: to produce traditional angiographic images or for flow quantification. Because time-of-flight (TOF) and contrast angiography are much faster sequences, phase contrast is rarely used to produce angiographic images. Instead, it is most often utilized to obtain physiologic information or to problem solve when other angiographic images give equivocal results.[3] Specifically, it is the most sensitive sequence for detecting slow-flowing blood, and unlike any other MR sequence, can give velocity, flow, and pressure data.[3-5]

Two types of information are acquired when an MR echo is recorded: magnitude and phase. It is analogous to a vector; the magnitude determines the length and the phase determines the direction (from 0° to 360°). To generate most images, the phase information is disregarded and only the magnitude information is displayed. However, there are scenarios when the phase information is useful. Phase information is utilized to localize signal in the phase-encoding direction. Protons along the phase-encoding gradient acquire different phases depending on their location along the gradient. For example, a proton at the weaker end of the gradient that experiences a 1.49T magnetic field will spin slightly slower than a proton in the middle of the gradient that experiences a 1.5T magnetic field. As the protons spin at different frequencies, they obtain different phase shifts, which can be used to map the location of the proton within the body. Phase-contrast sequences use this same principle, but employ special gradients to eliminate the phase differences between stagnant protons while accentuating the phase differences in moving protons. In phase-contrast sequences, moving protons experience a changing magnetic field and therefore accumulate a phase that is different from stationary protons, which experience a constant magnetic field. Since faster flowing protons travel a farther distance through the gradient than do slower moving protons, their phase difference (in comparison with stationary protons) will be greater than that of the slower flowing protons. In summary, in phase contrast, phase differences are proportional to a proton's velocity, which can be calculated.[3]

In addition to velocity, the phase shift is also proportional to the magnitude of the gradient, with larger gradients producing more phase shift per distance traveled. Therefore, for a given velocity, the degree of phase shift can be manipulated by adjusting the size of the gradient. To illustrate, consider a proton moving through a gradient with a constant velocity of 10 cm/sec. In a gradient ranging from 1.49T to 1.51T, the proton may accumulate +90° of phase shift. If the gradient were doubled to 1.48T to 1.52T, the proton would accumulate twice the phase shift, or +180°. The ability to adjust the gradient is important because phase shifts greater than ±180° result in aliasing, similar to Doppler ultrasound. As another example, consider a gradient that gives a proton with a velocity of

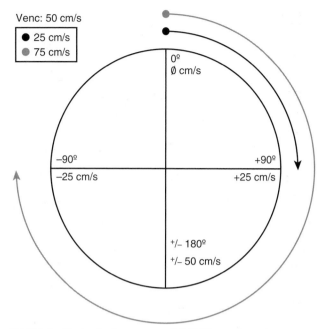

FIGURE 1. Aliasing in phase contrast. IF VENC set at 50 cm/sec, a proton with a velocity of 25 cm/sec will develop +90° of phase shift and be correctly calculated. However, a proton with a velocity of 75 cm/sec will develop +270° of phase shift and be incorrectly calculated as having a velocity of −25 cm/sec.

50 cm/sec a +180° phase and one with a velocity of −50 cm/sec a −180° phase. What if a proton has a velocity of 75 cm/sec? The proton will develop a +270° phase shift, which will be incorrectly labeled as a −90° phase shift. This is an example of aliasing as the proton is incorrectly calculated to have a −25 cm/sec velocity (Fig. 1).

Fortunately, we do not have to calculate the ideal size of the gradient ourselves. Instead, we enter a VENC value, or velocity encode value, which the computer uses to calculate the size of the gradient. The VENC value is the maximum velocity that can be correctly measured by the sequence before aliasing occurs. In other words, the computer sets the gradient so that the VENC value (maximum projected velocity) will result in a ±180° phase shift (in the example above, the VENC value would be 50 cm/sec). The closer the VENC is set to the measured velocity, the more accurate the measurement. If the VENC value is set too low (as in the example above), aliasing will occur. If the VENC value is set too high, slower velocities will not be measured accurately and the signal-to-noise ratio will decrease. The ideal VENC value for evaluating the venous sinus and veins is usually around 20 to 30 cm/sec.[3] For arterial blood, the VENC is usually greater than 100 cm/sec and can be as high as 300 or 400 cm/sec depending on the vessel that is being evaluated and on the degree of stenosis present.[3] Adjusting the VENC value is similar to adjusting the maximum velocity of Doppler ultrasound. The ability to manipulate the VENC value is one reason that phase contrast is the most sensitive MR sequence for the detection of slow-flowing blood. In Cases 1 and 2, the VENC was set to 30 cm/sec, resulting in successful detection of the slow-flowing blood in the iliac veins.

Phase contrast is a gradient-recalled echo (GRE) sequence that uses bipolar gradients to acquire signal. The two lobes of the bipolar gradient, often called the dephasing and rephasing lobes, are identical in magnitude and time, but exactly opposite in direction. Stationary protons experience two gradients that are exactly opposite to each other, resulting in a return to a net 0° phase. This occurs regardless of the position of the proton along the gradient. Moving protons, in contrast, will change locations in between the two lobes of the bipolar gradient, which results in two different magnetic field strengths influencing the phase of the proton. This difference results in an accumulation of a net change in phase relative to the stationary proton.[6]

In practice, a single bipolar gradient is not sufficient to account for magnetic field inhomogeneities, which lead to unwanted phase changes in nonmoving protons. To eliminate field inhomogeneities, a second mirror-image bipolar gradient is applied. This gradient is identical to the first, but in the opposite order. Echoes are recorded after each bipolar gradient and are then subtracted from each other. This results in a flow-sensitive sequence, similar to digital subtraction angiography (DSA). A stationary proton that accumulates phase during the first bipolar gradient (secondary to magnetic field inhomogeneities) will then acquire exactly the same phase during the second, reversed, bipolar gradient. Thus, when subtracted, the stagnant spin will have a net 0° phase. However, the moving spin will accumulate the same magnitude but the opposite direction of phase (e.g., +15° and −15°) during the second bipolar gradient as compared to the first. When subtracted, the opposite phase shifts will result in a net doubling of the phase shift (Fig. 2).

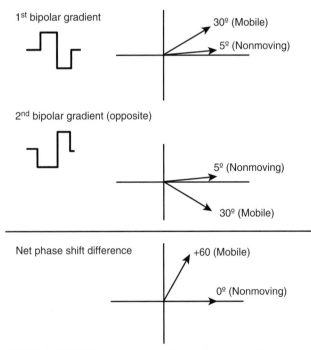

1st bipolar gradient

30º (Mobile)

5º (Nonmoving)

2nd bipolar gradient (opposite)

5º (Nonmoving)

30º (Mobile)

Net phase shift difference

+60 (Mobile)

0º (Nonmoving)

FIGURE 2. Field inhomogeneity correction in phase contrast. Stationary spins have a phase shift as a result of field inhomogeneities. When the bipolar gradient is flipped, field inhomogeneities will still produce the same phase shift (+5° in this case). However, the moving proton will have a −30° phase shift. By subtracting the two datasets, the phase shift of stationary protons cancel and the phase shift of the mobile protons is doubled. *(Adapted from Lee VS: Cardiovascular MRI: Physical Principles to Practical Protocols. Philadelphia: Lippincott Williams & Wilkins, 2006, p 207.)*

Unfortunately, obtaining echoes after each bipolar gradient makes the acquisition twice as long as TOF. In addition, flow is only detected in one dimension, the dimension oriented parallel to the axis of the gradient. To obtain flow in all three dimensions, as would be required to create a traditional angiographic image, the sequence must be repeated three times, making it prohibitively long.

As mentioned previously, flow quantification is the most common application of phase contrast. Flow quantification can be acquired in either one (through-plane flow) or two (in-plane flow) dimensions. With through-plane flow, the velocity-encoding gradient is oriented along the slice selection axis (craniocaudal for an axial scan) and information is obtained about flow that is moving through the plane of the image. For in-plane flow, the gradients are along the frequency- and phase-encoding axes (transverse and anteroposterior dimensions). Information is obtained about flow that occurs in the plane of the scan. Cases 1 and 2 illustrate through-plane flow, while Case 4 below illustrates in-plane flow.

Phase-contrast images have a characteristic angiographic appearance similar to fluoroscopic DSA images. This is because two separate datasets are obtained and then subtracted from each other in order to create the flow quantification image.[5] All stationary spins (0° phase shift) are assigned an intermediate gray signal. Mobile protons are then assigned either hypo- or hyperintense signal based upon the direction of flow, with an intensity level correlating to the velocity magnitude. Regions that contain air (and therefore are relatively devoid of signal), such as are found external to the patient, within the lungs, and within the facial sinuses, exhibit a static, or "snowstorm" appearance, which is secondary to background noise and random movement of protons.

As mentioned previously, one of the major advantages of phase-contrast techniques is the ability to calculate velocity and flow data. This information is typically acquired via through-plane images with the employment of cardiac gating to obtain dynamic information throughout the cardiac cycle. With the placement of a region of interest (ROI) and the use of commercially available computer software, one can determine both velocity and flow information in relation to time. These flow data can then be incorporated into the Bernoulli equation in order to determine intraluminal pressures, which can be used to evaluate the degree of a vessel stenosis (such as in aortic coarctation). Finally, higher order flow data such as pulsatility and jerk can be analyzed using more complex gradients. However, this application is rarely used.

There are several disadvantages to phase contrast that reduce its practicality and thereby its frequency of use. First, its long acquisition time (two to four times as long as TOF imaging) results in its relative rarity of use in MR angiographic imaging. Second, similar to DSA, phase contrast is very sensitive to motion degradation. In fact, if the patient moves during any of the acquisitions, the sequence is usually of non-diagnostic quality. Finally, regions of turbulent flow contain protons that swirl rather than moving in a single direction, resulting in a signal void that precludes the acquisition of velocity data. Turbulent flow most commonly occurs immediately distal to an area of high-grade stenosis or at the bifurcation of a vessel.

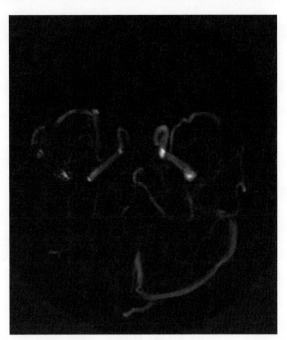

FIGURE 3. Axial phase-contrast slab image of the brain. There is absent signal in the right transverse and sigmoid sinuses signifying absence of flow.

Diagnosis: Right transverse and sigmoid sinus thrombosis.
Discussion: Phase contrast can be used in MR venograms to evaluate for venous sinus thrombosis. The lack of signal within the right transverse sinus and sigmoid sinus confirms venous sinus thrombosis.[7]

Physics Discussion

Phase-contrast angiography is acquired and displayed differently than phase contrast for use in flow quantification. Flow is detected in all three dimensions rather than simply one or two. In phase contrast, the net velocity is determined by the three-dimensional Pythagorean theorem (below) and is thus always positive (as the square of a negative number is positive).

$$V_{net} = \sqrt{V_x^2 + V_y^2 + V_z^2}$$

Signal intensity is based on net velocity of flow. The benefits of phase-contrast angiography are the excellent background suppression and the ability to detect flow in all three dimensions. Lengthy scanning times are phase contrast's biggest detraction as image acquisition is at least four times longer than that in TOF, which is already much more time intensive than gadolinium-enhanced contrast angiography.

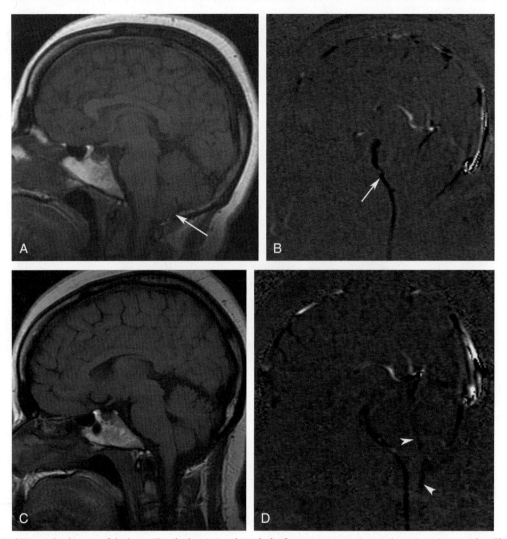

FIGURE 4A. Sagittal T1-weighted image of the brain. Tonsilar herniation through the foramen magnum is seen *(arrow)* consistent with a Chiari I malformation.

FIGURE 4B. Sagittal phase-contrast image of the brain. Black signal is seen anterior to the brainstem *(arrow)*. Little to no signal is seen in the region of the fourth ventricle, the foramen of Magendie, or dorsal to the cerebellum.

FIGURE 4C. Sagittal T1-weighted image of the brain. The patient is status post suboccipital craniotomy, which resulted in resolved tonsillar herniation.

FIGURE 4D. Sagittal phase-contrast image of the brain (status post suboccipital craniotomy). Redemonstrated is dark signal anterior to the brainstem. In addition, there is now black signal in the fourth ventricle, the foramen of Magendie, and dorsal to the cerebellum *(arrowheads)*.

Diagnosis: Chiari I malformation, pre- and postdecompression with improvement in cerebrospinal fluid (CSF) flow.

Discussion: In a Chiari I malformation, the cerebellar tonsils are low lying and can result in obstruction of CSF flow at the foramen magnum.[8] In the initial phase-contrast image, minimal to no flow is seen posterior to the brainstem. However, the phase-contrast image post suboccipital craniotomy demonstrates markedly improved flow in this region, which suggests resolution of the flow-limiting stenosis.

Physics Discussion

In addition to flow within vessels, phase contrast can be used to evaluate CSF flow.[8] CSF flow is even slower than venous flow and the VENC is set quite low, usually at 5 to 7 cm/sec for adults and 15 cm/sec for children. Additionally, CSF flow is complex, changing with the stage of the cardiac cycle.[9] Therefore, these sequences are displayed in cine mode to better characterize the flow. Normally, there is both to and fro flow within the subarachnoid space. Therefore, to confirm adequate bidirectional flow, one should ideally identify both dark and bright signal within the CSF spaces. Single static images (like the ones above) are not adequate for evaluating CSF flow dynamics in clinical practice, but are sufficient for illustrating points in MRI physics books.

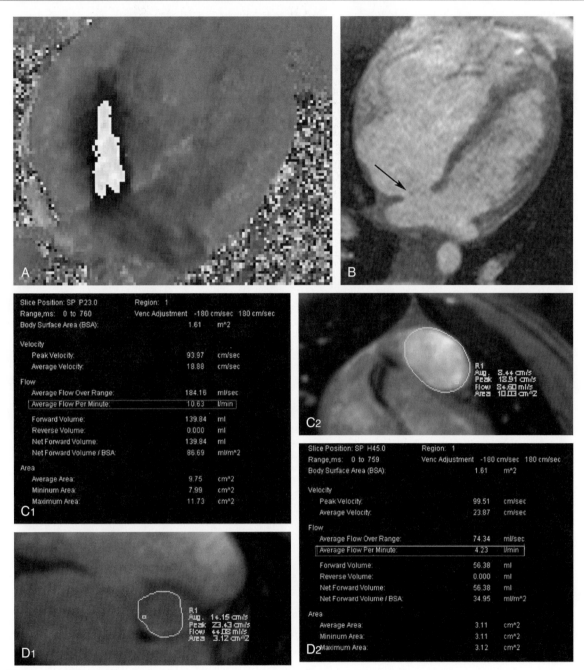

Slice Position: SP P23.0   Region: 1
Range,ms: 0 to 760   Venc Adjustment -180 cm/sec 180 cm/sec
Body Surface Area (BSA):   1.61   m^2

Velocity
    Peak Velocity: 93.97   cm/sec
    Average Velocity: 18.88   cm/sec

Flow
    Average Flow Over Range: 184.16   ml/sec
    Average Flow Per Minute: 10.63   l/min

    Forward Volume: 139.84   ml
    Reverse Volume: 0.000   ml
    Net Forward Volume: 139.84   ml
    Net Forward Volume / BSA: 86.69   ml/m^2

Area
    Average Area: 9.75   cm^2
    Mininum Area: 7.99   cm^2
    Maximum Area: 11.73   cm^2

C1

C2
R.1
Aug . 8.44 cm/s
Peak 18.91 cm/s
Flow 84.80 ml/s
Area 10.03 cm^2

Slice Position: SP H45.0   Region: 1
Range,ms: 0 to 759   Venc Adjustment -180 cm/sec 180 cm/sec
Body Surface Area (BSA):   1.61   m^2

Velocity
    Peak Velocity: 99.51   cm/sec
    Average Velocity: 23.87   cm/sec

Flow
    Average Flow Over Range: 74.34   ml/sec
    Average Flow Per Minute: 4.23   l/min

    Forward Volume: 56.38   ml
    Reverse Volume: 0.000   ml
    Net Forward Volume: 56.38   ml
    Net Forward Volume / BSA: 34.95   ml/m^2

Area
    Average Area: 3.11   cm^2
    Mininum Area: 3.11   cm^2
D2 Maximum Area: 3.12   cm^2

D1
R.1
Aug . 14.15 cm/s
Peak 23.43 cm/s
Flow 44.08 ml/s
Area 3.12 cm^2

FIGURE 5A. Four-chamber phase-contrast image of heart. A jet of flow is seen from the left atrium to the right atrium.

FIGURE 5B. Four-chamber magnitude image of heart. A large defect is seen between the right and left atrium *(arrow)* confirming atrial septal defect (ASD). Note the enlarged right heart from long-standing increased volume.

FIGURE 5C. Flow table (C1) from ROI over the main pulmonary artery (C2). There is an average flow of 10.63 L/min.

FIGURE 5D. Flow table (D2) from ROI over the aortic root (D1). There is an average flow of 4.23 L/min.

Diagnosis: Atrial septal defect (ASD) with left-to-right shunt.

Discussion: Phase contrast is an excellent method to noninvasively obtain flow information in patients with cardiac shunts.[10] In Case 5, the phase-contrast image (see Fig. 5A) nicely demonstrates the jet of flow from the left atrium to the right atrium, diagnostic of an ASD. However, many alternative sequences, including the magnitude image in Figure 5B, could have provided similar information. The true benefit of the phase contrast in this case is found in the flow tables, which demonstrate the severity of the left-to-right shunt. In this case, the Qp/Qs ratio is 10.63/4.23 or 2.5. While any value over 1 is consistent with a left-to-right shunt,[3] this particular case reveals a severe shunt as there is more than twice as much flow to the pulmonary circulation in comparison with the systemic circulation.

Physics Discussion

Flow dynamics are usually calculated with cardiac gated, through-plane phase contrast. An ROI is placed over the vessels of interest (in this case the aorta and main pulmonary artery) and the area of these vessels is traced. The computer automatically calculates the velocity based on the phase shift and the VENC value:

$$\text{Phase shift } (°) * VENC \ (cm/sec)/180° = velocity$$

Flow information is calculated by multiplying the average velocity by the cross-sectional area of the vessel[3]:

$$Velocity \ (cm/sec) * area(cm^2) * 60(sec/min)/1000(mL/L)$$
$$= flow(L/min)$$

Did you realize that Figure 5B is also a phase-contrast image? Remember, as per our earlier discussion, all echoes contain both magnitude and phase information. The magnitude data from the phase-contrast sequence can be displayed to give additional anatomic information. In actuality, the magnitude image is a GRE sequence as the protons are realigned using bipolar gradients. In this case, the magnitude image nicely displays the large ASD.

CASES 6 AND 7: COMPANION CASES

Case 6

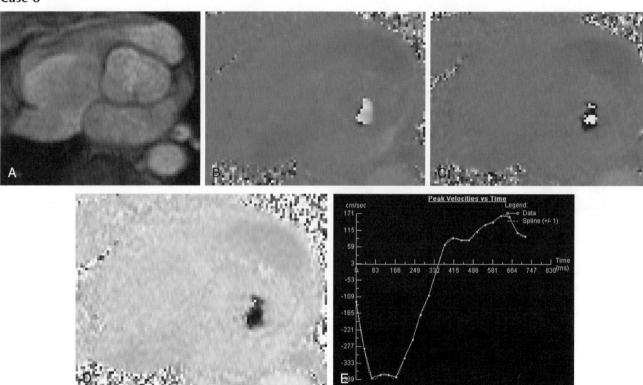

FIGURE 6A. Cross section through aortic valve, magnitude image. A dilated aortic root is seen.

FIGURE 6B. Cross section through aortic valve, phase-contrast image (VENC 250 cm/sec). Both hyper- and hypointense signal overlying the aortic valve are seen, signifying aliasing.

FIGURE 6C. Cross section through aortic valve, phase-contrast image (VENC 350 cm/sec). Persistent mixed signal and aliasing are seen.

FIGURE 6D. Cross section through aortic valve, phase-contrast image (VENC 400 cm/sec). Only black signal is seen, signifying no aliasing.

FIGURE 6E. Velocity graph from the aortic jet (VENC 400 cm/sec). There is high velocity during systole and reversal of velocities during diastole.

Diagnosis: Aortic stenosis with component of aortic insufficiency.

Discussion: Phase-contrast measurements of velocity have been validated with data from echocardiography.[11] The flow chart (see Fig. 6E) demonstrates high velocities during systole consistent with aortic stenosis. The reversed flow during diastole (the curve extends above the x-axis to the region corresponding to positive values on the y-axis) means there is also a component of aortic insufficiency. Determining jet velocities in aortic stenosis is important as it has both prognostic and treatment implications for the patient. Patients with jet velocities of less than 300 cm/sec are unlikely to have symptoms within the next 5 years. However, if the peak velocity is above 400 cm/sec, the patient is likely to experience symptoms within the next 2 years and there is an associated increased mortality rate.[12] The patient in Case 6 had a peak velocity of 382 cm/sec, which was equivocal. However, he was symptomatic and therefore underwent successful elective aortic valve repair.

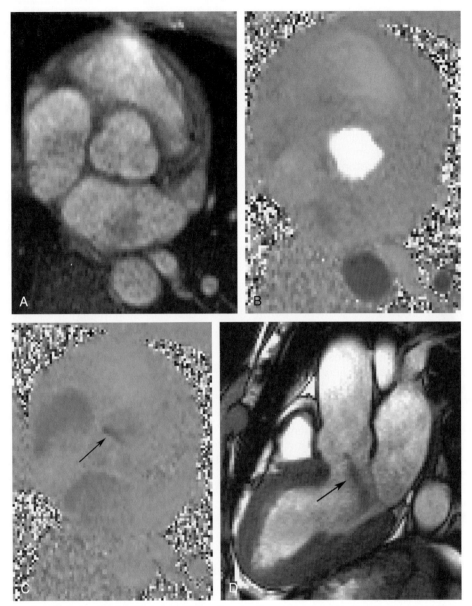

FIGURE 7A. Cross section through aortic valve, magnitude image. Normal aortic valve.

FIGURE 7B. Cross section through aortic valve, phase-contrast image, systole. Hyperintense signal is seen within the aortic root and hypointense signal within the descending aorta.

FIGURE 7C. Cross section through aortic valve, phase-contrast image, diastole. Slit of hypointense signal *(arrow)* over the aortic valve is consistent with reversed flow and aortic insufficiency.

FIGURE 7D. True fast imaging with steady-state precession (FISP) of the aortic outflow tract. A jet of dark signal *(arrow)* is seen extending back into the left ventricle, confirming aortic insufficiency.

Diagnosis: Aortic insufficiency.

Discussion: Complimentary to the previous case, this case demonstrates a jet of reversed flow during diastole on the phase-contrast images, confirming aortic insufficiency.

Physics Discussion

Case 6 is an example of how the VENC needs to be adjusted during the scan in order to eliminate aliasing. Normal aortic velocities are less than 250 cm/sec, which is usually the initial VENC setting. However, the initial phase-contrast image demonstrates both hyper- and hypointense signal within the aortic jet, signifying aliasing artifact. The series was repeated with an increased VENC of 350 cm/sec, which reduced, but did not eliminate, aliasing. Finally, a series with a VENC setting of 400 cm/sec was performed, which eliminated the aliasing artifact. The VENC was then set at 400 cm/sec to obtain the velocity graph.

Physics

1. All MR echoes contain both phase and magnitude information. Usually only the magnitude data are used to produce an image. Phase contrast makes use of the phase information.
2. Phase contrast relies on phase differences that result from protons moving through a complex magnetic field gradient.
3. The amount of phase a proton accumulates is proportional to its velocity and the size of the gradient (i.e., the faster a proton is moving and the larger the gradient applied, the more phase the proton will accumulate).
4. Phase shifts can be calculated from –180° to +180°. Protons that accumulate more phase than this result in aliasing.
5. Instead of directly calculating the appropriate size of the gradient, the physician or technologist enters a VENC value.
6. The VENC value is the maximum velocity that can be accurately measured by the sequence before aliasing occurs.
7. The closer the VENC value is to the measured velocity, the more accurate the measurement.
8. Phase contrast uses bipolar gradients (gradients with the same magnitude and phase, but opposite direction) to return stationary protons to 0° phase shift. Since moving protons change location between gradients, they do not experience the exact opposite magnetic field and thereby accumulate phase.
9. Mirror-image bipolar gradients (back-to-back bipolar gradients with reversed order) are used to eliminate phase differences that arise from magnetic field inhomogeneities.

Clinical

1. Phase contrast is a noncontrast MR angiographic technique that is used almost exclusively for the additional physiologic information it provides.
2. Phase contrast images have the appearance of DSA.
3. Stationary protons are represented by medium gray signal and flowing protons by either dark or bright signal (depending on the flow direction).
4. The magnitude data from a phase-contrast sequence can also be displayed to show anatomic information. It is effectively a GRE sequence.
5. Phase contrast is the most sensitive sequence for detecting flow. Thus, it is often used to differentiate slow flow from thrombus.
6. Phase contrast is particularly useful in providing physiologic data during cardiac imaging.
7. Phase-contrast velocity measurements are integral in making management decisions in the case of aortic stenosis.
8. Flow information from the aorta and pulmonary artery can be compared to evaluate the severity of a shunt.
9. Using Bernoulli's equation, pressure data can be obtained from velocity determinations, which can be useful in evaluating the significance of a vascular stenosis (such as in aortic coarctation).
10. Because of its extremely long acquisition time (three to four times that of TOF) as well as its sensitivity to patient motion, phase contrast is rarely used to produce traditional anatomic angiograms in clinical practice.

References

1. Spritzer CE, Norconk JJ, Sostman HD, Coleman RE: Detection of deep venous thrombosis by magnetic resonance imaging. *Chest* 104:54-60, 1993.
2. Catalano C, Pavone P, Laghi A, et al: Role of MR venography in the evaluation of deep venous thrombosis. *Acta Radiol* 38:907-912, 1997.
3. Lee VS: *Cardiovascular MRI: Physical Principles to Practical Protocols.* Philadelphia: Lippincott Williams & Wilkins, 2006, p 402.
4. Edelman R, Hesselink JR, Zlatkin MB: *Clinical Magnetic Resonance Imaging,* 2nd ed (Vol 1). Philadelphia: Saunders, 1996.
5. Brown MA, Semelka RC: *MRI Basic Principles and Applications,* 2nd ed. New York: Wiley-Liss, 1999, p 210.
6. Miyazaki M, Lee VS: Nonenhanced MR angiography. *Radiology* 248:20-43, 2008.
7. Provenzale JM, Joseph GJ, Barboriak DP: Dural sinus thrombosis: findings on CT and MR imaging and diagnostic pitfalls. *AJR Am J Roentgenol* 170:777-783, 1998.
8. Roldan A, Wieben O, Haughton V, et al: Characterization of CSF hydrodynamics in the presence and absence of tonsillar ectopia by means of computational flow analysis. *AJNR Am J Neuroradiol* 30:941-946, 2009.
9. Bhadelia RA, Bogdan AR, Kaplan RF, Wolpert SM: Cerebrospinal fluid pulsation amplitude and its quantitative relationship to cerebral blood flow pulsations: a phase-contrast MR flow imaging study. *Neuroradiology* 39:258-264, 1997.
10. Beerbaum P, Korperich H, Barth P, et al: Noninvasive quantification of left-to-right shunt in pediatric patients: phase-contrast cine magnetic resonance imaging compared with invasive oximetry. *Circulation* 103:2476-2482, 2001.
11. Kilner PJ, Manzara CC, Mohiaddin RH, et al: Magnetic resonance jet velocity mapping in mitral and aortic valve stenosis. *Circulation* 87:1239-1248, 1993.
12. Otto CM, Burwash IG, Legget ME, et al: Prospective study of asymptomatic valvular aortic stenosis: clinical, echocardiographic, and exercise predictors of outcome. *Circulation* 95:2262-2270, 1997.

Chapter 14

Diffusion MRI

Kimball L. Christianson, Allen W. Song, Elmar M. Merkle, and Ramsey K. Kilani

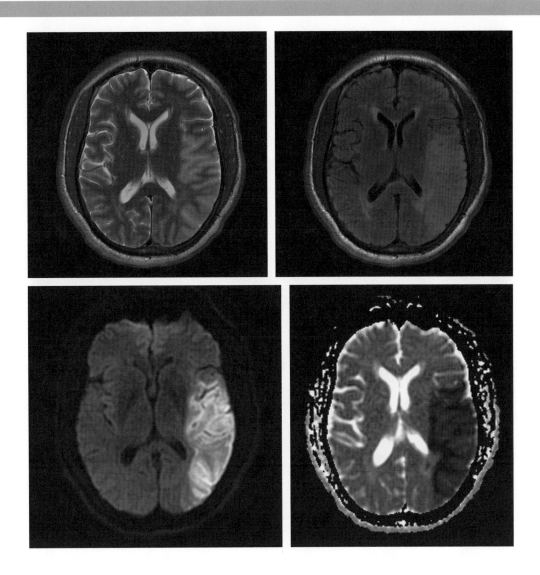

1. What is the diagnosis?

2. What causes the increased signal on the diffusion-weighted image?

3. Why is the apparent diffusion coefficient (ADC) map important?

4. How good is diffusion-weighted imaging at detecting acute stroke in comparison to conventional magnetic resonance imaging (MRI) sequences and computed tomography (CT)?

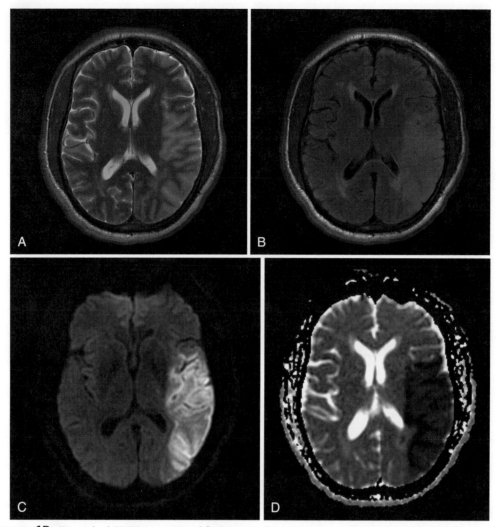

FIGURES 1A THROUGH 1D. T2-weighted (T2W) image (A) and fluid-attenuated inversion recovery (FLAIR) image (B) demonstrate areas of increased T2 signal with associated gyral swelling and sulcal effacement in the left middle cerebral artery (MCA) distribution. A diffusion-weighted image (C) demonstrates increased signal in the left MCA distribution with corresponding low signal in this region on the apparent diffusion coefficient (ADC) map (D) consistent with restricted diffusion.

1. Acute infarction in the left middle cerebral artery (MCA) distribution.

2. Increased signal on diffusion-weighted imaging (DWI) is primarily due to cytotoxic edema (cellular swelling). When neurons become ischemic and oxidative metabolism fails, the ATP-dependent ion transporters stop functioning. This results in an ion gradient across the cell membrane, which causes a shift of water molecules from the extracellular space into the intracellular space. As water increases within the cell (restricted diffusion), an overall decrease in the ability of water to move relative to the extracellular space occurs. Areas of cytotoxic edema, with restricted motion of water molecules, produce increased signal on diffusion-weighted images.

3. There is an element of T2 contrast within a diffusion-weighted image that can manifest as increased signal that is not attributable to restricted diffusion. Therefore, one must be able to distinguish increased signal resulting from restricted diffusion from increased signal resulting from

this T2 contrast or T2 shine-through. This is done by means of an apparent diffusion coefficient (ADC) map. If the area of increased signal on the diffusion-weighted image is low in signal on the ADC map, this confirms restricted diffusion. If the corresponding area on the ADC map is high in signal, then the increased signal is due to T2 shine-through, which is seen in facilitated diffusion (noncytotoxic edema) associated with many types of lesions.

4. The sensitivity of detecting acute stroke within the first 6 hours by using CT and conventional MRI alone is less than 50%. Application of diffusion weighting increases the sensitivity to about 95%.[1]

Diagnosis: Acute infarct in the left middle cerebral artery (MCA) distribution.

Discussion

Diffusion-weighted imaging (DWI) is based on the principle of "brownian" movement of water molecules. Because of its random nature, the diffusion process cannot be reversed in time. As such, the loss of coherence resulting from diffusion cannot be recovered even when a 180° refocusing pulse is used. The result is diffusion-related signal attenuation.[2]

Pulse sequences have been designed to make use of the capability of magnetic resonance imaging (MRI) to measure diffusion and apply it clinically. DWI can differentiate fast-moving protons (e.g., unrestricted diffusion) from slow-moving protons (e.g., restricted diffusion).[3] Spin echo echo-planar imaging is typically the most commonly used imaging sequence in DWI primarily because of its speed, which helps minimize macroscopic motion artifact. The distinguishing feature of a diffusion-weighted sequence is that two strong equal and opposite gradients are applied on either side of the 180° refocusing pulse. The first gradient pulse dephases the protons and the second gradient pulse rephases the protons. If the protons remain static throughout the course of the pulse sequence, then they will be simply rephased by the second gradient and this will result in no change in phase coherence and signal. If the protons undergo diffusion during the pulse sequence, then they will not be completely rephased by the gradient pair and the result will instead be loss of phase coherence and signal.[3]

Signal intensity from a diffusion-weighted sequence is generated according to the following equation (Stejskal-Tanner sequence):

$$S = S_o e^{-bD}$$

Where:
S = measured signal
S$_o$ = signal without diffusion gradients
b = b factor
D = diffusion coefficient

$$\textbf{b factor} = \gamma^2 G^2 \delta^2 (\Delta - \delta/3)$$

Where:
γ = 42 MHz/T
G = strength of the diffusion gradients
δ = duration of diffusion gradient pulses
Δ = time between diffusion gradient radiofrequency (RF) pulses

As stated in the above equation, So is the original signal in the image. This signal intensity is made up of T1, T2, and proton density contrast; however, in a spin echo echo-planar sequence the T2 contrast predominates. Therefore, some of the bright signal seen on diffusion-weighted images can be due to T2 contrast. This is often referred to as "T2 shine-through." An apparent diffusion coefficient (ADC) map is generated to distinguish between bright signal resulting from areas of restricted diffusion and areas of T2 shine-through. An ADC map is generated by combining two sequences, which are performed at different b values; however, all other factors, including T1, T2, and proton density contrast, are kept exactly the same. Typically, one spin echo echo-planar sequence is performed where the b factor is 0 and the image appears as a T2-weighted image. A second sequence is performed where the b factor is greater than 0 and is a diffusion-weighted image. The ADC map is then calculated by taking the negative logarithm of the ratio of those two image sets according to the equation:

$$D = -(1/b)\ln(S/S_o)$$

ADC mapping effectively eliminates the contribution of all other contrast except that resulting from diffusion. Restated, the contrast of an ADC map is purely dependent on the diffusion coefficient of the acquired tissues and not T1 or T2* values.

Diffusion tensor imaging (DTI) is a variant of DWI that illustrates molecular diffusion along axonal tracts and is discussed in greater detail later in this chapter.

CASES 2 AND 3: COMPANION CASES

Case 2

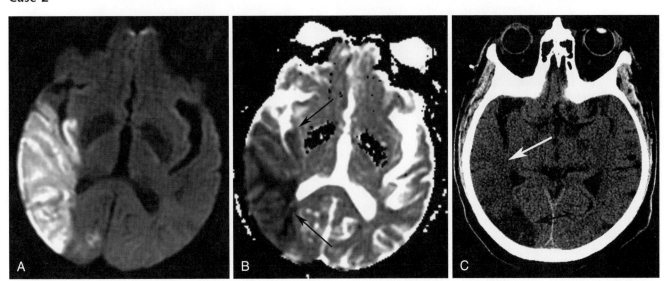

FIGURES 2A AND 2B. Diffusion-weighted (A) and ADC (B) images demonstrating restricted diffusion in the right MCA territory (*black arrows,* B).

FIGURE 2C. Axial computed tomography (CT) image that shows a corresponding area of low density and sulcal effacement in the right MCA distribution (*white and black arrows*).

Diagnosis: Acute infarct in the right MCA territory.

Case 3

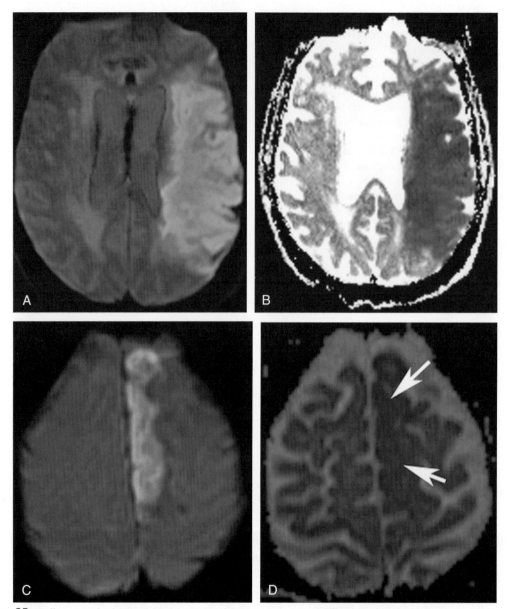

FIGURES 3A AND 3B. Diffusion-weighted (A) and ADC (B) images demonstrating restricted diffusion in the left MCA territory.

FIGURES 3C AND 3D Diffusion-weighted (C) and ADC (D) images that demonstrate restricted diffusion in the left anterior cerebral artery (ACA) territory (*white arrows,* D).

Diagnosis: Left MCA and anterior cerebral artery (ACA) infarcts of different ages.

Discussion

On T2-weighted images, it is often difficult to distinguish between new stroke, old stroke, and new extension of a previous stroke because all appear as increased signal. The aging of infarcts can also be problematic on diffusion-weighted images alone, as the increased signal can be present for months. This increased signal is due to restricted diffusion in the acute phase of an infarct and is increasingly due to T2 shine-through as the infarct ages. Unfortunately, the diffusion-weighted image does not reliably discriminate between causes of increased signal. The ADC map, in contrast, is quantitative and can be used to help age an infarct. In general, within the first 3 days of an infarct the ADC value is decreased about 50% compared to normal parenchyma. Within the second half of the first week, the ADC value is decreased about 25% to 50% and then 0% to 25% within 7 to 12 days. After 10 to 12 days, the signal inverts from low (dark) signal to high (bright) signal on the ADC map. Therefore, increased signal on both the diffusion-weighted image and the ADC map in a patient with known stroke is suggestive of a chronic infarct.[4-6]

The black arrows in Figure 2B delineate the area of infarction on the ADC map. Visually, there is no significant difference between the decreased signal within the anterior and posterior aspect of the region of infarction. However, when the ADC values were measured, they were decreased by 50% in the anterior aspect of the infarct (*white arrow* in Fig. 2C) and decreased by 20% in the posterior aspect of the infarct (*black arrow* in Fig. 2C). This suggests the anterior region of the infarct is acute and the posterior aspect of the infarcted region is subacute. This is consistent with the findings on CT with the very low density posteriorly (*black arrow*) representing subacute infarct and the more subtle area of low density and sulcal effacement anteriorly (*white arrow*) representing acute infarct.

The ADC values taken from the left MCA infarct in Figures 3A and 3B demonstrate a decrease in the ADC value of 50% consistent with an acute infarct. The measured ADC value decrease in the left ACA infarct in Figures 3C and 3D is decreased by 20%, consistent with a subacute stroke.

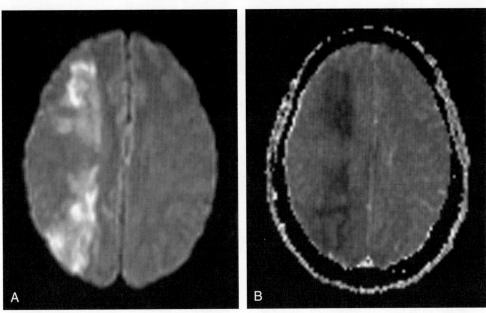

FIGURES 4A AND 4B. Diffusion-weighted (A) and ADC (B) images demonstrate wedge-shaped areas of restricted diffusion extending both anteriorly and posteriorly in the right hemisphere. These areas of restricted diffusion do not correlate to one vascular distribution but instead lie between the vascular distributions of more than one artery and are called "watershed" infarctions. Anteriorly, the area of restricted diffusion lies in a watershed distribution between the MCA and ACA territories. Posteriorly, the area of restricted diffusion lies between the vascular territories of the MCA, ACA, and posterior cerebral artery (PCA).

Diagnosis: Watershed infarction.
Discussion: The watershed areas of the brain are categorized as cortical and internal (or superficial-to-deep white matter). The cortical watershed zone is illustrated by Case 4 and represents the area over the brain surface that is supplied by end arteries from more than one artery. Internal watershed zone infarcts are characterized as infarcts that occur in the corona radiata between the superficial and deep perforators of the MCA and in the centrum semiovale between the superficial perforators of the MCA and ACA. Classically bilateral watershed infarcts are thought to be due to etiologies that result in hemodynamic compromise and severe hypotension. The etiology of unilateral watershed infarcts is unclear. Current hypotheses include superimposed hypotension on severe carotid disease, and microemboli from severe carotid disease.[7] In many cases, there may be synergy between these two hypotheses, with a hypotensive episode impairing the normal washout of microemboli.

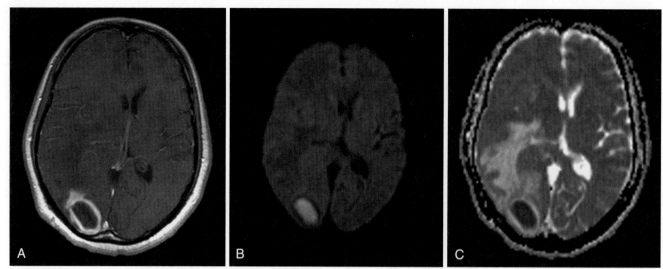

FIGURE 5A. Axial postcontrast T1-weighted (T1W) images demonstrates a rim-enhancing lesion in the right occipital lobe.

FIGURES 5B AND 5C. Diffusion-weighted (B) and ADC (C) images demonstrate restricted diffusion within the lesion.

Diagnosis: Right occipital lobe abscess.

Discussion

The differential diagnosis of a rim-enhancing lesion is extensive and includes glioma, abscess, demyelinating disease, metastatic disease, radiation, infarct, and evolving hematoma. Clinical history is often very helpful in narrowing the differential, as the appearance on the conventional MRI sequences can be nonspecific. Diffusion-weighted imaging with ADC mapping can be particularly helpful in distinguishing between an abscess and a necrotic primary brain tumor or metastatic lesion. Demonstration of restricted diffusion within the central portion of the lesion strongly suggests abscess as the diagnosis. Most commonly, the central areas of necrotic tumors demonstrate increased diffusion and are dark on diffusion-weighted images. Infarct is in the differential, but rim enhancement of an infarct is uncommon and often these two entities (abscess and infarct) can be distinguished clinically.[6]

It is hypothesized that an abscess has restricted diffusion centrally because of the physical characteristics of pus. The increased viscosity and cellularity of pus limit the motion of a water molecule and result in restricted diffusion, with increased signal on diffusion-weighted images and corresponding decreased signal on ADC maps.[6]

In Case 5, there is increased T2 signal seen on the ADC image surrounding the lesion consistent with vasogenic edema. This region of vasogenic edema in the periatrial white matter is isointense to white matter on the diffusion-weighted image. Vasogenic edema is an example of unrestricted diffusion and should appear dark on the diffusion-weighted image; however, the decreased signal resulting from the unrestricted diffusion of the vasogenic edema is being counterbalanced by the T2 shine-through effect, resulting in an isointense appearance.

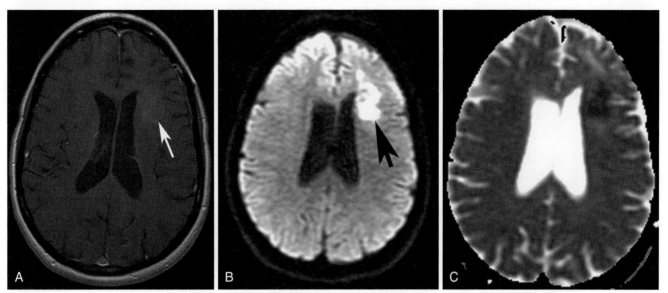

FIGURE 6A. Axial postcontrast T1W image that demonstrates a subtle area of focal hyperenhancement in the left anterior corona radiata *(white arrow)* along the inferior aspect of a resection cavity for a glioblastoma multiforme (GBM).

FIGURES 6B AND 6C. Increased signal is seen on the diffusion-weighted image (B, *black arrow*) with low signal seen in this region on the ADC image (C) consistent with restricted diffusion corresponding to the area of hyperenhancement on the postcontrast T1W image.

Diagnosis: Recurrent glioblastoma multiforme (GBM).

Discussion

Many different benign and malignant lesions can produce restricted diffusion. These include acute infarct, abscess, tumors, demyelinating disease, epidermoid cyst, granulomas, hyperacute and late subacute hematomas, and Creutzfeldt-Jakob disease.[6]

Diffusion of water in both primary and metastatic brain lesions varies from restricted to unrestricted. When restricted diffusion is noted, it is hypothesized that this is due to increased cellularity and high nuclear-to-cytoplasmic ratio of the tumor, resulting in decreased extracellular space and increased intracellular ions, respectively. Lymphoma is a particularly highly cellular tumor that appears to demonstrate restricted diffusion on a more consistent basis than other tumors.

One of the common diagnostic dilemmas in brain tumor imaging is distinguishing between post-therapeutic changes and recurrent or residual tumor status post tumor resection. Enhancement appears in Case 6 along the inferior aspect of the resection cavity, concerning for recurrent or residual disease. Restricted diffusion in this region strongly suggests the presence of residual or recurrent tumor in this case, though a rim of cytotoxic edema (caused by injury to adjacent small arteries) can be seen in the setting of a recent resection. Follow-up imaging can be used in the postresection period to distinguish restricted diffusion caused by cytotoxic edema (which evolves) from that of tumor hypercelluarity (which does not evolve in the absence of therapy).[6]

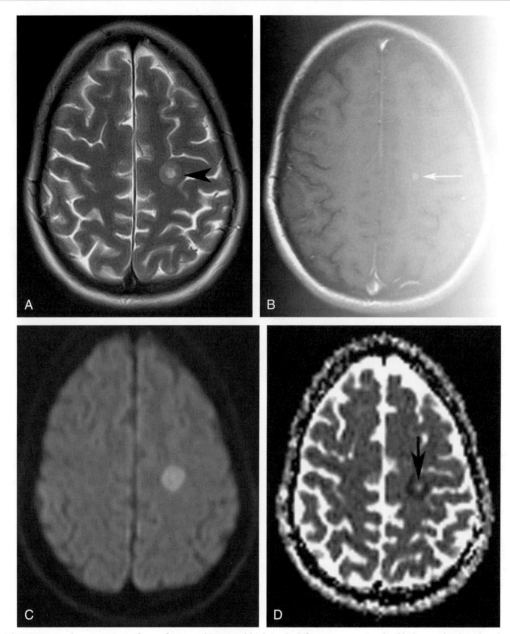

FIGURE 7A. Axial T2W image demonstrating a focus of increased T2 signal high in the left centrum semiovale *(black arrowhead)* with a thin low-T2-signal rim and a larger, circumferential area of increased T2 signal external to the thinner low-T2-signal area.

FIGURE 7B. Postcontrast T1W image demonstrates a small focus of enhancement corresponding with the lesion in the T2W image *(white arrow)*.

FIGURE 7C. Diffusion-weighted image that demonstrates increased signal throughout the lesion.

FIGURE 7D. On the ADC map, increased signal centrally *(black arrow)* with a low-signal peripheral rim can be appreciated. The central area of increased signal on both the diffusion-weighted and ADC images most likely represents T2 shine-through, whereas the peripheral, circumferential region demonstrates characteristics consistent with restricted diffusion.

Diagnosis: Multiple sclerosis (MS) plaque.

Discussion: This patient has of history of MS with numerous other lesions not demonstrated on these images. The enhancement seen on the postcontrast image (see Fig. 7B) suggests active demyelination in this plaque. Diffusion signal intensity varies in MS plaques. Increased signal on diffusion-weighted images is most often due to T2 shine-through. However, when restricted diffusion is present, active disease is presumed, though the precise cause is unclear. In this case, the more peripheral area of restricted diffusion may represent a zone of cytotoxic edema or inflammatory cell infiltrate.[6]

Case 8

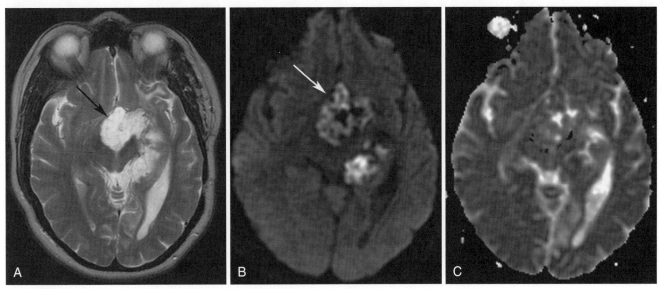

FIGURE 8A. Axial T2W image demonstrating a lobulated high-T2-signal mass in the third ventricle *(black arrow).*

FIGURE 8B. Diffusion-weighted image demonstrating increased signal within the periphery of the lesion *(white arrow).*

FIGURE 8C. The signal on the ADC image is similar but slightly darker otherwise it's not really restricted to the surrounding brain parenchyma. The postcontrast images (not shown) demonstrated no enhancement.

Diagnosis: Epidermoid cyst.

Case 9

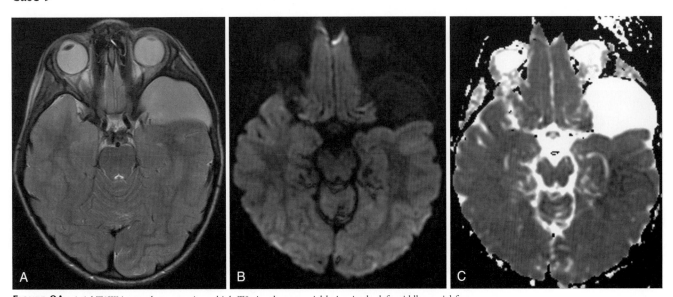

FIGURE 9A. Axial T2W image demonstrating a high-T2-signal, extra-axial lesion in the left middle cranial fossa.

FIGURE 9B. Diffusion-weighted image shows low signal in the corresponding location seen on the T2W image.

FIGURE 9C. ADC image demonstrates increase increased signal consistent with unrestricted diffusion.

Diagnosis: Arachnoid cyst.

Discussion

Epidermoid cyst versus arachnoid cyst is a classic differential. While it can be difficult to distinguish the two entities on conventional MRI sequences, DWI allows for a specific diagnosis. As is illustrated by Cases 8 and 9, epidermoid cysts demonstrate increased signal on diffusion-weighted images (restricted diffusion) in comparison to cerebrospinal fluid (CSF) secondary to the internal contents (debris, keratin, cholesterol). Arachnoid cysts follow CSF on all sequences, including diffusion imaging.

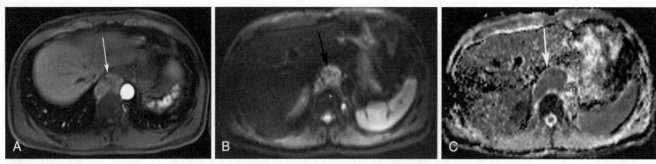

FIGURE 10A. Postcontrast volumetric interpolated breath-hold examination (VIBE) sequence in the arterial phase that demonstrates enhancing retrocrural lymph nodes *(white arrow)*.

FIGURES 10B AND 10C. Diffusion-weighted (B) and ADC (C) images that demonstrate restricted diffusion within these retrocrural lymph nodes *(black arrow* in B, *white arrow* in C).

Diagnosis: The patient was status post left nephrectomy for renal cell carcinoma with retrocrural lymph nodes very concerning for metastatic disease.

Discussion: The extent to which diffusion-weighted imaging in abdominal MRI may be useful is still undergoing investigation. The utilization of diffusion weighting was limited in abdominal MRI because of technical factors. However, with the advent of echo-planar imaging, which is significantly faster, its applications in the abdomen remain to be seen. The abdominal organ ADC values, in decreasing order, are the kidneys, liver, pancreas, and spleen. Case 10 illustrates the differences in ADC values nicely. The liver, which has a high ADC value, is relatively low in signal on the diffusion-weighted image. The spleen has a low ADC value and is increased in signal on the diffusion-weighted image and darker on the ADC image. Currently, the main application of diffusion weighting in the abdomen—identifying lymph nodes from both benign and malignant etiologies—is also illustrated in this case. Lymph nodes have a low ADC value and demonstrate increased signal on diffusion-weighted imaging. This increased signal on diffusion-weighted images can sometimes help otherwise inconspicuous-appearing lymph nodes appear obvious.[8]

CASES 11 AND 12: COMPANION CASES

Case 11

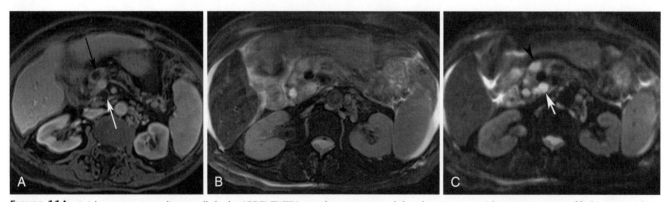

FIGURE 11A. Axial postcontrast gradient-recalled echo (GRE) T1W image demonstrates a subtle enhancing mass with a necrotic center *(black arrow)*, with upstream pancreatic ductal dilation that is not well visualized. There is a second even more subtle low-signal lesion in the uncinate process of the pancreas *(white arrow)*.

FIGURE 11B. Axial T2W image. The two pancreatic lesions seen in A are again seen but are only mildly T2 hyperintense, and the borders are difficult to distinguish from the surrounding signal.

FIGURE 11C. Axial diffusion-weighted image. The pancreatic neck lesion *(black arrowhead)* and the uncinate process lesion *(white arrow)* appear very bright and are easily distinguished from the surrounding parenchyma.

Diagnosis: Adenocarcinoma in the neck of the pancreas and multilobulated cystic lesion in the uncinate process that could represent an intraductal papillary mucinous neoplasm (IPMN) or mucinous cystic neoplasm.

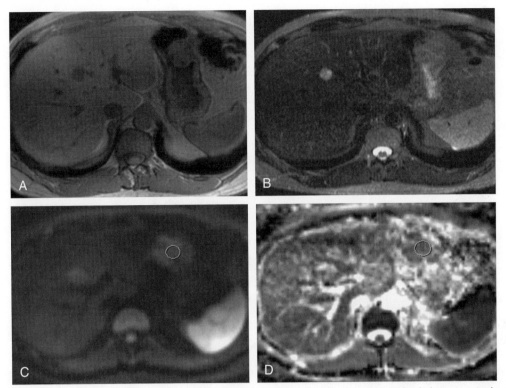

FIGURES 12A AND 12B. Axial precontrast GRE T1W image (A) and axial T2W image (B). There is a small T2 bright lesion seen in the right hepatic lobe. What is your differential?

FIGURES 12C AND 12D. Corresponding axial diffusion-weighted (C) and ADC (D) images demonstrate the focal, bright liver lesion, which is a hemangioma. Of greater importance is a large area of restricted diffusion in the region of the stomach. Did you note that in Figures 12A and 12B?

Diagnosis: Gastric adenocarcinoma and hepatic hemangioma.

Discussion: DWI can be very helpful in abdominal imaging both in lesion detection and as a screening tool, especially in difficult-to-evaluate areas such as the stomach. In Case 11, the adenocarcinoma and the cystic lesion in the uncinate process are both visible on the routine sequences; however, the very bright signal on the diffusion-weighted image makes detecting the lesions much more straightforward. In Case 12, the mass in the stomach was an unknown finding. Like Case 11, the mass can be seen on the routine sequences, but could be easily overlooked as the stomach is usually not part of the standard reading pattern in hepatic MRI. DWI is crucial in this case because the large area of restricted diffusion is very difficult to overlook.

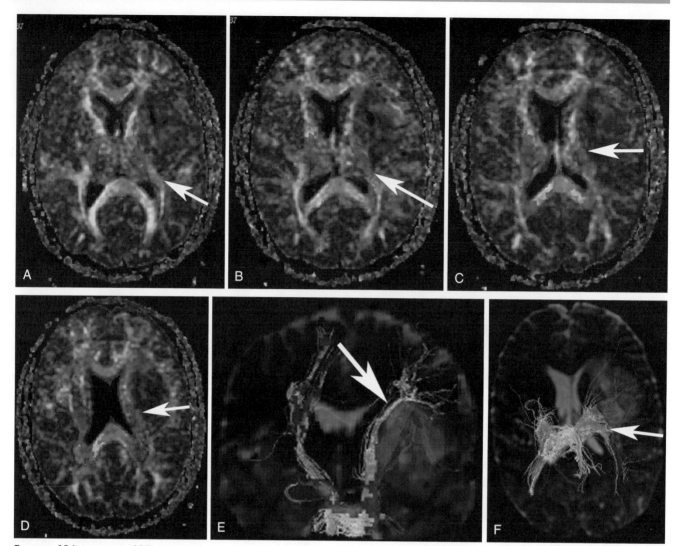

FIGURES 13A THROUGH 13D. Fractional anisotropy (FA) images that demonstrate medial deviation of the left internal capsule *(white arrows)*.

FIGURES 13E AND 13F. Tractography images that again demonstrate medial deviation of the internal capsule *(white arrows)* but also demonstrate a high-signal mass centered in the left basal ganglia, which is the cause of the deviation. *(See Color Plate.)*

Diagnosis: Mass centered in the left basal ganglia resulting in medial deviation of the left internal capsule.

Discussion: This is an example of how diffusion tensor imaging (DTI) can be clinically helpful. DTI measures anisotropic diffusion often seen along white matter tracts such as the internal capsule in this case. Knowing the relationship of the important white matter tracts to the mass can be helpful to the surgeon prior to surgery. The fractional anisotropy (FA) images are color-coded maps that indicate the orientation of the direction of diffusion. In this case, the internal capsule appears to be predominantly blue in color, corresponding with a direction along the *z*-axis. The magnetic resonance (MR) tractography images substantiate the findings seen in the FA images but also delineate the fiber connections among different brain regions based on the direction of diffusion.

Physics Discussion

The ADC value is generally dependent on the direction of the gradient. It is only invariant if one assumes that molecular movement is isotropic (the molecules move the same in all directions) with a Gaussian distribution. In this case, the diffusion distance would have a spatial distribution resembling a sphere. In general, however, in order to optimize the accuracy of the ADC value and remove its dependence on the gradient direction, measurements from three orthogonal gradients from a voxel are averaged and this number is assigned as the ADC value.

There are parts of the brain, such as within axonal bundles, where the structure of the tissue influences the direction of diffusion. For example, molecules are more likely to diffuse in the direction of an axon rather than perpendicular to it. This is called anisotropic diffusion (molecules do not move the same in all directions). Anisotropic diffusion changes the shape of the three-dimensional diffusion distribution from a sphere to a cigar or ellipsoid shape. DTI is a technique that measures anisotropic diffusion and, thereby, obtains directional information. With anisotropic diffusion there are six degrees of freedom as opposed to one with isotropic diffusion. Thus, as opposed to the ADC image, where two acquisitions are necessary, six acquisitions as well as a reference image are needed to perform DTI. The mathematical properties of the diffusion tensor are beyond the scope of this book. However, in simplistic terms, six noncollinear gradient-encoding directions are acquired to fully characterize the diffusion ellipsoid (i.e., the three eigenvectors). The average of the diffusivities along the eigenvectors (eigenvalues) is termed the *Trace* of the diffusion tensor. The Trace image appears very similar to an ADC image, and it is rotational invariant.

In practice, FA is the method most often used to characterize the anisotropy of diffusion. This scalar constant is calculated from the eigenvalues of the diffusion tensor for each voxel and then displayed in an image format. A color-coded image is then obtained to indicate the orientation of the longitudinal direction of diffusion (i.e., along the direction of the largest eigenvector). For example, red represents diffusion along the x-axis, blue represents diffusion along the y-axis, and green represents diffusion along the z-axis. The intensity of the color is representative of the FA. DTI works well when the axonal fibers are aligned in one direction, but this technique is not helpful in areas where there are crossing fibers because it cannot be used to separate multiple diffusion ellipsoids at a time.[9]

With a fully resolved diffusion tensor model throughout the brain, MR tractography can be carried out to delineate the fiber connections among different brain regions. It can take the orientation information from either DTI or diffusion spectrum imaging and apply different computer tracking algorithms to map out the connectivity of the brain.[9]

KEY POINTS

1. Diffusion-weighted imaging (DWI) is based on the principle of "brownian" movement of water molecules.
2. Increased signal on DWI is primarily due to cytotoxic edema (cellular swelling).
3. There is an element of T2 contrast within a diffusion-weighted image that can manifest as increased signal called "T2 shine-through." This is distinguished from restricted diffusion by means of an ADC map. If the area of increased signal on the diffusion-weighted image is low in signal on the ADC map, this confirms restricted diffusion. If the corresponding area on the ADC is high in signal, then the increased signal is due to T2 shine-through, which is seen in facilitated diffusion (noncytotoxic edema) associated with many types of lesions.
4. The distinguishing feature of a diffusion-weighted sequence is that two strong equal and opposite gradients are applied on either side of the 180° refocusing pulse.
5. The ADC map is quantitative and can be helpful in aging infarcts.
6. DWI can be helpful in narrowing the differential diagnosis of a rim-enhancing lesion and in distinguishing between an arachnoid cyst and an epidermoid cyst.
7. DWI is primarily helpful in abdominal imaging in identifying lymph nodes, as a screening tool, and in lesion detection.
8. Diffusion tensor imaging (DTI) is unique in that is measures anisoptropic diffusion as seen along white matter tracts.

References

1. Srinivasan A, Goyal M, Al Azri F, Lum C: State-of-the-art imaging of acute stroke. *RadioGraphics* 26(Suppl 1):S75-S95, 2005.
2. Stadnik TM, Luypaert R, Jager T, Osteaux M: Diffusion imaging: from basic physics to practical imaging. *RSNA EJ/RadioGraphics* April, 1999.
3. Bitar R, Leung G, Perng R, et al: MR pulse sequences: what every radiologist wants to know but is afraid to ask. *RadioGraphics* 26:513-537, 2006.
4. Schlaug G, Siewert B, Benfield A, et al: Time course of the apparent diffusion coefficient (ADC) abnormality in human stroke. *Neurology* 49:113-119, 1997.
5. Fiebach J, Jansen O, Schellinger P, et al: Serial analysis of the apparent diffusion coefficient time course in human stroke. *Neuroradiology* 44:294-298, 2002.
6. Stadnik TW, Demaerel P, Luypaert RR, et al: Imaging tutorial: differential diagnosis of bright lesions on diffusion-weighted MR images. *RadioGraphics* 23:e7, 2003.
7. Momjian-Mayor I, Baron J-C: The pathophysiology of watershed infarction in internal carotid artery disease: review of cerebral perfusion studies. *Stroke* 36:567-577, 2005.
8. Saremi F, Knoll AN, Bendavid OJ, et al: Characterization of genitourinary lesions with diffusion-weighted imaging. *RadioGraphics* 29:1295-1317, 2009.
9. Hagmann P, Jonasson L, Maeder P, et al: Understanding diffusion MR imaging techniques: from scalar diffusion-weighted imaging to diffusion tensor imaging and beyond. *RadioGraphics* 26(Suppl 1):S205-S223, 2006.

Chapter 15

Perfusion Magnetic Resonance Imaging

Wells I. Mangrum, Mustafa R. Bashir, Elmar M. Merkle, Allen W. Song, and Michael J. Paldino

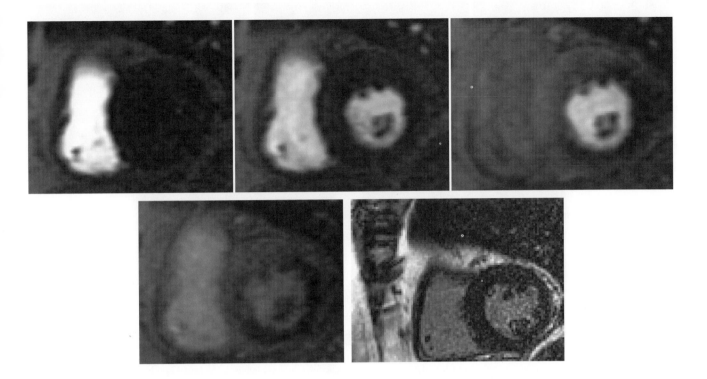

1. What type of a study is this?

2. How soon were these images obtained after giving contrast?

3. What is the diagnosis if the first four images were obtained during stress (and the rest images were normal)?

4. What is the diagnosis if the first four images were obtained during rest?

5. How can you tell that this patient has had prior surgery?

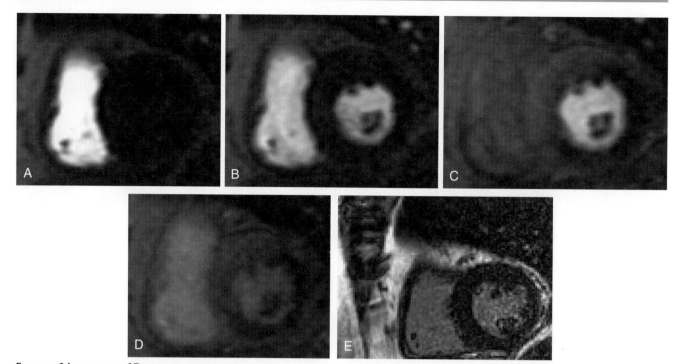

FIGURES 1A THROUGH 1D. Four short-axis images of the heart during a stress cardiac perfusion study. The images are of the same axial slice shown over time (A to D). Contrast progresses from the right ventricle to the left ventricle, then perfuses the myocardium, as evidenced by a blush of myocardial enhancement. There is no perfusion of the subendocardial muscle in the lateral and inferior walls.

FIGURE 1E. Delayed postcontrast short-axis view of the heart. No delayed enhancement is seen in the myocardium.

1. The first four images are from a cardiac magnetic resonance imaging (MRI) perfusion study. The last image is a delayed postcontrast image.

2. The cardiac perfusion study (see Figs. 1A through 1D) is performed during the first minute after the injection of contrast. The delayed image (see Fig. 1E) is obtained 10 minutes after the injection of contrast.

3. Ischemia in the lateral and inferior walls of the heart (see discussion below).

4. Hibernating myocardium in the lateral and inferior walls of the heart (see discussion below).

5. Linear susceptibility artifact in the sternum is from sternotomy wires from prior coronary artery bypass graft (CABG) surgery.

Diagnosis: Ischemia in the lateral and inferior walls of the heart.

Discussion

The perfusion of an organ is a basic physiologic process that can be altered by disease. The main utilities of perfusion imaging include providing information about the presence or absence of ischemia (as shown in Case 1), assessing the metabolic activity of the tissue of interest, and evaluating the status of relevant vasculature.[1] Magnetic resonance imaging (MRI) is one of many available techniques to measure perfusion.

Cardiac MRI perfusion studies are primarily used to evaluate the cardiac vasculature and myocardium. They are analogous to nuclear cardiac perfusion studies. Cardiac stress perfusion studies in MRI are generally performed with the same pharmacologic stress agents used in nuclear medicine perfusion studies.[1] Ischemic and infarcted myocardium both exhibit the absence of subendocardial enhancement on stress perfusion images. However, on delayed imaging, only infarction will show delayed subendocardial enhancement, because of the presence of fibrotic scar that continues to accumulate contrast agent for several minutes after contrast administration.[2]

Rest perfusion images are helpful in distinguishing ischemic from hibernating myocardium. Hibernating myocardium has decreased blood flow even at rest, differentiating it from exercise-induced ischemia. Consequently, hibernating myocardium will demonstrate no subendocardial enhancement on rest perfusion studies, whereas ischemic myocardium will appear normal at rest.[3] Hibernating myocardium can be differentiated from infarcted myocardium by the fact that hibernating myocardium will not enhance on delayed images, whereas infarcted myocardium will enhance.

Several MRI techniques are used to maximize detection of ischemia in cardiac perfusion imaging.[1] First, a preparatory inversion recovery pulse is applied with the effective time to inversion (TI) set to null the signal from nonenhancing myocardium. Then, multiple postcontrast short-axis images are obtained of the heart. These images are electrocardiographically gated to reduce cardiac motion. A fast gradient echo technique is used to rapidly acquire an image series of the heart during diastole. At our institution, during first-pass perfusion stress testing, images are obtained at three or four levels from base to apex during every R-R interval. The sequence is repeated for first-pass perfusion and washout over approximately 1 minute. When viewing the acquired images in cine mode, gadolinium is seen to pass from the right heart to the left heart, and then to equilibrate in the blood pool. The normal myocardium will show rapid uptake of contrast agent followed by rapid washout.

CASE 2

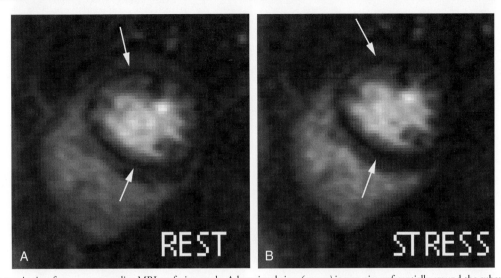

FIGURE 2A. Short-axis view from a stress cardiac MRI perfusion study. A low-signal ring *(arrows)* is seen circumferentially around the subendocardium.

FIGURE 2B. Short-axis view from a rest cardiac MRI perfusion study. Again, a low-signal ring *(arrows)* is seen circumferentially around the subendocardium.

Diagnosis: Ring artifact.

Clinical Discussion: Theoretically, a circumferential infarct could also have this appearance. However, it would be unusual for an infarct to involve the entire heart so uniformly. Additionally, the clinical presentation, cardiac wall motion, and ejection fraction would all be different in these two patient populations.

Physics Discussion

Transient hypointense artifacts are frequently seen along the myocardium–blood pool interface that can mimic diffuse subendocardial hypoperfusion. This artifact is manifested as a low-signal-intensity ring encircling the subendocardium and is likely due to susceptibility effects from the divergent magnetic susceptibility of intravascular gadolinium and the adjacent myocardium. To differentiate this artifact from true hypoperfusion, resting perfusion images can be obtained. On the resting studies, if the transient hypointense subendocardial signal persists, the finding is likely artifactual. Because cardiac perfusion imaging is T1 weighted, the times to echo (TEs) are shorter and the sequence is less sensitive to susceptibility effects than a T2* sequence (such as T2*-weighted dynamic susceptibility perfusion images in the brain).[1] However, susceptibility artifact can still be an issue in cardiac perfusion imaging, as illustrated by this case.

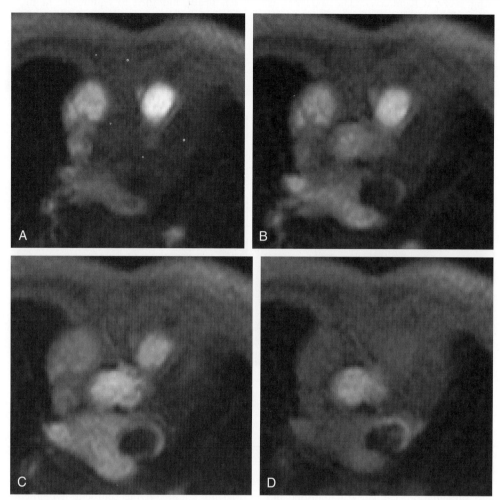

FIGURE 3. Axial cardiac perfusion images centered at the level of the left atrium. The images are of the same level shown over time (A to D). There is a predominantly low-signal-intensity mass abutting the posterior wall of the left atrium. The lateral aspect of the mass shows mild enhancement in the last perfusion image (D).

Diagnosis: Metastasis from gastric adenocarcinoma

Clinical Discussion: The differential diagnosis of an intra-atrial mass includes both thrombus and neoplasm. If there is muscular invasion, a neoplasm is likely. Another clue is that atrial myxomas often have a pedicle attaching them to the fossa ovalis. However, in some cases, such as this one, the diagnosis is difficult to make based on structural features alone. Perfusion imaging can be helpful, since enhancement of the lesion excludes bland thrombus. This lesion was found to be a metastasis from gastric adenocarcinoma. On these images, it is unclear whether the nonenhancing portion of the mass represents nonenhancing (necrotic) tumor or bland thrombus on the tumor.

Physics Discussion

Cardiac MRI perfusion analysis is generally qualitative. Qualitative analysis means that the raw perfusion data are analyzed visually and no quantitative analysis is performed. In this example, the perfusion of the atrial mass is assessed by simply observing the signal change of the mass over time. In *quantitative* perfusion analysis, a single computational image is created mathematically that represents perfusion. Examples of quantitative perfusion analysis are shown later in this chapter.

It is also important to note that cardiac MRI perfusion uses gadolinium-based contrast material as the perfusion agent and assesses the concentration of gadolinium with T1-weighted imaging. This is referred to as *dynamic contrast enhancement.* Alternate methods used in other organ systems to acquire MRI perfusion images are briefly explored later in this chapter.

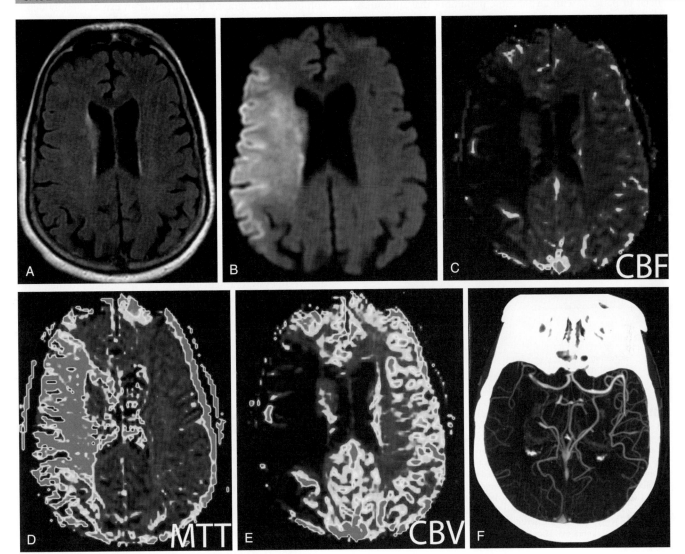

FIGURE 4A. Axial fluid-attenuated inversion recovery (FLAIR) image of the brain. There is subtle increased T2 signal in the periventricular white matter, right worse than left.

FIGURE 4B. Axial diffusion-weighted image. Restricted diffusion is noted in the right frontal and parietal lobes in the distribution of the right middle cerebral artery (MCA).

FIGURE 4C. Axial cerebral blood flow (CBF) calculation from an MRI perfusion study. Decreased blood flow in the right MCA distribution matches the diffusion abnormality.

FIGURE 4D. Axial mean transit time (MTT) calculation from an MRI perfusion study. Increased mean transit time is noted in the right MCA distribution.

FIGURE 4E. Axial cerebral blood volume (CBV) calculation from an MRI perfusion study. Decreased cerebral blood volume is noted in the right MCA distribution.

FIGURE 4F. Axial computed tomographic angiogram (CTA) maximal intensity projection (MIP) image. There is an abrupt cutoff of the right M1 segment. Very little flow is documented in the right MCA distribution. (*See Color Plate.*)

Diagnosis: Right MCA distribution infarct with no ischemic penumbra.

Discussion

MRI perfusion imaging in the brain is probably best known for its use in acute stroke imaging. A brief review of stroke imaging and therapy will help explain the current role of perfusion imaging in stroke. Intravenous administration of a thrombolytic has been shown to improve clinical outcomes in patients treated within the first 3 to 4.5 hours of ischemic stroke onset (assuming patients do not meet exclusion criteria).[4,5] After 4.5 hours, the risks of giving intravenous thrombolytics may outweigh the benefits.[5]

Unfortunately, many patients do not present to the hospital within the first 4.5 hours of symptom onset. However, it is possible that some of these late-presenting patients would benefit from thrombolytics. How can we determine which patients would benefit from thrombolytics? One popular hypothesis states that intravenous thrombolytics would be beneficial in patients with an ischemic penumbra that surrounds the infarct core, even if those patients present after the 4.5-hour time window. The ischemic penumbra refers to that ischemic brain tissue that is at risk to progress to infarction, but that is potentially salvageable[2] (Fig. 1). If there is no penumbra, theoretically the ischemic tissue is not salvagable and there is minimal benefit to giving thrombolytics. Conversely, if there is a large penumbra, then intervention is needed to salvage the portion of the brain that is at risk but not yet infarcted.

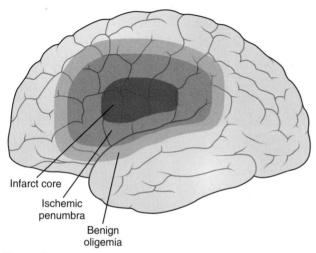

FIGURE 1. Illustration depicting the concept of the ischemic penumbra. An arterial occlusion causes an area in the adjacent brain to undergo irreversible infarction. This area is known as the *infarct core*. Additionally, there is a surrounding portion of the brain that is at risk for infarction but not yet irreversibly damaged. This separate area is termed the *ischemic penumbra*.[6] Finally, there is a third area around the ischemic penumbra that has abnormal perfusion but will never undergo infarction; this area is termed *benign oligemia*.[7] Experimental models have shown that the penumbra remains viable for hours; these studies also show that the infarct core gradually expands into the ischemic penumbra.[6,8] Early intervention to reperfuse the penumbra may prevent the ischemic tissue from progressing to complete infarction.

Vital to this management strategy is the idea that MRI (or computed tomography [CT]) perfusion can accurately depict the infarct core and the ischemic penumbra. The problem is that MRI and CT cannot yet definitively predict the areas of infarct core and ischemic penumbra.[7] In order to explain the current problems with penumbra imaging, one must first explain the classical theory behind perfusion imaging.

Classically, the infarct core is considered to be the area of the brain that has restricted diffusion on MRI while areas of the brain with reduced perfusion and normal diffusion are classically thought to represent the ischemic penumbra.[9] Identifying an area of restricted diffusion is relatively straightforward by MRI. However, characterizing perfusion defects is more complex. One way to assess perfusion is by analyzing the raw data that depict perfusion over time. This technique is referred to as *qualitative analysis* and is the same method used in cardiac perfusion studies shown earlier in this chapter. The main advantage of qualitative analysis is that it is fast.[10]

Alternatively, *quantitative analysis* of the perfusion data can provide further insights to the underlying pathology. In quantitative analysis, mathematical models are applied to the perfusion data to calculate hemodynamic parameters that describe the physiologic character of tissue vasculature. Common hemodynamic parameters that can be derived from perfusion imaging include cerebral blood volume (CBV), mean transit time (MTT), and cerebral blood flow (CBF). CBV is the volume of blood within the vasculature in a given volume of the brain. MTT is the time it takes for blood to traverse the capillary bed. CBF is the volume of blood flowing through a given volume of tissue per unit time. The physiologic changes assessed by MTT, CBF, and CBV at various stages of ischemic stroke are summarized in Figure 2.[10]

Applying the classic ischemic penumbra theory to Case 4, we see that the perfusion defects in the right middle cerebral artery (MCA) distribution (characterized by reduced CBF, reduced CBV, and increased MTT) are similar in size to the diffusion defect. Consequently, this patient has no ischemic penumbra and theoretically would not benefit from intravenous thrombolytics.

MTT	CBF	CBV	Physiology
↑	—	↑	Preserved autoregulation
↑	↓	↑	Impaired autoregulation
↑	↓	↓	Lost autoregulation

FIGURE 2. A summary of the physiologic changes in MTT, CBF, and CBV during ischemic stroke. The first mechanism of compensation during ischemia is dilation of the arterioles through autoregulation. At first, this autoregulation is sufficient to restore normal CBF and the CBF is unchanged. The CBV and MTT go up because the arteriolar dilation results in increased blood volume in the capillary microcirculation (Row 1 in chart).[11] Eventually, the limits of the autoregulatory mechanism are overcome and CBF begins to decrease (Row 2).[10] CBV continues to be elevated because there still is maximal arteriolar dilation through autoregulation. Finally, the body's ability to **autoregulate is overcome and autoregulation fails resulting in a fall in CBV (Row 3).**[10]

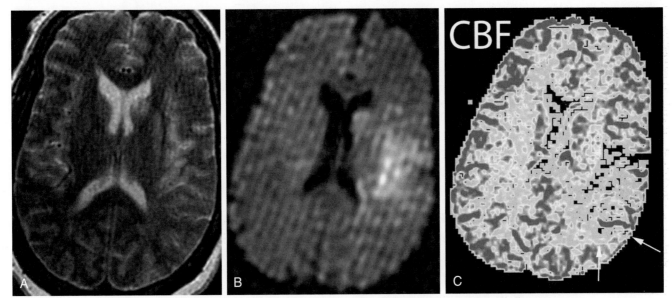

FIGURE 5A. Axial T2-weighted image of the brain. High T2 signal is present in the left caudate, the putamen, and the cortex of the left sylvian region.

FIGURE 5B. Axial diffusion-weighted image. High signal in the region of the left perisylvian region represents restricted diffusion (confirmed by apparent diffusion coefficient [ADC] map, not shown). Also note that this image has stripe artifact (see "Other Artifacts" section in Chapter 9 for a more detailed discussion of this artifact).

FIGURE 5C. Cerebral blood flow (CBF) map. There is decreased flow in the left perisylvian region extending posteriorly into the posterior left parietal lobe. The CBF defect is slightly larger than the diffusion defect (mismatch shown by *white arrows*). (*See Color Plate.*)

MTT	CBF	CBV	Physiology	Viability
↑	—	↑	Preserved autoregulation	Tissue may or may not be at risk?
↑	↓	↑	Impaired autoregulation	Ischemic penumbra?
↑	↓	↓	Lost autoregulation	Infarct core?

FIGURE 3. The challenges associated with using MTT, CBF, and CBV to predict benign oligemia, ischemic penumbra, and infarct core. It has been shown that changes in CBF better represent the final infarct size (ischemic penumbra + infarct core) than do changes in MTT or CBV[12,13]; MTT perfusion defects can overestimate the area of ischemic penumbra[7,12]; and CBV most closely follows restricted diffusion changes.[10] Using these principles, one may conclude that the infarct core is represented by a marked decline in CBV with associated restricted diffusion (Row 3); and that the ischemic penumbra is represented by reduced CBF with normal CBV (Row 2); and that areas with increased MTT and normal CBF may or may not go on to infarction (Row 1). However, such a conclusion would be at times erroneous because these general principles do not always hold in the individual patient. For example, areas of the brain with restricted diffusion and decreased CBV do not always go on to infarction.[7,14] Additionally, changes in CBF are not 100% sensitive for areas of the brain that go on to infarction. Another seeming contradiction to the above theory is the demonstration that MTT can occasionally underestimate infarct expansion.[12] Thus, MRI and CT cannot yet definitively characterize areas of ischemic penumbra or infarct core in the human brain during ischemic stroke.[7]

Diagnosis: Left perisylvian infarct in the left MCA distribution with small ischemic penumbra in the posterior left parietal lobe.

Discussion

If this patient presented 5 hours after symptom onset and did not meet exclusion criteria, should this patient receive intravenous thrombolytics? The answer is controversial, in part because there are some problems with the ischemic penumbra hypothesis (Fig. 3). Empirical evidence has shown that areas of restricted diffusion can at times return to normal.[14] Thus, restricted diffusion does not always mean irreversible infarct. Other studies have shown that perfusion defects can be reversible even when vessel occlusion persists.[15]

In other words, perfusion imaging can overestimate tissue at risk.

Another reason why this question is controversial is the mixed evidence provided by randomized controlled trials. While some earlier trials found a benefit of intravenous thrombolytics to late-presenting patients with ischemic penumbra defined by imaging,[16] more recent studies have shown no improvement and possibly even worse outcomes in similar patient populations who receive intravenous thrombolytics versus placebo.[17]

In conclusion, patients with a larger penumbra might benefit more from thrombolytic therapy, even outside of the traditional time window. For now, however, the practice of using MRI penumbra imaging to guide therapy remains a matter of debate.

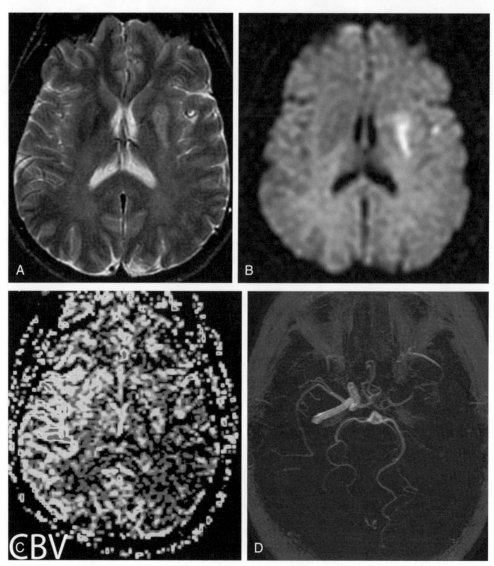

FIGURE 6A. Axial fast spin echo (FSE) T2-weighted image. High T2 signal is seen in the left putamen.

FIGURE 6B. Axial diffusion-weighted image. Restricted diffusion is noted in the left putamen and in the perisylvian left frontal lobe (confirmed on apparent diffusion coefficient [ADC] maps not shown).

FIGURE 6C. Axial cerebral blood volume (CBV) map. There is decreased CBV in the left middle cerebral artery (MCA) distribution involving the left parietal more than left frontal lobes.

FIGURE 6D. Maximal intensity projection (MIP) image from a two-dimensional time-of-flight sequence. There is no flow in the left internal carotid artery. There is some flow in the bilateral anterior cerebral arteries and the left M1 segment, likely from collateral flow via the circle of Willis. There is an abrupt termination of the left M1 segment. (*See Color Plate.*)

Diagnosis: Left internal carotid artery (ICA) dissection resulting in a left MCA distribution ischemic stroke.

Clinical Discussion: In this case, the majority of the posterior distribution of the left MCA demonstrates decreased CBV, but the corresponding area of restricted diffusion is relatively small. This is in contradistinction to the hypothesis that both the CBV and diffusion-weighted imaging (DWI) maps can be used interchangeably to represent infarct core. (One example of the use of this hypothesis is the fact that many use CBV to represent infarct core in CTA perfusion cases where no DWI is available.[7]) Some argue that the presence of a CBV-DWI mismatch is strong evidence for the existence of an ischemic penumbra and that these patients would benefit the most from therapy.[18] This patient was treated conservatively and recovered with relatively few long-term sequelae from this left ICA dissection.

Physics Discussion

There are two general methods by which magnetic resonance (MR) perfusion can be performed: bolus techniques and arterial spin labeling. Bolus perfusion techniques include dynamic susceptibility-weighted (DSC) and dynamic contrast-enhanced (DCE) MRI. These bolus techniques derive physiologic information from assessment of the concentration of gadolinium passing through the tissue microcirculation over time. This is done by repeatedly scanning the volume of interest, typically every second or so, prior to and after the administration of contrast agent.

DSC-MRI is based on the sequential acquisition of T2*-weighted images following contrast administration. Gadolinium's paramagnetic properties cause heterogeneity in the local magnetic field as it passes through the vasculature and/or tissues. These field heterogeneities cause dephasing of protons, resulting in a shortened T2* time and signal loss (see Chapter 2 and Chapter 8 for discussions on T2* and suscepitility artifact, respectively). Since these susceptibility effects extend several millimeters beyond the actual gadolinium molecules (i.e., adjacent to a vessel), this method is particularly sensitive to the presence of contrast in areas of low vascular density, for example, in capillary beds. Figure 4 shows an example of the effects of gadolinium on the T2*-weighted signal of a region of interest of the brain over time.

Because the signal intensity over time reflects the concentration of gadolinium over time, a concentration-over-time curve (CTC) can be calculated from the signal intensity curve[19] (Fig. 5). Physiologic parameters can then be calculated from the CTC as follows: the area under the CTC provides an estimate of the CBV within the voxel; MTT is estimated from the width of the contrast bolus; and regional CBF is calculated using the central volume theorem: CBF = CBV/MTT.

The shape of the concentration-time curve (CTC) is affected by various factors, including infusion rate, cardiovascular function, and vascular stenoses. These variations can invalidate direct interindividual (or even interscan) comparison of the derived parameters. One approach to this problem is to measure the concentration of arterial contrast agent over time (the arterial input function) from a large nearby artery and use this information to calculate CBF (Fig. 6). This process, known as "deconvolution," estimates the CTC in each voxel that would be seen if the input were a bolus of infinitely short duration. By controlling for some of the variability in contrast delivery, deconvolution can be used as the basis for absolute

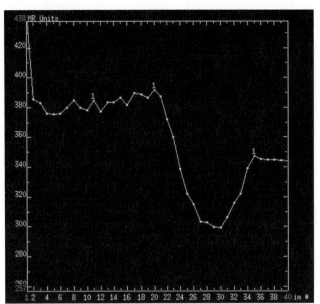

FIGURE 4. Signal intensity curve over time of a region of interest in the brain during a DSC perfusion study. The *y*-axis represents the net T2*-weighted signal intensity. The *x*-axis represents the image number (in this case 40 images were obtained of the region of interest over a period of 1 minute). Note that, during the first 21 images, the T2*-weighted signal in the selected region of interest is relatively unchanged. Then, the contrast agent enters the region of interest and the signal begins to fall as a result of the T2* shortening effects of gadolinium. The T2* signal hits a trough when the gadolinium concentration from the first pass reaches a maximum. Then, as the contrast agent washes out, the T2* signal begins rising again. The new baseline is lower than the precontrast images because the intravascular gadolinium has not yet been totally cleared from the intravascular pool.

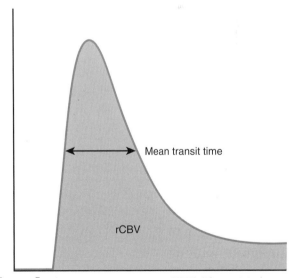

FIGURE 5. The concentration-time curve (CTC). The y-axis is the concentration of contrast in a voxel; the x-axis is time. The CTC is mathematically derived from the signal intensity curve shown in Figure 4. The CBV is estimated from the CTC by calculating the area underneath the curve. MTT is estimated as the width of the contrast bolus. CBF can then be derived by dividing the CBV by the MTT.

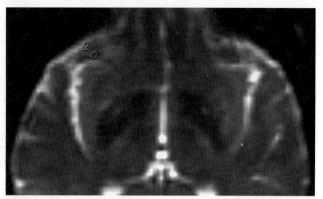

FIGURE 6. Region of interest drawn over the right MCA to calculate an arterial input. The changes in signal over time in the artery reflect the changes from various parameters that are otherwise difficult to quantify, such as cardiovascular function and contrast bolus technique. This measurement is then used to calculate a more accurate CBF, CBV, and MTT (see text for more detailed discussion).[19]

measurements of CBF.[20] In Case 6, the provided CBV map is "normalized" to the reference arterial inflow. CBF and MTT can also be normalized in this way.[20]

In contrast to DSC-MRI, DCE-MRI uses T1-weighted sequences to characterize the CTC. The cardiac perfusion cases shown in the beginning of this chapter are examples of MRI perfusion using DCE-MRI. In comparison to susceptibility-related signal loss, gadolinium-induced T1 shortening is less susceptible to relatively remote alterations of the magnetic field outside of the vasculature, resulting in an extremely short radius of action. It is therefore particularly suitable to characterize the passage of contrast agent between the intravascular space and the extracellular-extravascular spaces. There are many ways to characterize the CTC in DCE-MRI, including subjective, semiquantitative, and quantitative methods. Although more technically demanding, pharmacokinetic modeling can be used to extract quantitative physiologic information about the microcirculation. Commonly modeled parameters include the fractional plasma volume, fractional volume of the extracellular-extravascular space, and K^{trans} (the transfer coefficient between the intravascular and extravascular spaces). The last parameter, which provides a measure of vessel permeability, is of particular interest in characterizing the effects of antiangiogenesis treatment in patients with high-grade primary brain tumors.

Arterial spin labeling (ASL) perfusion imaging does not require an exogenous contrast agent, but rather uses a radiofrequency pulse to invert the spins of protons in flowing blood proximal to the areas of interest (e.g., while blood is in the neck prior to cerebral perfusion imaging). Inflow of these protons into a given voxel, therefore, results in a reduction in its signal intensity. The labeled image volume can then be subtracted from the dataset obtained using an identical MR sequence performed without the labeling pulse. The result is an image with contrast that is based primarily on tissue perfusion. This technique is completely noninvasive, avoids the use of contrast agent, and is inherently quantitative, advantages that make it particularly well suited for certain populations. ASL perfusion techniques are thus under active development to be translated to routine clinical use.

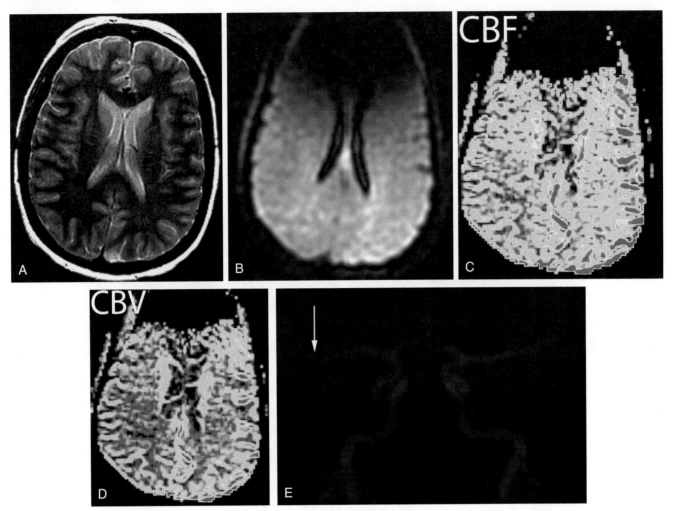

FIGURE 7A. Axial fast spin echo (FSE) T2-weighted image of the brain. No abnormality is seen.

FIGURE 7B. Axial diffusion-weighted image. No focus of restricted diffusion is identified.

FIGURES 7C AND 7D. Color-coded cerebral blood flow (CBF) and cerebral blood volume (CBV) maps demonstrate large perfusion defects in the right frontal and parietal lobes.

FIGURE 7E. Anterior-projection magnetic resonance angiography maximal intensity projection (MIP) image. Irregular and discontinuous flow is seen in the right middle cerebral artery (MCA) with an abrupt cutoff in the distal right M1 segment *(arrow)*. (*See Color Plate.*)

Diagnosis: Air embolism resulting in large ischemic penumbra.

Clinical Discussion: This patient developed acute onset of left-sided weakness during bronchoscopy. The patient was rushed to the MR scanner and the large ischemic penumbra was identified, presumably due to an air embolus at the time of bronchoscopy. The patient was treated in a hyperbaric chamber and went on to complete recovery.

Incidentally, this case supports the hypothesis that the ischemic penumbra, as measured by perfusion and diffusion-weighted images, can predict portions of the brain that are potentially salvageable. Presumably, the hyperbaric chamber relieved the air embolus and allowed reperfusion of the ischemic penumbra before any of the brain underwent infarction. This presumption is supported by the clinical findings that the patient had a full recovery after the treatment.

Physics Discussion

Case 7 also demonstrates the potentially deleterious effects of susceptibility artifact in perfusion MRI. Perfusion MRI in the brain is commonly performed with echo-planar imaging, taking advantage of the technique's short acquisition time. However, echo-planar sequences are highly sensitive to T2* effects. While this is useful when measuring the T2* effects of gadolinium, it can be deleterious in cases in which susceptibility artifact is present. This patient's orthodontic braces cause large signal voids in the perfusion images in the bilateral frontal lobes. Similarly, the diffusion-weighted image, which is also based on echo-planar imaging, also shows a large region of signal loss in the same area. The fast spin echo T2-weighted image is normal and does not have any susceptibility artifact because the 180° refocusing pulse counters the dephasing caused by the local magnetic field heterogeneity (see Chapter 8 for a more detailed explanation).

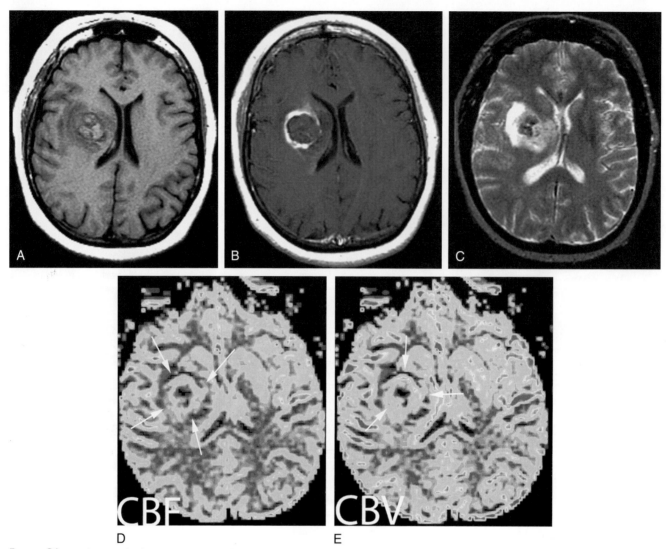

FIGURE 8A. Axial T1-weighted precontrast image. A heterogeneous mass with areas that are intrinsically bright on T1-weighted imaging is centered in the right basal ganglia.

FIGURE 8B. Axial T1-weighted postcontrast image. The mass demonstrates rim enhancement.

FIGURE 8C. Axial T2-weighted image. The mass is heterogeneous on T2 with areas of low and high T2-weighted signal.

FIGURES 8D AND 8E. Cerebral blood flow (CBF) (D) and cerebral blood volume (CBV) perfusion images. There is increased CBF and increased CBV around the rim of the mass *(white arrows)*. (*See Color Plate.*)

Diagnosis: Hemorrhagic glioblastoma multiforme.
Clinical Discussion: Hypertensive hemorrhage is the most common cause of spontaneous (nontraumatic) intraparenchymal hemorrhage in the adult brain. The diagnosis of hypertensive hemorrhage is often suggested by its location and a clinical history of hypertension. In this case, imaging demonstrates a heterogeneous lesion centered in the right basal ganglia with signal characteristics consistent with blood products. There is a smooth rim of peripheral enhancement, a finding commonly seen as a parenchymal hematoma resolves. In this case, the adjacent increased CBV is the only indicator that this bleed may not be hypertensive in etiology. Although definitive data are lacking, a recent case series evaluated CBV maps in patients with confirmed hypertensive hemorrhage: Five of six patients had decreased ipsilateral hemispheric perfusion; none of those examinations demonstrated increased ipsilateral perfusion.[21] The patient in Case 8 was ultimately diagnosed with glioblastoma multiforme.

Physics Discussion
While perfusion imaging is useful to evaluate for ischemia, it also has a role in nonischemic disease, such as the characterization of neoplasms.[22] For example, perfusion imaging can help differentiate a highly vascular, high-grade tumor (relatively high CBV) from a low-grade tumor (low CBV),[23] although this does not always hold (some low-grade tumors can have high CBV values, and some clinically benign intracranial tumors are highly vascular, such as meningiomas and choroid plexus tumors).[23] Perfusion imaging can also help to differentiate tumor recurrence (high CBV) from radiation necrosis (low

CBV).[24] This indication is particularly useful because tumor recurrence and radiation necrosis can have a similar appearance on conventional MRI techniques, manifesting as a mass with variable degrees of surrounding edema and ring enhancement on serial MRI evaluation.[24]

Less commonly, perfusion imaging is used to evaluate the status of the intracranial vasculature. For example, it can be used to evaluate overall brain perfusion before and after an extraintracranial bypass procedure.[25] Perfusion imaging can also be used to characterize the vasculature of the brain adjacent to a mass, prior to functional MRI. In this situation, perfusion imaging can warn of possible false-negative results on functional MRI caused by tumor-induced failure of autoregulation (see Chapter 17 for a more thorough explanation).[26]

CASE 9

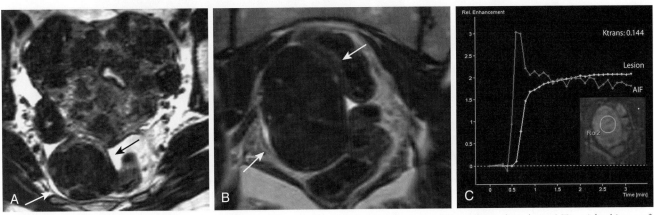

FIGURE 9A. Axial reconstructed SPACE (sampling perfection with application-optimized contrasts using different flip angle evolutions) T2-weighted image of the pelvis. There are multiple uterine fibroids. Additionally, there is a low-signal mass posterior to the uterus and adjacent to the uterus and rectum *(arrows)*.

FIGURE 9B. Coronal reconstructed SPACE T2-weighted image centered over the low-signal mass in the posterior pelvis. The low T2-weighted signal mass is ovoid in shape and surrounded by multiple loops of bowel *(arrows)*.

FIGURE 9C. Graph depicting relative enhancement of the lesion *(white curve)* following contrast administration. The *gray curve* measures the enhancement in the aorta and thereby depicts the arterial input function or AIF (note that the region of interest for the aorta is not included in the field of view on these images). The inset coronal T1 dynamic contrast-enhanced image in the right lower quadrant shows the region of interest drawn to acquire the perfusion data. The calculated K^{trans} for the region of interest was 0.144.

Diagnosis: Pedunculated leiomyoma.

Clinical Discussion: Subserosal pedunculated uterine fibroids and ovarian fibromas can be difficult to differentiate on conventional MRI because they can both be low in signal on T1- and T2-weighted images. One study has shown that dynamic contrast enhancement can be used to distinguish these masses. Uterine leiomyomas have greater maximal enhancement and higher rates of enhancement than ovarian fibromas.[27] In Case 9, a subserosal leiomyoma was favored given the lesion's brisk, homogeneous enhancement, similar to the patient's other intramural leiomyomas (not shown), and its apparent connection with the uterus on the axial image (see Fig. 9A).

Physics Discussion

In addition to cardiac and neurologic evaluations, perfusion imaging is also being used to study genitourinary and gastro-intestinal diseases. Perfusion imaging in these organ systems is frequently performed using T1-weighted dynamic contrast enhancement (the same technique used in the cardiac cases shown in the beginning of this chapter). Intravenous gadolinium is given and multiple image volumes are acquired over time. A graph can then be generated describing the relative enhancement of the area of interest (see Fig. 9C). Using the arterial input as a control, the concentration of gadolinium over time can then be computed.

Quantitative perfusion analysis is also frequently performed in body imaging. K^{trans} is one quantitative parameter often measured. K^{trans} measures the rate of diffusion of contrast between the intravascular space and the extravascular-extracellular space. K^{trans} is proportional to both the rate of flow in the vessels and their permeability.[28] As flow increases, there is more contrast to diffuse into the extravascular space; similarly, if the vessels are "leaky" (as in tumor vascularity), a higher percentage of contrast will leak into the extravascular space. K^{trans} can be a useful quantitative parameters in oncology. As a malignant tumor grows, it promotes the growth of additional small vessels through angiogenesis. In general, the vessels recruited by tumor angiogenesis are abnormal in that they are especially fragile and "leaky." Measuring this property as expressed by K^{trans} can yield useful diagnostic information about the physiology of the lesion of interest.[28]

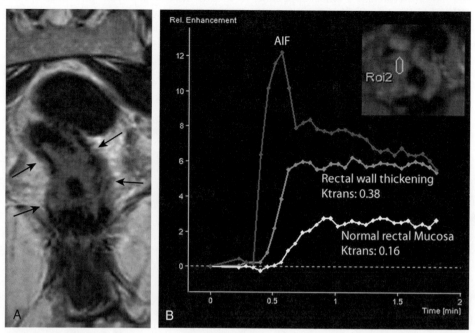

FIGURE 10A. Coronal reconstructed SPACE T2-weighted image of pelvis. There is mass-like circumferential rectal wall thickening that is intermediate in T2-weighted signal intensity *(arrows)*.

FIGURE 10B. Graph depicting relative enhancement over time. The dark gray curve represents the arterial input function (AIF). The medium gray curve is the enhancement of the mass-like area of rectal wall thickening. The white curve is derived from a region of interest selected over normal rectal mucosa (not shown). Inset in the right upper corner is a coronal T1-weighted dynamic contrast-enhanced image showing the region of interest drawn over the rectal wall thickening. Qualitatively, the mass-like area enhances much more quickly and reaches a higher peak than the normal rectal mucosa. Quantitatively, the perfusion is also increased in the area of rectal wall thickening. The measured K[trans] of the area of wall thickening was 0.38, whereas the normal rectal mucosa K[trans] measured 0.16.

Diagnosis: Rectal carcinoma.

Discussion: Inflammatory conditions, such as diverticulitis, can also cause colorectal wall thickening. However, perfusion is not typically as elevated in these conditions.[29] Rectal carcinoma requires angiogenesis to ensure continued growth. Dynamic contrast enhancement has been shown to predict the degree of rectal carcinoma angiogenesis,[30] which can be used for diagnostic purposes. For example, one study has shown that colon cancer and diverticulitis can be accurately distinguished using perfusion imaging; this differentiation can be difficult using anatomic criteria alone. Colorectal cancer has significantly higher levels of blood flow, blood volume, and vascular permeability.[29]

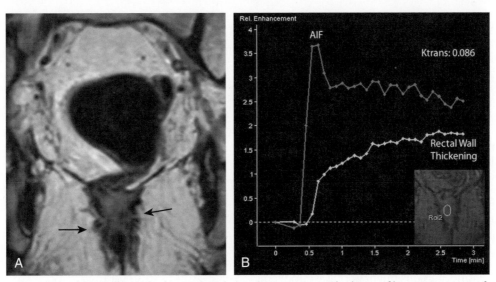

FIGURE 11A. Coronal reconstructed SPACE T2-weighted image through the pelvis in a patient with a history of low anterior resection for rectal carcinoma and coloanal anastomosis. Colonic wall thickening is noted at the anatomosis *(arrows).*

FIGURE 11B. Graph depicting relative enhancement over time. The gray curve is the arterial input. The white curve is the enhancement of the area of rectal wall thickening. The inset coronal T1-weighted dynamic contrast-enhanced image in the right lower quadrant shows the region of interest used to calculate the curve. Qualitatively, the perfusion of the area of wall thickening appears low. This is supported by quantitative data that calculated K^{trans} for the area of abnormality at 0.086 (for perspective, this is less than 25% of the K^{trans} measured in the rectal carcinoma shown in Case 10).

Diagnosis: Rectal wall scarring from prior surgery.

Discussion: This patient is status post low anterior resection for rectal carcinoma. The primary imaging dilemma is whether the rectal wall thickening seen in Figure 11A represents postoperative scar or recurrent tumor. On conventional imaging, this can be a difficult distinction because both entities enhance and can be morphologically identical. Perfusion imaging can help by characterizing the enhancement pattern in further detail. One study has shown that recurrent tumor demonstrates increased perfusion in comparison to scar.[31] That study specifically found that the relative enhancement of the wall thickening with respect to the arterial input was less in scar than in tumor.[31] Another as-yet unproven but possible distinction is that the enhancement curve for fibrosis continues to increase over time (as shown in Fig. 11B), whereas tumor enhancement plateaus, then washes out.

Defining Perfusion

1. The perfusion of an organ is an inherent physiologic parameter that can be altered in disease states. Perfusion can be measured with many different techniques, including MRI.
2. MRI perfusion can be assessed by two main types of techniques: Bolus techniques that use a gadolinium-based contrast agent and arterial spin labeling.
   a. Dynamic contrast enhancement is a T1-weighted bolus technique used frequently in cardiac perfusion imaging and body perfusion imaging.
   b. Dynamic susceptibility contrast is a T2*-weighted bolus technique used frequently in brain perfusion imaging.
   c. Arterial spin labeling does not use any contrast. Flowing intravascular protons are instead labeled using radiofrequency pulses applied upstream to the images.

Cardiac Perfusion Imaging

1. Cardiac perfusion imaging is a useful tool to evaluate for stress-induced myocardial ischemia.
2. Electrocardiographically gated T1-weighted images are obtained postcontrast. Cardiac perfusion analysis is usually qualitative: the raw images are analyzed visually.
3. Occasionally, cardiac perfusion imaging can also be helpful to distinguish between tumor and thrombus.

Brain Perfusion Imaging

1. The penumbra is the area of the brain that is ischemic but not yet infarcted. This is the area of the brain that is potentially salvageable with intervention.
2. MRI seeks to define the penumbra. In theory, a diffusion defect represents the infarcted core and the perfusion defect is the entire ischemic area. The difference between the diffusion and perfusion images is the penumbra.
3. Brain perfusion analysis uses quantitative techniques. Perfusion parameters such as cerebral blood flow (CBF), cerebral blood volume (CBV), and mean transit time (MTT) are mathematically computed and displayed in a series of color-coded images.
   a. The CBV is the volume of blood within the small vessels and capillary bed in a given area of the brain.
   b. The MTT is the time it takes for blood to traverse the capillary bed.
   c. CBF = CBV/MTT.
4. Brain perfusion imaging can also be used to characterize the grade of tumors, to distinguish between radiation necrosis and tumors, and to characterize blood flow.

Body Perfusion Imaging

1. Dynamic contrast enhancement can be used in the genitourinary and gastrointestinal systems to characterize lesions.
2. Malignant tumors rely on angiogenesis to grow. This angiogenesis creates fragile and leaky vessels. The leakiness of these vessels can be measured using K^{trans}, a quantitative parameter derived from perfusion imaging.

References

1. Lee VS: *Cardiovascular MRI: Physical Principles to Practical Protocols.* Philadelphia: Lippincott Williams & Wilkins, 2006.
2. Kim RJ, Fieno DS, Parrish TB, et al: Relationship of MRI delayed contrast enhancement to irreversible injury, infarct age, and contractile function. *Circulation* 100:1992-2002, 1999.
3. Tadamura E, Yamamuro M, Kubo S, et al: Hibernating myocardium identified by cardiovascular magnetic resonance and positron emission tomography. *Circulation* 113: e158-e159, 2006.
4. The National Institute of Neurological Disorders and Stroke rt-PA Stroke Study Group: Tissue plasminogen activator for acute ischemic stroke. *N Engl J Med* 333:1581-1588, 1995.
5. Lees KR, Bluhmki E, von Kummer R, et al, for the ECASS, ATLANTIS, NINDS and EPITHET rt-PA Study Group Investigators: Time to treatment with intravenous alteplase and outcome in stroke: an updated pooled analysis of ECASS, ATLANTIS, NINDS, and EPITHET trials. *Lancet* 375:1695-1703, 2010.
6. Schlaug G, Benfield A, Baird AE, et al: The ischemic penumbra: operationally defined by diffusion and perfusion MRI. *Neurology* 53:1528, 1999.
7. Kidwell C, Alger J, Saver J: Evolving paradigms in neuroimaging of the ischemic penumbra. *Stroke* 35:2662-2665, 2004.
8. Heiss WD, Graf R, Wienhard K, et al: Dynamic penumbra demonstrated by sequential multitracer PET after middle cerebral artery occlusion in cats. *J Cereb Blood Flow Metab* 14:892-902, 1994.
9. Srinivasan A, Goyal M, Al Azri F, Lum C: State-of-the-art imaging of acute stroke. *RadioGraphics* 26(Suppl 1):S75-S95, 2006.
10. de Lucas ME, Sánchez E, Gutiérrez A, et al: CT protocol for acute stroke: tips and tricks for general radiologists. *RadioGraphics* 28:1673-1687, 2008.
11. Zaharchuk G, Mandeville J, Bogdanov A, et al: Cerebrovascular dynamics of autoregulation and hypoperfusion: an MRI study of CBF and changes in total and microvascular cerebral blood volume during hemorrhagic hypotension. *Stroke* 30:2197-2205, 1999.
12. Parsons M, Yang Q, Barber A, et al: Perfusion magnetic resonance imaging maps in hyperacute stroke. *Stroke* 32:1581-1587, 2000.
13. Rohl L, Ostergaard L, Simonsen C, et al: Viability thresholds of ischemic penumbra of hyperacute stroke defined by perfusion-weighted MRI and apparent diffusion coefficient. *Stroke* 32:1524-1628, 2001.
14. Kranz PG, Eastwood JD: Does diffusion-weighted imaging represent the ischemic core? An evidence-based systematic review. *AJNR Am J Neuroradiol* ajnr.A1547, 2009.
15. Kucinski T, Naumann D, Knab R, et al: Tissue at risk is overestimated in perfusion-weighted imaging: MR imaging in acute stroke patients without vessel recanalization. *AJNR Am J Neuroradiol* 26:815-819, 2005.
16. Hacke W, Albers G, Al-Rawi Y, et al: The Desmoteplase in Acute Ischemic Stroke Trial (DIAS): a Phase II MRI-based 9-hour window acute stroke thrombolysis trial with intravenous desmoteplase. *Stroke* 36:66-73, 2005.
17. Hacke W, Furlan AJ, Al-Rawi Y, et al: Intravenous desmoteplase in patients with acute ischaemic stroke selected by MRI perfusion-diffusion

weighted imaging or perfusion CT (DIAS-2): a prospective, randomised, double-blind, placebo-controlled study. *Lancet Neurol* 8:141-150, 2009.

18. Schaefer P, Hunter G, He J, et al: Predicting cerebral ischemic infarct volume with diffusion and perfusion MR imaging. *ANJR Am J Neuroradiol* 23:1785-1794, 2002.

19. Atlas SW: *Magnetic Resonance Imaging of the Brain and Spine*, 4th ed. Philadelphia: Lippincott Williams & Wilkins, 2009.

20. Rempp KA, Brix G, Wenz F, et al: Quantification of regional cerebral blood flow and volume with dynamic susceptibility contrast-enhanced MR imaging. *Radiology* 193:637-641, 1994.

21. Kidwell CS, Saver JL, Mattiello J, et al: Diffusion-perfusion MR evaluation of perihematomal injury in hyperacute intracerebral hemorrhage. *Neurology* 57:1611-1617, 2001.

22. Wintermark M, Sesay M, Barbier E, et al: Comparative overview of brain perfusion imaging techniques. *Stroke* 36:e83-e99, 2005.

23. Cha S, Knopp EA, Johnson G, et al: Intracranial mass lesions: dynamic contrast-enhanced susceptibility-weighted echo-planar perfusion MR imaging. *Radiology* 223:11-29, 2002.

24. Barajas RF, Chang JS, Segal MR, et al: Differentiation of recurrent glioblastoma multiforme from radiation necrosis after external beam radiation therapy with dynamic susceptibility-weighted contrast-enhanced perfusion MR imaging. *Radiology* 253:486-496, 2009.

25. Caramia F, Santoro A, Pantano P, et al: Cerebral hemodynamics on MR perfusion images before and after bypass surgery in patients with giant intracranial aneurysms. *AJNR Am J Neuroradiol* 22:1704-1710, 2001.

26. Hou BL, Bradbury M, Peck KK, et al: Effect of brain tumor neovasculature defined by rCBV on BOLD fMRI activation volume in the primary motor cortex. *Neuroimage* 32:489-497, 2006.

27. Thomassin-Naggara I, Daraï E, Nassar-Slaba J, et al: Value of dynamic enhanced magnetic resonance imaging for distinguishing between ovarian fibroma and subserous uterine leiomyoma. *J Comput Assist Tomogr* 31:236-242, 2007.

28. Yankeelov TE, Gore JC: Dynamic contrast enhanced magnetic resonance imaging in oncology: theory, data acquisition, analysis, and examples. *Curr Med Imaging Rev* 3:91-107, 2007.

29. Goh V, Halligan S, Taylor SA, et al: Differentiation between diverticulitis and colorectal cancer: quantitative CT perfusion measurements versus morphologic criteria—initial experience. *Radiology* 242:456-462, 2007.

30. Zhang XM, Yu D, Zhang HL, et al: 3D dynamic contrast-enhanced MRI of rectal carcinoma at 3T: correlation with microvascular density and vascular endothelial growth factor markers of tumor angiogenesis. *J Magn Reson Imaging* 27:1309-1316, 2008.

31. Dicle O, Obuz F, Cakmakci H: Differentiation of recurrent rectal cancer and scarring with dynamic MR imaging. *Br J Radiol* 72:1155-1159, 1999.

Chapter 16

Magnetic Resonance Spectroscopy

Wells I. Mangrum, Allen W. Song, and Jeffrey R. Petrella

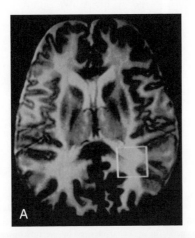

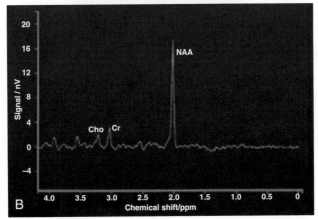

1. What are differential considerations for the findings in A?

2. What type of graph is represented in B?

3. What is *N*-acetyl aspartate (NAA)?

4. Would the NAA chemical shift peak of 2.0 ppm change if the magnet field strength was increased to 3 Tesla?

5. What is the diagnosis?

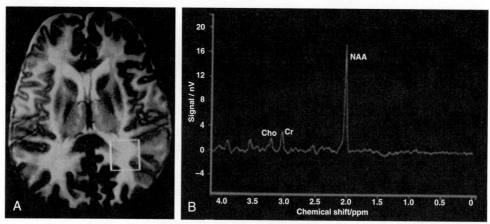

FIGURE 1A. Axial T2-weighted magnetic resonance (MR) image. There is diffusely increased T2 signal in the white matter, including the subcortical white matter. The *square* overlying the left parietal white matter marks the area characterized by spectroscopy.

FIGURE 1B. Point-resoved single-voxel spectroscopy (PRESS) waveform (time to echo [TE] = 30 msec). NAA, choline (Cho), and creatine (Cr) peaks are labeled. The NAA peak is markedly elevated with respect to the choline and creatine peaks.

1. There is diffuse white matter T2 prolongation. Broad differential considerations include dysmyelinating conditions (Alexander disease, Canavan disease, metachromatic leukodystrophy), demyelinating conditions (acute disseminated encephalomyelitis or multiple sclerosis), infections (human immunodeficiency virus), and toxicities (chemotherapy or radiation therapy).

2. This is a spectroscopy waveform. The voxel of interest is demarcated by the *square* shown in the left parietal lobe in Figure 1A.

3. NAA is a molecule associated with neurons and axons. Its function is unknown. It is used as a marker of neurons/axons.

4. No, the chemical shift does not change with field strength. NAA has a chemical shift of 2.0 parts per million (ppm) at 1.5 Tesla and 3 Tesla. Similarly, choline is always 3.2 ppm and lactate is always 1.33 ppm. Shift peaks are useful to memorize as most charts do not come labeled. (I labeled this one for you to be merciful.)

5. The spectroscopy waveform is very characteristic of Canavan disease. The key finding is the marked elevation of the NAA peak. Canavan disease is one of the few conditions that result in an elevation of the NAA level. There is an elevation in NAA because of a deficiency in the myelin synthesis pathway.[1]

Diagnosis: Canavan disease.

Clinical Discussion: Canavan disease is an autosomal recessive dysmyelinating disease that is thought to result from a deficiency of aspartoacylase, leading to elevated *N*-acetyl aspartate (NAA) levels in the brain, serum, and urine. Patients present in the first year of life with macrocephaly and spasticity. Death usually occurs within the first few years of life. Imaging findings include diffuse, symmetrical increased T2 signal in the cerebral subcortical and deep white matter. The elevated NAA peak on spectroscopy is a characteristic finding of Canavan disease.[1]

Physics Discussion

Instead of producing an image, magnetic resonance spectroscopy (MRS) creates a waveform on a graph. The waveform represents the chemical environment of protons in the voxel of interest. Knowing the chemical environment can be useful to help make the diagnosis.

Spectroscopy identifies the chemicals in a voxel by measuring the effect that these chemicals have on a proton's precession frequency. A proton in pure free water precesses at a frequency defined by the Larmour equation (at 1.5 Tesla, the precession frequency of a proton in water is ~64 MHz). If that proton is not free in water but instead in a chemically different molecule, such as NAA, then the precession frequency of that proton is slightly altered. This alteration of frequency is measured in units of Hertz and is therefore expressed in parts per million (ppm) with respect to the precession frequency of water (which is measured in MHz). For example, the chemical shift for NAA is 2.02 ppm. This means that a proton in NAA in a 1.5-Tesla magnet has a precession frequency that is shifted from that of water by 128 Hz (64 million × 2 per million = 128).

Each molecule has a specific chemical shift: the chemical shift of NAA is 2.02 ppm, lactate is 1.33 ppm, choline is 3.22 ppm, and so forth. By measuring the precession frequency of a proton, and by calculating the chemical shift, one can determine the relative quantity and type of molecules in a given voxel. This molecular environment is represented graphically by the spectroscopy waveform. The x-axis of the waveform represents the chemical shift in ppm. The y-axis measures the relative number of protons with that chemical shift. The area under the curve of each peak represents the relative concentration of the molecule of interest.

In order to interpret MRS, one needs to understand the function of the different molecules being measured (Table 1).[2,3] **NAA** is synthesized in the mitochondria of neurons, and its function is unknown. Clinically, NAA serves as a marker for the presence of neurons, including neuronal axons in white matter. **Creatine** (Cr) is used clinically as a marker for energy metabolism. Low levels of creatine suggest that the area of

Table 16-1	Description of Common Spectroscopy Molecules: Their Chemical Shifts, Main Functions, and Classic Associations		
MOLECULE	**CHEMICAL SHIFT**	**FUNCTION**	**CLASSIC ASSOCIATION (↑ INCREASED; ↓ DECREASED)**
Lipids	0.8–1.5 ppm	Fat	↑: Dipolic space and subcutaneous fat
Lactate	1.33 ppm	Anaerobic activity	↑: Ischemia, infarction, seizures, metabolic disorders, necrotic tumors …
NAA	2.02 ppm	Neuronal/axonal marker	↓ Leukodystrophy, malignant neoplasm, multiple sclerosis, infarction … ↑ Elevated in Canavan disease
Creatine	3.02 ppm	Marker of metabolic activity	Assumed to be unchanged and used to calculate ratios (Cho:Cr and NAA:Cr) ↓ Tumors.
Choline	3.22 ppm	Cellular turnover	↑ Increased in tumors, inflammation, infection, multiple sclerosis …
Myoinositol	3.56 ppm	Glial marker	↑ Gliosis, astrocytosis, Alzheimer's disease

interest is highly metabolically active. Creatine is also often assumed to be stable and is used for calculating metabolite ratios (e.g., Cho:Cr and NAA:Cr). **Choline** (Cho) is found in the cell membrane. It serves as a marker for the cellular turnover of a lesion. Choline is elevated both in the setting of increased cellular production, such as in a tumor, and in the setting of cellular breakdown, such as in leukodystrophy and multiple scleorsis. **Lactate** is a marker for anaerobic metabolism. Normally, lactate levels in the brain are so low that they cannot be measured by spectroscopy. Increased anaerobic metabolism, such as with ischemia or tumor necrosis, results in lactate peaks. **Myoinositol** is a sugar. It is absent from neurons but present in glial cells. It is used as a marker for glial proliferation or an increase in glial size. **Lipids** are markers for fat, as is seen in the subcutaneous tissues or in the diploic space of the calvarium.

It is important to know a few of the limitations of spectroscopy. First, the chemical levels are often not specific. For example, a novice may see a lactate peak in a lesion and use that information to conclude that the lesion is due to an infarct. While it is true that lactate peaks can be seen in infarcts, there are many other conditions that can cause lactate peaks, including tumors, seizures, metabolic conditions, inflammatory conditions, and so forth.[4] Similarly, an increase in the choline level may cause one to conclude that the lesion in question is a tumor. However, increased choline levels are also noted in infarctions, inflammation, and multiple sclerosis.[4] One must therefore always interpret the MRS finding in the context of conventional magnetic resonance imaging (MRI) findings.

A second limitation to spectroscopy is low signal-to-noise ratio; this is because we are measuring chemicals with extremely low concentrations. To overcome the low signal-to-noise ratio, voxel size needs to be large (i.e., on the order of centimeters), resulting in low spatial resolution. This can at times be a limiting factor clinically, where we are often concerned about lesions smaller than 1 cubic centimeter in size.

CASE 2

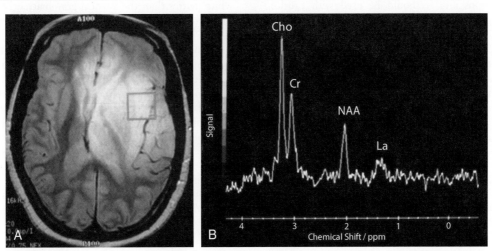

FIGURE 2A. Axial fluid-attenuated inversion recovery (FLAIR) image of brain. Increased T2 signal is centered in the left frontal lobe but seen to extend into the left basal ganglia and via the corpus callosum into the right frontal lobe and basal ganglia. There is relative preservation of the normal brain architecture. A small amount of mass effect with left-to-right midline shift is noted. The *square* overlying the left perisylvian region demarcates the single voxel measured in the corresponding spectroscopy waveform.

FIGURE 2B. PRESS waveform (TE = 30 msec). Spectroscopy images demonstrate elevation of the Cho:Cr ratio and decrease of the NAA:Cr ratio. A small, poorly defined peak at 1.2 to 1.4 ppm is consistent with a lactate peak.

Diagnosis: Gliomatosis cerebri; the elevated choline and lactate portend a poor prognosis.[5]

Clinical Discussion: Gliomatosis cerebri is a diffusely infiltrating neoplasm associated with a poor prognosis that occurs predominantly in middle-aged adults (40s to 50s). MRI usually reveals diffuse and contiguous infiltration of the white matter of at least two lobes that is isointense on T1-weighted images and hyperintense on T2-weighted images. The overlying brain structure is preserved. Frequently, there is bihemispheric extension through the corpus callosum into the basal ganglia.[5,6]

Gliomatosis cerebri usually has a decrease in the NAA peak on spectroscopy.[5] The choline peak can be variable. There is some evidence that elevation of the choline peak is inversely related to patient prognosis.[5,7] Elevation of the lactate peak is another concerning finding.[5]

Physics Discussion

In order to know whether a peak is abnormally elevated or decreased, one must first know the appearance of a normal spectroscopy waveform. The spectroscopy waveform of the normal human brain is predominantly made up of NAA, creatine, choline, and myoinositol peaks. In the normal brain, a line can usually be drawn connecting the peaks of these four molecules. This line makes a 45° angle with the x-axis, an angle referred to as "Hunter's angle." An alteration in the angle or a peak outside the line is a cause for concern (Fig. 1).

Hunter's angle can help interpret the changes in the molecular peaks of a spectroscopy waveform. In Case 2, the choline peak at 3.2 ppm is higher than the creatine peak at 3.0 ppm. Assuming that creatine is unchanged, and recalling that in the normal situation choline is less than creatine (think of Hunter's angle), we can conclude that choline is elevated in this case. Similarly, we can see that NAA is less than creatine, a reversal of the normal relationship, indicating a decrease in levels of NAA. A lactate peak is always abnormal.

Hunter's angle is a useful visual aid for beginners as they introduce themselves to spectroscopy but, like many rules, it has many exceptions and it should be used with caution. Hunter's angle generally applies to images obtained of the cortex with a stimulated echo aquisition mode, or STEAM, sequence and a short time to echo (TE). (The STEAM sequence is an alternative to the PRESS sequence and is further discussed in Case 3.) Changing any of these factors, even in the normal brain, can cause a disruption of Hunter's angle.[8]

Another factor complicating the understanding of the normal spectrum is that it is not always the same. The normal spectrum changes with age (infant compared to adult). At

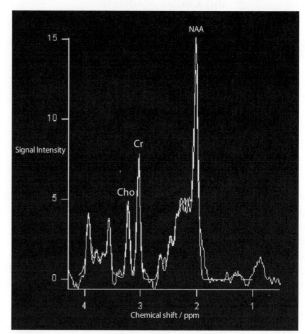

FIGURE 1. Spectroscopy waveform in normal brain (TE = 135 msec). A peak of the waveform at 2.02 ppm means that NAA is abundant in the area of interest; conversely, a trough of the waveform at 1.33 ppm means that there are relatively few molecules of lactate in the area of interest. Note that a line forming a 45° angle to the x-axis can be drawn connecting the peaks of choline, creatine, and NAA. The angle that this line forms is known as "Hunter's angle."

birth, the NAA levels are low, and the choline and myoinositol are high. By 4 years of age, the spectra have a more adult appearance.[3,9] The normal spectrum also differs within specific regions of the brain. Above the level of the ventricles, choline is higher in the frontal than parietal lobes and higher in the white matter than the cortical gray matter. Below the level of the third ventricle, choline levels are elevated in the insular cortex, thalamus, and hypothalamus.[3,10]

Because the normal spectrum changes with age, regional location within the brain, and imaging technique, it is often difficult to predict what it should look like. For this reason, it is often of utility to obtain a spectrum of the contralateral normal hemisphere for purposes of comparison. Fortunately, metabolites are highly symmetrical between the left and right hemispheres in normal patients.[11]

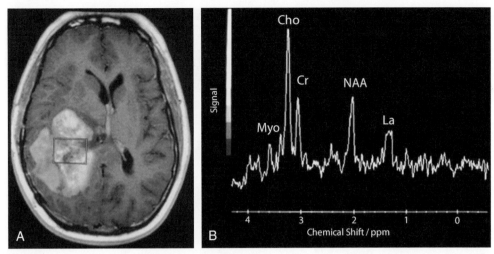

FIGURE 3A. Axial T1-weighted postcontrast MR image. A heterogeneously enhancing mass is centered in the right parietal periventricular white matter. There is associated mass effect with mild right-to-left midline shift. The *square* within the mass in the right parietal lobe marks the area characterized by spectroscopy.

FIGURE 3B. PRESS waveform (TE = 30 msec). There is a small but abnormal lactate peak. The NAA levels are decreased and the choline levels are markedly increased. Myoinositol levels are also decreased.

Discussion: Glioblastoma multiforme (GBM).
Clinical Discussion: In general, the higher the grade of the primary brain tumor, the greater the Cho:NAA and Cho:Cr ratios and the lower the myoinositol level.[12,13] This case of a GBM with markedly elevated choline and decreased myoinositol supports the spectroscopy grading hypothesis. However, it should be noted that some low-grade tumors have elevated choline levels and some high-grade tumors can have low choline levels, so it is difficult to assign a grade to an individual tumor based on spectroscopy alone.[3] However, MRS combined with conventional imaging is quite effective at distinguishing high- from low-grade tumors.[4]

Physics Discussion

Spectroscopy techniques can be divided into single-voxel and multivoxel techniques. In the single-voxel technique (the technique used to produce the waveform in the preceding cases), the spectrum is generated from a single region of the brain. Three 90° slice-selective pulses are used to select the voxel of interest (Fig. 2). This technique is called "point-resolved" single-voxel spectroscopy (PRESS). The selected voxel size is usually on the order of 8 cm³ (2 × 2 × 2 cm). Even though the voxel of interest is specifically selected, signal from outside the voxel can still manifest. To minimize this outside noise, "crusher" gradients and "outer-volume suppression" pulses are also used. An alternative to the PRESS technique is the stimulated echo acquisition mode (STEAM) technique. The STEAM sequence uses three 90° pulses to generate a stimulated echo (which only captures half of the available signal), and the corresponding three slice-selective gradients along three different axes to localize the voxel of interest. STEAM is seldom used today in clinical practice, in part because PRESS has higher signal-to-noise ratio.[3]

The advantages of single-voxel technique include short scan times and the relative ease with which short echo time studies can be performed. The main disadvantage of single-voxel

"POINT-RESOLVED" SPECTROSCOPY

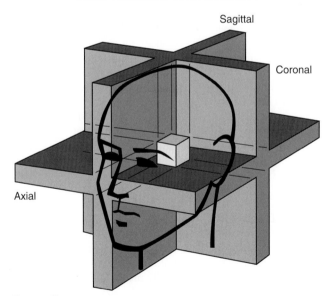

FIGURE 2. Image representing voxel selection in single-voxel point-resolved spectroscopy (PRESS). The voxel of interest is defined by the cube created by the intersection of the three 90° slice selection pulses.

technique is that only one voxel is measured, limiting the ability to determine changes in metabolite concentration over different areas in the brain. Of course, the single-voxel technique can be performed multiple times to get different samples over space, but such a strategy often exceeds the time constraints of a normal clinical MRI.[3] The other disadvantage of the single-voxel technique is its large voxel size. A large voxel size makes it difficult to get an accurate spectrum from smaller regions, such as the enhancing rim of a centrally necrotic tumor, because of partial volume averaging with adjacent areas.

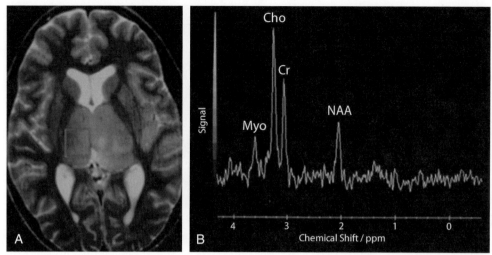

FIGURE 4A. Axial fast spin echo (FSE) T2-weighted MR image. There is high T2 signal and mass-like expansion involving the bilateral thalami. The lesion is well defined and there is relatively little vasogenic edema in the surrounding white matter. A *square* demarcates the voxel of interest for the spectroscopy waveform.

FIGURE 4B. PRESS waveform (TE = 30 msec). The NAA:Cr ratio is low and the Cho:Cr ratio is high. A myoinositol peak at 3.6 ppm is noted.

Diagnosis: Well-differentiated astrocytoma.

Clinical Discussion: The diagnosis of a tumor is supported by the spectroscopy waveform, but the spectroscopy results are equivocal with respect to tumor grade. In a well-differentiated astrocytoma, we would expect to see an elevated myoinositol-to-creatine ratio. For example, one study found the myoinositol:Cr ratio to average 0.8 in low-grade astrocytomas, 0.5 in normal control patients, 0.3 in anaplastic astrocytomas, and 0.15 in GBM.[13] At the same time, the lack of a lactate peak argues against a high-grade tumor such as a GBM. The equivocal spectroscopy findings in this case demonstrates the point that it is difficult to discern the grade of an astrocytoma based on the spectroscopy waveform alone, and that such findings need to be interpreted in the context of conventional MRI findings.[14]

Physics Discussion

The MRS spectrum changes with the field strength and the TE used. With higher field strength, the signal-to-noise ratio increases and the spectral resolution improves. The spectral resolution improvement is visually manifested as a narrowing of the molecule peak width. This allows for improved resolution of molecules with similar chemical shifts. For these reasons, spectroscopy is often preferred in magnets with higher field strength.[3]

The MRS spectrum changes with TE because of the different T2 times of each compound measured. At long echo times (140 to 280 msec), only choline, creatine, and NAA are detected in normal patients. Lactate, alanine, or other molecules may be detectable if their concentrations are abnormally elevated. Compounds with short T2 relaxation times such as myoinositol and lipids are not visible with long TE times. This is because the short T2 relaxation time of these molecules causes these molecules to lose all of their signal with long echo times. At short TE times (35 msec or less), all of the aforementioned molecules can be visualized.[3] Spectroscopy protocols need to be created with these TE effects in mind. If the myoinositol level is important for the diagnosis, then a short TE time is required. If one is only interested in the NAA, choline, and creatine peaks, then a long TE should be used because there will be less noise caused by the molecules with a short T2 relaxation time.

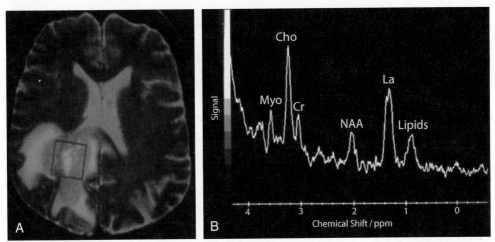

FIGURE 5A. Axial FSE T2-weighted MR image of the brain. A mass is centered in the right periventricular white matter. T2 prolongation is seen in the surrounding white matter. The *square* demarcates the area of interest for spectroscopy.

FIGURE 5B. PRESS waveform (TE = 30 msec). Lactate is elevated, NAA is reduced, choline is elevated, and myoinositol is decreased.

Diagnosis: Glioblastoma multiforme.

Clinical Discussion: This patient has a GBM. The elevated lactate levels are presumably secondary to the central ischemia and necrosis. Under normal conditions, the lactate levels in the brain are so low that they are not detectable. However, local hypoxia or ischemia can result in anaerobic metabolism in the brain and the production of lactate. Elevated lactate levels can be seen in brain tumors (such as in this case), mitochondrial disease, infarcts, and other disease.

Physics Discussion

The lactate peak has a characteristic double peak at 1.33 ppm. This double peak is a useful marker to remember because sometimes lipid peaks, which range from 0.8 to 1.55 ppm, can overlap in appearance with lactate peaks. However, it would be unusual for a lipid to have a similar double peak at 1.33 ppm. Another way to distinguish between lactate and lipid peaks is to change the TE. Lipids have a short T2 relaxation time and are only seen on short TE times. If a long TE time is used, the lipid signal will be eliminated and only the lactate peak will remain. It is interesting to note that, if an intermediate TE time is used (144 msec), the lactate peak will invert along the y-axis and result in a negative double peak! The reason for this inversion of the lactate peak is scalar coupling between methyl groups in the lactate molecule.[15]

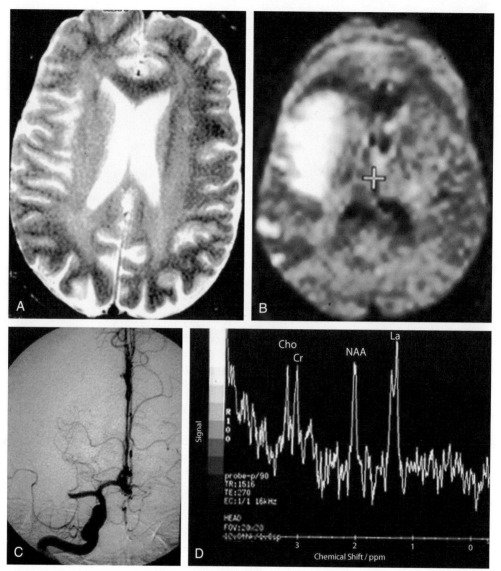

FIGURE 6A. Axial FSE T2-weighted MR image. There is poorly defined increased T2 signal in the right perisylvian cortex in the right middle cerebral artery (MCA) distribution.

FIGURE 6B. Axial diffusion-weighted MR image. Restricted diffusion is seen in the right basal ganglia and right frontal and parietal lobes in the right MCA distribution.

FIGURE 6C. Right internal carotid arteriogram. An abrupt cutoff of flow is seen in the M1 segment of the right MCA.

FIGURE 6D. PRESS waveform (TE = 270 msec). The lactate doublet peak is the dominant peak. There is also a slight increase in the Cho:Cr ratio and a decrease in the NAA:Cr ratio.

Diagnosis: Right middle cerebral artery (MCA) distribution infarct.

Clinical Discussion: The MRI and angiography images are diagnostic of an acute stroke. The MRS spectrum demonstrates the changes of an acute stroke. NAA is decreased as a result of neuronal loss, and lactate levels are elevated as a result of increased anaerobic metabolism. (Note that, at a TE of 270 msec, the lactate doublet peak is now again positive. See discussion of Case 5 regarding inversion of the lactate peak at intermediate TE values.) Choline levels in ischemic stroke are less predictable.[16] While elevated lactate peaks can also be seen in high-grade tumors (as shown in previous cases), the lactate peaks in infarctions tend to be more pronounced.[2] Notice that in this case the lactate peak is the dominant peak of the spectrum.

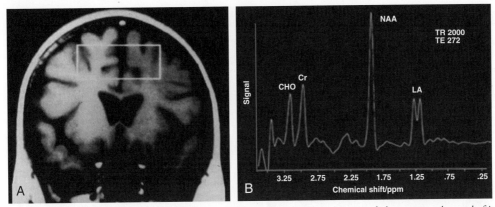

FIGURE 7A. Normal coronal T1-weighted MR image used for localization of spectroscopy volume. A *rectangle* demonstrates the voxel of interest.

FIGURE 7B. PRESS waveform (TE = 272 msec). A prominent lactate peak is identified. The NAA:Cr and Cho:Cr ratios are normal.

Diagnosis: Abnormally elevated lactate peak.

Discussion: This is a patient with a rare mitochondrial disorder (Kearns-Sayre syndrome). The typical MRI appearance of this disorder is high T2 signal in the subcortical cerebral white matter, brainstem, globus pallidus, and thalamus.[17] The abnormal elevation of the lactate peak is likely secondary to the dysfunctional mitochondria resulting in impaired oxidative metabolism. Serial studies have empirically demonstrated that the lactate peak in this condition precedes T2 signal abnormalities, suggesting that metabolic dysfunction precedes parenchymal damage.[18]

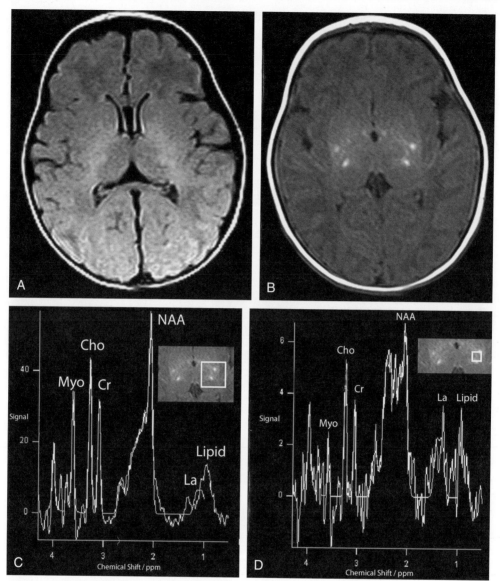

FIGURE 8A. Axial FLAIR image. Normal brain.

FIGURE 8B. Axial T1-weighted MR image without contrast: Increased T1 signal is seen in the bilateral thalami and putamen.

FIGURE 8C. PRESS waveform (TE = 30 msec). Axial T1-weighted MR image in right upper corner with a *large white square* over the left basal ganglia demarcates the voxel of interest for the waveform. The NAA:Cho ratio is decreased. The suggestion of a small lactate peak is identified.

FIGURE 8D. PRESS repeated but now with smaller voxel of interest (note the *small white box* overlying the left basal ganglia). TE = 30 msec. Again, the NAA:Cho peak is decreased. A peak at 1.3 ppm likely represents a lactate peak. Note that there is increased fluctuation in the waveform as a whole compared to the prior spectroscopy study.

Diagnosis: Hypoxic-ischemic encephalopathy.

Clinical Discussion: Neonatal hypoxic-ischemic encephalopathy (HIE) is an acquired condition caused by reduced cerebral perfusion and oxygenation in both preterm and term infants. One classic sign of HIE with conventional imaging is foci of increased T1 signal in the basal ganglia, thalami, and posterior limb of the internal capsule. Infarctions are best seen with diffusion-weighted imaging. FLAIR sequences and post-contrast sequences are less sensitive sequences for HIE.[19] Spectroscopy is occasionally used to attempt to characterize the severity of the HIE. Lower NAA:Cr and lower NAA:Cho ratios are thought to have a poor prognosis.[20] Additionally, elevated lactate levels are thought to portend a poor prognosis.[21]

Physics Discussion

This case also demonstrates the effect of voxel size on the spectroscopy waveform. A larger voxel size allows for higher signal-to-noise ratio and results in a smoother spectrum. However, the downside of this large voxel size is low spatial resolution. In this case, the MRI technician repeated the PRESS sequence with a smaller voxel size trying to better capture the molecular changes in the small T1 bright foci in the left putamen and thalamus. The smaller voxel size did more clearly show a lactate peak, possibly because of decreased partial volume averaging. However, the smaller voxel size also resulted in significantly increased noise within the waveform as manifested by the irregular appearance of the waveform.

CASE 9

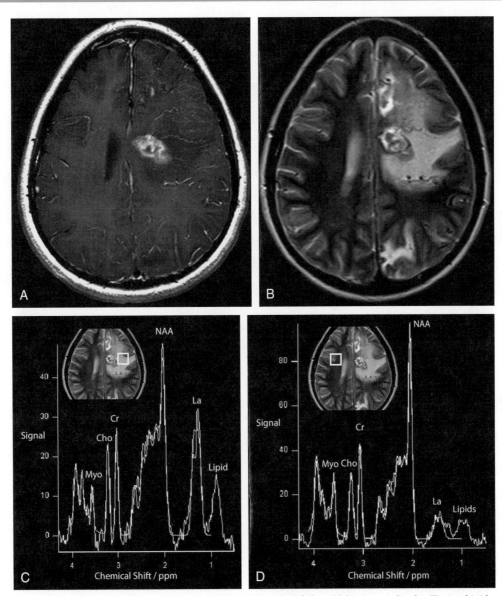

FIGURE 9A. Axial T1 postcontrast MR image. Rim-enhancing mass is identified in the left frontal lobe. Surrounding low T1 signal is identified. A separate site of low T1 signal is seen in the medial left parietal lobe.

FIGURE 9B. Axial T2-weighted MR image. The rim-enhancing mass is heterogeneous on T2 weighting, with areas of high and low signal. There is surrounding T2 prolongation in the left frontal lobe white matter. A separate T2 bright area is seen posteriorly in the left parietal lobe.

FIGURE 9C. PRESS waveform (TE = 30 msec). The voxel of interest is shown in the *white square* on the inset axial T2-weighted MR image. The voxel is in the T2 bright white matter surrounding the left frontal lobe lesion. There is an elevated lactate peak. The other levels are within normal limits.

FIGURE 9D. PRESS waveform of contralateral hemisphere (TE = 30 msec). There may be trace elevation of lactate levels. Otherwise, the spectrum is within normal limits.

Diagnosis: Biopsy-proven primary angiitis of the central nervous system (PACNS).

Clinical Discussion: PACNS is a vasculitis of unknown etiology that affects cerebral arteries and veins. Although PACNS can have a multitude of appearances on conventional MRI, it most commonly presents as multiple enhancing masses with surrounding edema.[22] On spectroscopy, the enhancing lesions and edema may have an elevation in lactate. However, the real value diagnostic value of spectroscopy is the absence of an abnormally elevated choline peak. Most neoplasms will have an elevated choline level, so a normal choline level (as shown in this case) should at least raise the possibility that the enhancing lesion is not a neoplasm.[22]

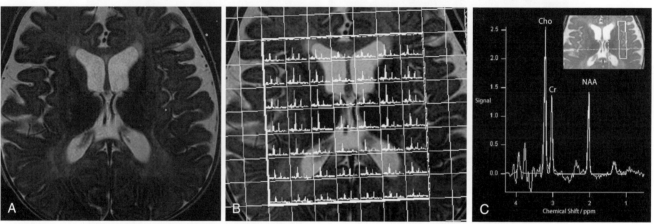

FIGURE 10A. Normal axial T2-weighted image of the brain.

FIGURE 10B. Normal axial T2-weighted image of the brain with an overlying grid from a multivoxel technique.

FIGURE 10C. Spectroscopy data combining multiple voxels in the left frontal lobe. Cho:Cr is elevated and NAA:Cr is decreased. Myoinositol is slightly increased.

Diagnosis: Krabbe's disease.

Clinical Discussion: Krabbe's disease is a leukodystrophy caused by a deficiency in the lysosomal enzyme galactocerebrosidase. Conventional MRI classically demonstrates extensive bilateral symmetrical abnormal T2 signal in the white matter of the bilateral cerebral hemispheres. Spectroscopy shows elevation in choline and myoinositol and a decrease in NAA. These spectroscopy findings are thought to be due to gliosis and loss of axons in the areas of demyelination.[23]

Physics Discussion

Spectroscopy data can also be acquired using a multivoxel technique (also called chemical shift imaging). In this technique, data from multiple voxels are acquired simultaneously. This is achieved by using phase-encoding gradients to resolve spatial information (two phase-encoding gradients for two-dimensional [2D] spectroscopic imaging and three phase-encoding gradients for three-dimensional [3D] spectroscopic imaging). Even in the case of multivoxel spectroscopy, the volume of interest is usually still selected using the PRESS sequence. The PRESS sequence selects a large area and then the phase-encoding gradients allow data collection from multiple voxels within the area of interest. (In Case 10, the PRESS selection is identified as the *large white square* in Figure 10B while each voxel of interest is shown by the *small squares* in Figure 10B. Note that each small square has its own spectrum.) The main advantage of the multivoxel technique is that it allows multiple samples to be acquired simultaneously.[3,24] This often alleviates the need to accurately localize a single voxel to the area of pathology prior to the spectroscopy acquisition. In addition, the multivoxel spectroscopic imaging technique allows for a smaller voxel size, which reduces partial volume averaging (see physics discussion of Case 8). One disadvantage of the multivoxel technique is that acquisition time is much longer.

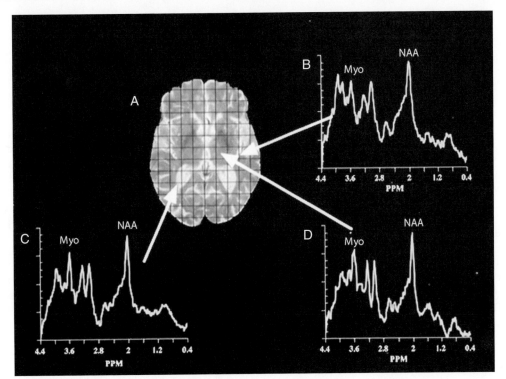

FIGURE 11A. Axial FSE T2-weighted MR image. Overlying grid demonstrates the voxels captured by multivoxel spectroscopy.

FIGURE 11B. MRS spectrum of a voxel in left perisylvian cortex. Myoinositol levels are elevated.

FIGURE 11C. Spectrum of a voxel in right periatrial white matter. Myoinositol levels are elevated.

FIGURE 11D. Spectrum of a voxel in left thalamus. Myoinositol levels are elevated. Case 11 courtesy of Cecil Charles, PhD.

Diagnosis: Increased myoinositol levels and mildly decreased NAA levels.

Clinical Discussion: This is a patient with Alzheimer's disease. Conventional MRI of Alzheimer's disease reveals global or focal atrophy involving the frontal, temporal, and parietal lobes and limbic systems. Volumetric studies of the hippocampus or entorhinal cortex have been performed to assess whether a patient with mild cognitive impairment will progress to Alzheimer's disease, but it is not clear whether a volumetric study is more reliable than common cognitive tests.[25] Spectroscopy in Alzheimer's disease shows a decrease in the NAA levels and an increase in myoinositol levels.[3] These changes are most pronounced in the mesial temporal lobe, hippocampus, parietotemporal region, frontal lobe, and occipital lobe. Presumably these spectroscopy changes correspond to the known pathologic changes of neuronal loss (decreased NAA) and increased gliosis (increased myoinositol). Despite the advances of spectroscopy and volumetric MRI, in clinical practice, Alzheimer's disease remains a clinical diagnosis. However, new criteria have been proposed in which volumetric and molecular imaging techniques will likely play a central role in early diagnosis and therapeutic assessment.[26]

1. MRS measures the relative quantity of molecules in a given voxel.
2. Chemical shift: Molecules cause adjacent protons to undergo a change in precession frequency. This frequency change, measured in parts per million, is known as the chemical shift. Each molecule has a specific chemical shift.
3. MRS spectrum: The *x*-axis represents the chemical shift measured in parts per million. The *y*-axis measures the relative number of molecules at each chemical shift.
4. Hunter's angle: A line can be drawn on the spectroscopy waveform of the normal brain that connects the prominent molecular peaks. This line creates a positively shaped 45° angle, known as Hunter's angle, with the *x*-axis.
5. Common molecules depicted in the spectroscopy waveform:
   a. NAA: neuronal marker
   b. Choline: cellular turnover
   c. Creatine: reference molecule
   d. Myoinositol: glial marker
   e. Lactate: anaerobic metabolism
6. Clinical pitfalls of MRS:
   a. Low specificity
   b. Low spatial resolution
7. Effects of TE on spectroscopy: Lipids, myoinositol, and some amino acids have a short T2 time and will consequently lose signal and not be visualized on studies with a long TE. Lactate doublet peak inverts at intermediate TEs (140 msec).
8. Single-voxel spectroscopy: Three 90° slice-selective pulses select a single voxel of interest. Advantages include shorter scan time and the relative ease with which short TE scans can be acquired.
9. Multivoxel spectroscopy (spectroscopic imaging): Multiple voxels in a plane (2D) or volume (3D) of interest are obtained simultaneously using multiple phase-encoding gradients. This is useful in disorders for which multiple areas of the brain need to be sampled at greater spatial resolution.

References

1. Michel SJ, Given CA: Case 99: Canavan disease. *Radiology* 241:310-324, 2006.
2. Soares DP, Law M: Magnetic resonance spectroscopy of the brain: review of metabolites and clinical applications. *Clin Radiol* 64:12-21, 2009.
3. Barker P, Bizzi A, Stefano N, et al: *Clinical MR Spectroscopy.* New York: Cambridge University Press, 2010.
4. Hollingworth W, Medina LS, Lenkinski RE, et al: A systematic literature review of magnetic resonance spectroscopy for the characterization of brain tumors. *AJNR Am J Neuroradiol* 27:1404-1411, 2006.
5. Guzman-de-Villoria JA, Sanchez-Gonzalez J, Munoz L, et al: ¹H MR spectroscopy in the assessment of gliomatosis cerebri. *AJR Am J Roentgenol* 188:710-714, 2007.
6. del Carpio-O'Donovan R, Korah I, Salazar A, Melancon D: Gliomatosis cerebri. *Radiology* 198:831-835, 1996.
7. Bendszus M, Warmuth-Metz M, Klein R, et al: MR spectroscopy in gliomatosis cerebri. *AJNR Am J Neuroradiol* 21:375-380, 2000.
8. Lin A, Ross BD, Harris K, Wong W: Efficacy of proton magnetic resonance spectroscopy in neurological diagnosis and neurotherapeutic decision making. *Neuroradiology* 2:197-214, 2005.
9. Kreis R, Ernst T, Ross BD: Development of the human brain: *in vivo* quantification of metabolite and water content with proton magnetic resonance spectroscopy. *Magn Reson Med* 30:424-437, 1993.
10. Pouwels PJW, Frahm J: Regional metabolite concentrations in human brain as determined by quantitative localized proton MRS. *Magn Reson Med* 39:53-60, 1998.
11. Nagae-Poetscher LM, Bonekamp D, Barker PB, et al: Asymmetry and gender effect in functionally lateralized cortical regions: a proton MRS imaging study. *J Magn Reson Imaging* 19:27-33, 2004.
12. Law M, Yang S, Wang H, et al: Glioma grading: sensitivity, specificity, and predictive values of perfusion MR imaging and proton MR spectroscopic imaging compared with conventional MR imaging. *AJNR Am J Neuroradiol* 24:1989-1998, 2003.
13. Castillo M, Smith JK, Kwock L: Correlation of myo-inositol levels and grading of cerebral astrocytomas. *AJNR Am J Neuroradiol* 21:1645-1649, 2000.
14. Panigrahy A, Krieger MD, Gonzalez-Gomez I, et al: Quantitative short echo time ¹H-MR spectroscopy of untreated pediatric brain tumors: preoperative diagnosis and characterization. *AJNR Am J Neuroradiol* 27:560-572, 2006.
15. Lange T, Dydak U, Roberts TPL, et al: Pitfalls in lactate measurements at 3T. *AJNR Am J Neuroradiol* 27:895-901, 2006.
16. Saunders DE: MR spectroscopy in stroke. *Br Med Bull* 56:334-345, 2000.
17. Chu BC, Terae S, Takahashi C, et al: MRI of the brain in the Kearns-Sayre syndrome: report of four cases and a review. *Neuroradiology* 41:759-764, 1999.
18. Kapeller P, Offenbacher H, Stollberger R, et al: Magnetic resonance imaging and spectroscopy of progressive cerebral involvement in Kearns Sayre syndrome. *J Neurol Sci* 135:126-130, 1996.
19. Liauw L, van der Grond J, van den Berg-Huysmans AA, et al: Hypoxic-ischemic encephalopathy: diagnostic value of conventional MR imaging pulse sequences in term-born neonates. *Radiology* 247:204-212, 2008.
20. Graham SH, Meyerhoff DJ, Bayne L, et al: Magnetic resonance spectroscopy of N-acetylaspartate in hypoxic-ischemic encephalopathy. *Ann Neurol* 35:490-494, 1994.
21. Malik GK, Pandey M, Kumar R, et al: MR imaging and in vivo proton spectroscopy of the brain in neonates with hypoxic ischemic encephalopathy. *Eur J Radiol* 43:6-13, 2002.
22. Panchal NJ, Niku S, Imbesi SG: Lymphocytic vasculitis mimicking aggressive multifocal cerebral neoplasm: MR imaging and MR spectroscopic appearance. *AJNR Am J Neuroradiol* 26:642-645, 2005.
23. Zarifi MK, Tzika AA, Astrakas LG, et al: Magnetic resonance spectroscopy and magnetic resonance imaging findings in Krabbe's disease. *J Child Neurol* 16:522-526, 2001.
24. Atlas SW: *Magnetic Resonance Imaging of the Brain and Spine,* 4th ed. Philadelphia: Lippincott Williams & Wilkins, 2009.
25. Fleisher AS, Sun S, Taylor C, et al: Volumetric MRI vs clinical predictors of Alzheimer disease in mild cognitive impairment. *Neurology* 70:191-199, 2008.
26. Dubois B, Feldman HH, Jacova C, et al: Research criteria for the diagnosis of Alzheimer's disease: revising the NINCDS-ADRDA criteria. *LANEUR* 6:734-746, 2007.

Chapter 17

Functional Magnetic Resonance Imaging

Wells I. Mangrum, Christopher J. Roth, Allen W. Song, James T. Voyvodic, and Jeffrey R. Petrella

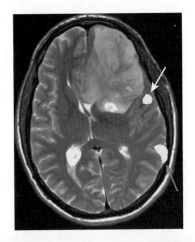

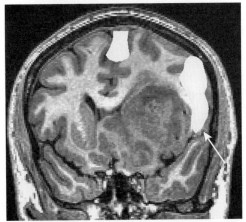

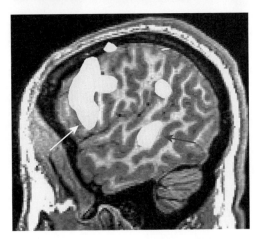

1. What type of task does a patient typically perform in "language mapping"?

2. When a particular brain area activates or functions, how does local blood flow change?

3. How do oxyhemoglobin and deoxyhemoglobin appear on T2*-weighted images?

4. Are functionally active areas of the brain hyperintense or hypointense on T2*-weighted images?

5. What cortical areas of the brain are depicted by the different arrows?

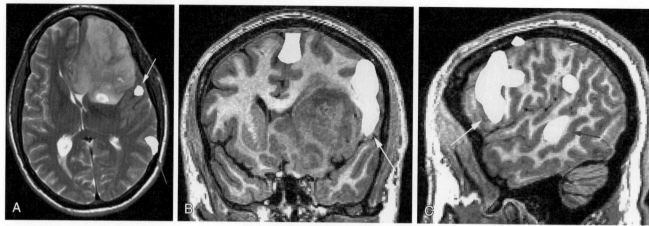

FIGURES 1A THROUGH 1C. Functional magnetic resonance imaging (fMRI) data obtained during language mapping. Color-coded statistical data from the fMRI has been co-registered to axial (A), coronal (B), and sagittal (C) T1- and T2-weighted images for anatomic localization. A large mass (biopsy-proven glioblastoma multiforme [GBM]) is identified in the left frontal lobe. The left inferior frontal gyral activation *(white arrows)* is consistent with the dominant expressive speech area. This lies within 1 cm of the posterolateral border of the left frontal mass. The left posterior superior temporal gyrus activation *(dark arrows)* is consistent with the dominant receptive speech area and is separated from the mass by the sylvian fissure. *(See Color Plate.)*

1. There are many language paradigms. One common method involves asking patients to read an incomplete sentence and mentally complete the sentence. Other common methods include verb generation paradigms and picture-naming paradigms (pictures are especially useful in pediatric patients).

2. Blood flow increases to areas of the brain that are functionally active.

3. Deoxyhemoglobin has a lower signal than oxyhemoglobin on T2*-weighted images. This is because deoxyhemoglobin is paramagnetic, which destroys the homogeneity of the field and leads to a lower signal.

4. Functionally active areas of the brain have increased blood flow and as a result have less deoxyhemoglobin. Consequently, functionally active areas of the brain are brighter on T2*-weighted fMRI.

5. *White arrows* depict the expressive speech cortex; *dark arrows* depict the receptive speech cortex.

Diagnosis: Left-dominant expressive and receptive speech. The expressive speech cortex is within 1 cm of the left frontal glioblastoma multiforme (GBM).

Clinical Discussion: Intraoperative cortical mapping confirmed the finding of an expressive speech area in the upper part of the inferior frontal gyrus, immediately adjacent to the mass. A limited resection of the anterior and medial aspect of the tumor was performed. The patient had no postsurgical neurologic deficit.

Physics Discussion

Functional MRI (fMRI) is used to identify the regions of the brain that are functionally active during performance of a particular sensorimotor or cognitive task. In the clinical setting, fMRI is often used to anatomically localize eloquent cortex. Examples of eloquent cortex include sensory and motor cortices, language areas (Wernicke's, Broca's), and visual and auditory cortices (Fig. 1). Precise localization of eloquent cortex is

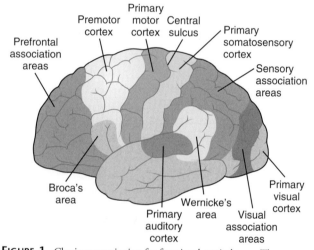

FIGURE 1. Classic anatomic sites for functional cortical areas. The expressive speech area (Broca's area) is classically located in the inferior frontal gyrus (pars opercularis and pars triangularis). The receptive speech area (Wernicke's area) is classically located in the posterior aspect of the superior temporal gyrus. In most patients, the expressive and receptive speech areas are in the left cerebral hemisphere, but this is not always the case. The primary motor and sensory cortical areas lie anterior and posterior to the central sulcus. The visual areas in the occipital lobes are additional cortical areas that are frequently activated in fMRI scans.

often needed in the preoperative management of patients with tumors near eloquent cortex to avoid postoperative neurologic deficits; fMRI has been documented to change neurosurgical treatment planning in this regard.[1,2]

Alternatives to fMRI include the Wada test and intraoperative cortical stimulation. In the Wada test, a barbiturate is administered into one of the internal carotid arteries, resulting in temporary anesthetization and functional loss of a large portion of the cerebral hemisphere supplied by that artery. The patient is then asked to perform simple tasks that require language or memory. The Wada test is helpful to lateralize the side of dominant memory and language function. fMRI is generally preferred to the Wada test because it is less invasive and because it gives additional spatial information about the lesion and the language/memory areas.[3,4]

Intraoperative cortical stimulation is performed by the neurosurgeon during an awake craniotomy with local anesthesia. First, the patient is asked to repeatedly perform a simple task such as raising and lowering her leg. Then the neurosurgeon uses a probe to electrically stimulate the cortex. The neurosurgeon marches down the cortex with his or her neurostimulator until the patient suddenly is no longer able to raise her leg. If the patient is now unable to raise her leg, then the neurosurgeon knows that the portion of the brain just stimulated is in the leg portion of the motor cortex. The electrical stimulation overloads the local neurons, causing them to temporarily be unable to function. Among tests to localize functional cortex, intraoperative cortical stimulation is the gold standard. fMRI is not yet accurate enough spatially to replace intraoperative cortical mapping, but it can be useful for preoperative planning and reducing the duration of and extent of the craniotomy.[3] Additionally, fMRI can at times be complimentary to the cortical mapping studies, revealing cortical activity that is not revealed during intraoperative cortical mapping.

fMRI works by taking advantage of the differences in oxyhemoglobin and deoxyhemoglobin. Oxyhemoglobin has no unpaired electrons and thus essentially no magnetic moment. Conversely, deoxyhemoglobin has unpaired electrons and a significant magnetic moment. As a result of its significant paramagnetism, deoxyhemoglobin disrupts the magnetic field uniformity in its vicinity and leads to a faster decay of transverse magnetization in its surroundings (i.e., as a result of destructive addition). Subsequently, the immediately adjacent regions will appear darker on T2*-weighted imaging. This effect of oxygen levels on MRI images is known as the blood oxygenation level–dependent (BOLD) effect.[5]

Intuitively, one may think that functionally active areas of the brain will produce more deoxyhemoglobin and will thus appear dark on fMRI images. However, functionally active areas of the brain appear bright on fMRI images. This seeming paradox can be explained by describing how the brain responds to increased functional demands. Increased functional activity of the neuron results in an increased demand for oxygen. The body responds to this increased demand for oxygen by causing arteriolar dilation and increased supply of oxyhemoglobin. The vasodilation response, known as the hemodynamic response, leads to an excessive increase of arterial blood flow and actually results in a net increase of the oxygenation level and a decrease of deoxyhemoglobin in the activated brain regions (Fig. 2). As a result, functionally active areas of the brain actually increase in overall signal on fMRI images.

The color-coded fMRI images are statistical representations of the fMRI data. fMRI images are frequently obtained with gradient-recalled echo–based echo-planar imaging (EPI), a sequence particularly sensitive to the T2* effects of deoxyhemoglobin. A statistical model is then applied to the EPI image to determine which voxels have an increase in signal beyond a chosen statistically significant threshold during the task compared to the rest period. Typically, the BOLD effect results in

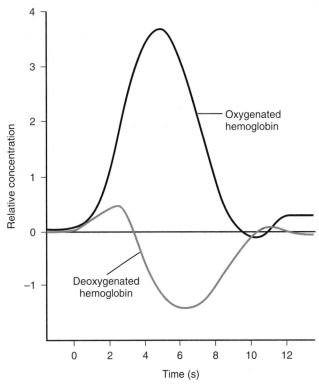

FIGURE 2. Changes in the oxygenated-to-deoxygenated hemoglobin ratio following neuronal activation.[6,7] It is interesting to note that, initially, there is a transient rise in the deoxyhemoglobin level from baseline. However, the hemodynamic response quickly activates and the increased blood flow is so robust that the deoxyhemoglobin levels actually fall. The fall in the deoxyhemoglobin levels causes an increase in MRI signal as a result of the BOLD effect (described in the text). (Data in this figure are based on a study performed on the visual cortex of a cat using high-resolution optical imaging to measure oxyhemoglobin and deoxyhemoglobin levels.[7]) (Adapted from Huettel SA, Song AW, McCarthy G: *Functional Magnetic Resonance Imaging,* 2nd ed. Sunderland, MA: Sinauer Associates, Inc., 2009.)

a signal change from baseline that is up to 3% at 1.5T and up to 6% at 3T for voxel volumes of about $3 \times 3 \times 3$ mm.[8] This signal change can be detected using various statistical methods. These voxels are then color coded according to the degree of statistical significance of the increased signal. Finally, the color-coded statistical maps are overlaid on a higher resolution anatomic sequence such as a fast spin echo T2-weighted sequence.

The final fMRI images need to be co-registered with an anatomic MRI reference because they typically have poor spatial resolution. The spatial resolution of fMRI is poor because of the low signal-to-noise ratio associated with the BOLD effect (and because of the high temporal resolution demands of fMRI). Large voxels are used to counter the poor signal-to-noise ratio. These large voxels result in poor spatial resolution. Spatial resolution may also be limited by the vascular system and the hemodynamic response: The area of the brain with the increased perfusion can often be larger than the neuronally active area of the brain.[6]

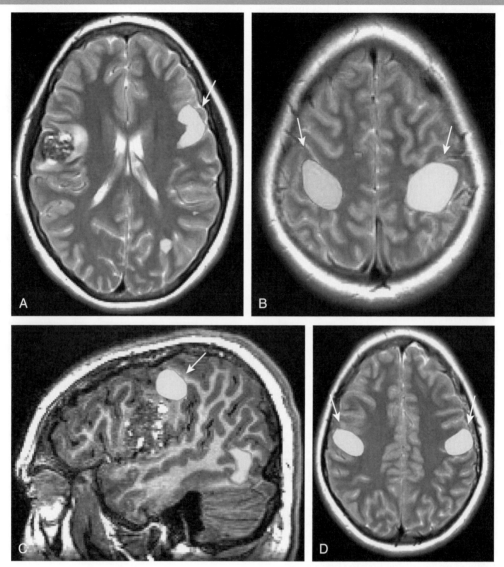

FIGURE 2A. Language mapping fMRI overlaid on axial T2-weighted image. The active area in the inferior left frontal lobe *(arrow)* represents Broca's expressive speech area. A cavernoma is centered in the inferior right frontal gyrus, on the contralateral side of the expressive speech area.

FIGURE 2B. Hand motor mapping fMRI overlaid on axial T2-weighted image. The active areas *(arrows)* correspond to the hand motor and sensory cortex.

FIGURES 2C AND 2D. Mouth motor mapping fMRI overlaid on sagittal T1-weighted (C) and axial T2-weighted (D) images. The mouth motor strips *(arrows)* are lateral and inferior to the hand motor strips. The mouth motor strip in the right frontal lobe is within 1 cm of the cavernoma. *(See Color Plate.)*

Diagnosis: Left-dominant speech; the mouth motor cortex is immediately adjacent to the cavernoma.

Clinical Discussion: The cavernoma was resected shortly after the fMRI because of recurrent and progressive seizures. Intraoperative cortical stimulation confirmed the face motor cortex to lie just posterior to the cavernoma. The cavernoma was then completely resected with careful attention paid to not dissect into the face cortex area. At 2 years of follow-up, the patient is seizure free and has no motor deficits.

Physics Discussion

Multiple different tasks can be performed by the patient to activate different portions of their cortex for fMRI. Language mapping can be done with multiple paradigms.[3] As mentioned previously, one common method involves asking patients to read an incomplete sentence and mentally complete the sentence. Reading and comprehending the sentence activates the receptive speech areas, while mentally completing the sentence activates expressive speech areas. In motor hand tasks, one paradigm involves having the patient alternately squeeze each hand. Note that squeezing the hand will activate both sensory and motor cortices (as shown in Case 2) because the hand is sensing the act of squeezing. To elicit motor mouth function, as in this example, the patient is asked to repetitively pucker her mouth. One functional paradigm often performed on patients unable to cooperate (paralyzed or comatose patients) involves rubbing a feather over a hand in order to determine the sensory cortices. In general, the sensory cortices are homologously aligned with the motor areas across the central sulcus. Functional paradigms also exist for many other areas of eloquent cortex, including memory cortex and visual cortex, with varying degrees of clinical applicability.[8]

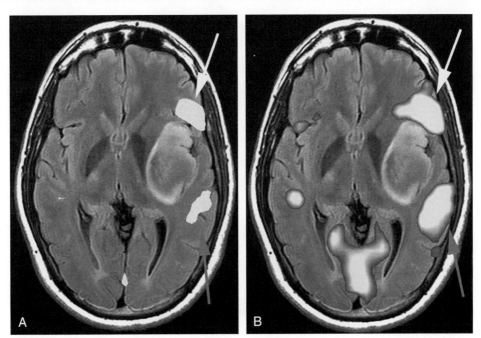

FIGURE 3A. fMRI data obtained with a threshold *t*-value greater than 6.0. The fMRI data are then color-coded and overlaid on an anatomic fluid-attenuated inversion recovery (FLAIR) image. A mass is centered in the left putamen. The dominant expressive speech area *(white arrow)* and receptive speech area *(gray arrow)* are marked.

FIGURE 3B. fMRI data recalculated with a lower threshold *t*-value (*t*-value > 3.0) and overlaid on the same anatomic FLAIR image. Even though the threshold value has been changed, the data in both Figure 3A and Figure 3B are statistically significant (*p* < 0.005). With the lower threshold value, the dominant expressive *(white arrow)* and receptive *(gray arrow)* speech areas are larger and appear to have closer approximation with the mass. (*See Color Plate.*)

Diagnosis: Left-dominant speech; a well-differentiated astrocytoma (grade II) is in close proximity to the dominant motor and receptive speech areas.

Clinical Discussion: The patient was taken for an awake craniotomy and the tumor was resected. When the posterior aspect of the tumor was resected, the patient did develop slow speech. In particular, the patient had difficulty understanding questions. The resection was then discontinued. At clinical follow-up, the patient had no speech difficulties.

Discussion

The statistical analysis of the fMRI data is critical in the production of the fMRI image. The activation maps are generated by calculating the *t*-value statistic of how different the BOLD signal is during the active language condition compared to the rest condition at each voxel. The activation map is thresholded to only show voxels that exceed the statistical significance level.

In Figures 3A and 3B, the *t*-value threshold was chosen to be 6.0 and 3.0, respectively. Both of these levels are statistically significant but, by setting the higher threshold, only the most significant voxels are included, thus potentially missing some truly active voxels that may be closer to the lesion. The problem with setting the threshold too low is that the map will then include some less active voxels, which show a BOLD signal but may not be directly involved in language function. There is no *a priori* way to determine the optimal cutoff threshold because the activation statistical signal is dependent on task duration, patient attention levels, BOLD signal amplitude, and physiologic noise levels, all of which can be highly variable. In practice, thresholds are typically adjusted by an experienced user based on the relative overall strength of the fMRI signal plus knowledge of the task properties and the relevant functional brain anatomy.

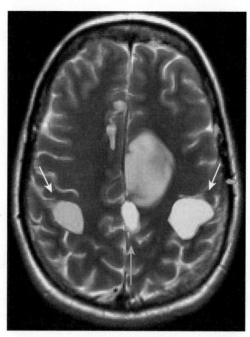

FIGURE 4. fMRI data obtained during hand motor mapping overlaid on axial T2-weighted image. A mass (biopsy-proven anaplastic astrocytoma) is seen along the medial aspect of the left frontal lobe. The hand motor and sensory cortex is marked by the *white arrows*. Additionally, a focus of activity is noted in the cortex along the superior and medial aspect of the mass *(gray arrow)* that is likely due to a left supplementary motor area. (*See Color Plate.*)

Diagnosis: The anaplastic astrocytoma is in close proximity to the left hemisphere motor cortex, and the mass immediately abuts a left supplementary motor area.

Clinical Discussion: The patient was taken for an awake craniotomy. Intraoperative cortical mapping demonstrated the cortical strip along the posterior aspect of the exposed brain. The tumor was then removed until the patient began to "get slow with naming." At this point, it became clear to the surgeons that they were in or immediately adjacent to the supplementary motor area. The surgical resection was then discontinued.

Discussion

This case demonstrates the complexity of cortical function. The primary motor strip has a critical role in motor function. However, other areas of the brain are also used during motor function, and loss of these other areas may or may not also result in loss of motor function. In this example, an area of cortex separate from the precentral gyrus is activated during the functional MRI. Because this area is active during the motor task, the implication is that this area is used in the execution of motor function. In this example, this additional area of activation represents the supplementary motor area. The supplementary motor area is used for "higher" motor function such as the planning and preparation for motor function.

fMRI is of particular value in demonstrating the supplementary motor area[9] because often intraoperative cortical stimulation is not successful in eliciting responses from the supplementary motor area.[10] As a result, if only intraoperative cortical stimulation is used, the supplementary motor area may be inadvertently excised, resulting in at least temporary paralysis after the procedure.

In this particular case, the intraoperative cortical mapping did not reveal the site of the supplementary motor area. However, the existence of the area on the fMRI scan was confirmed by the onset of symptoms when the supplementary motor area was approached during dissection.

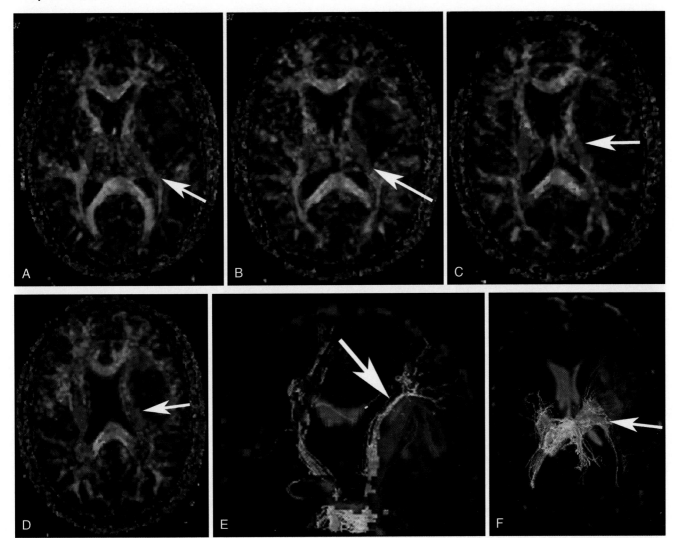

FIGURES 13A THROUGH 13D. Fractional anisotropy (FA) images that demonstrate medial deviation of the left internal capsule *(white arrows)*.

FIGURES 13E AND 13F. Tractography images that again demonstrate medial deviation of the internal capsule *(white arrows)* but also demonstrate a high-signal mass centered in the left basal ganglia, which is the cause of the deviation.

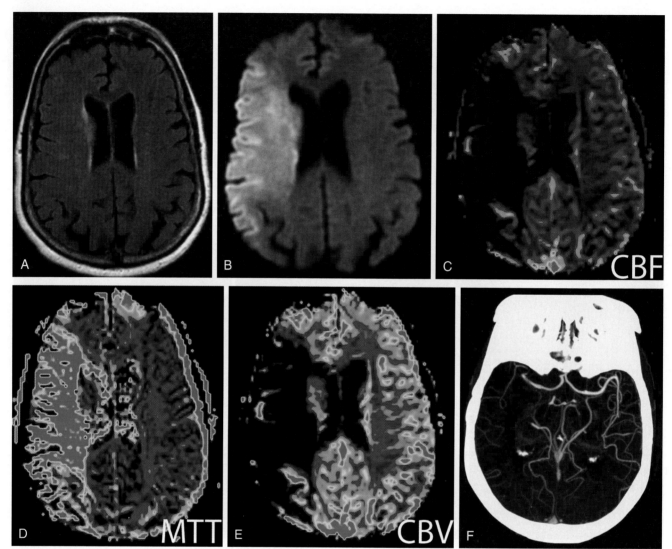

FIGURE 4A. Axial fluid-attenuated inversion recovery (FLAIR) image of the brain. There is subtle increased T2 signal in the periventricular white matter, right worse than left.

FIGURE 4B. Axial diffusion-weighted image. Restricted diffusion is noted in the right frontal and parietal lobes in the distribution of the right middle cerebral artery (MCA).

FIGURE 4C. Axial cerebral blood flow (CBF) calculation from an MRI perfusion study. Decreased blood flow in the right MCA distribution matches the diffusion abnormality.

FIGURE 4D. Axial mean transit time (MTT) calculation from an MRI perfusion study. Increased mean transit time is noted in the right MCA distribution.

FIGURE 4E. Axial cerebral blood volume (CBV) calculation from an MRI perfusion study. Decreased cerebral blood volume is noted in the right MCA distribution.

FIGURE 4F. Axial computed tomographic angiogram (CTA) maximal intensity projection (MIP) image. There is an abrupt cutoff of the right M1 segment. Very little flow is documented in the right MCA distribution.

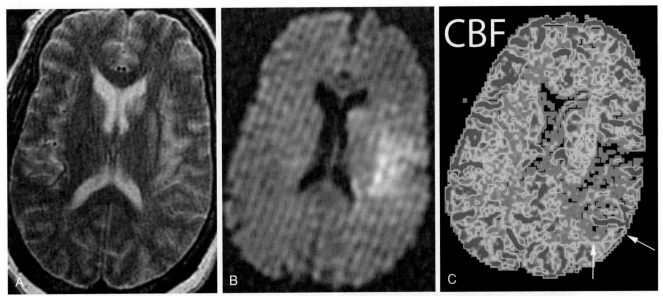

FIGURE 5A. Axial T2-weighted image of the brain. High T2 signal is present in the left caudate, the putamen, and the cortex of the left sylvian region.

FIGURE 5B. Axial diffusion-weighted image. High signal in the region of the left perisylvian region represents restricted diffusion (confirmed by apparent diffusion coefficient [ADC] map, not shown). Also note that this image has stripe artifact (see "Other Artifacts" section in Chapter 9 for a more detailed discussion of this artifact).

FIGURE 5C. Cerebral blood flow (CBF) map. There is decreased flow in the left perisylvian region extending posteriorly into the posterior left parietal lobe. The CBF defect is slightly larger than the diffusion defect (mismatch shown by *white arrows*).

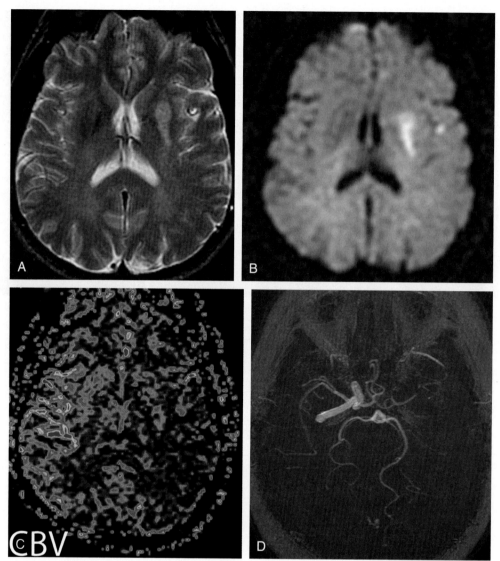

FIGURE 6A. Axial fast spin echo (FSE) T2-weighted image. High T2 signal is seen in the left putamen.

FIGURE 6B. Axial diffusion-weighted image. Restricted diffusion is noted in the left putamen and in the perisylvian left frontal lobe (confirmed on apparent diffusion coefficient [ADC] maps not shown).

FIGURE 6C. Axial cerebral blood volume (CBV) map. There is decreased CBV in the left middle cerebral artery (MCA) distribution involving the left parietal more than left frontal lobes.

FIGURE 6D. Maximal intensity projection (MIP) image from a two-dimensional time-of-flight sequence. There is no flow in the left internal carotid artery. There is some flow in the bilateral anterior cerebral arteries and the left M1 segment, likely from collateral flow via the circle of Willis. There is an abrupt termination of the left M1 segment.

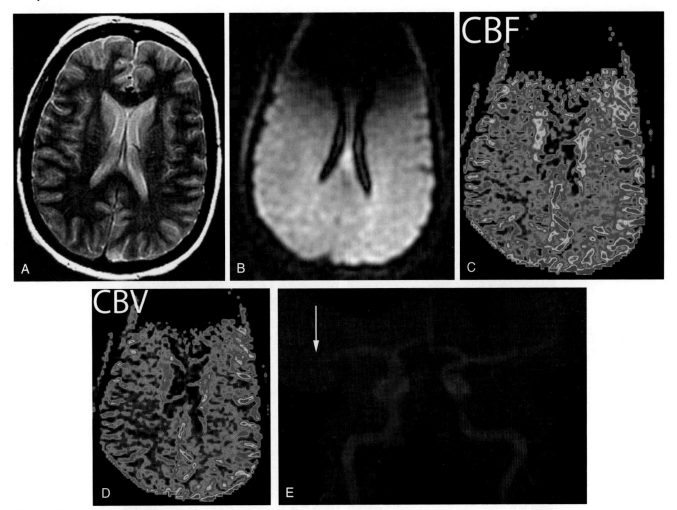

FIGURE 7A. Axial fast spin echo (FSE) T2-weighted image of the brain. No abnormality is seen.

FIGURE 7B. Axial diffusion-weighted image. No focus of restricted diffusion is identified.

FIGURES 7C AND 7D. Color-coded cerebral blood flow (CBF) and cerebral blood volume (CBV) maps demonstrate large perfusion defects in the right frontal and parietal lobes.

FIGURE 7E. Anterior-projection magnetic resonance angiography maximal intensity projection (MIP) image. Irregular and discontinuous flow is seen in the right middle cerebral artery (MCA) with an abrupt cutoff in the distal right M1 segment *(arrow)*.

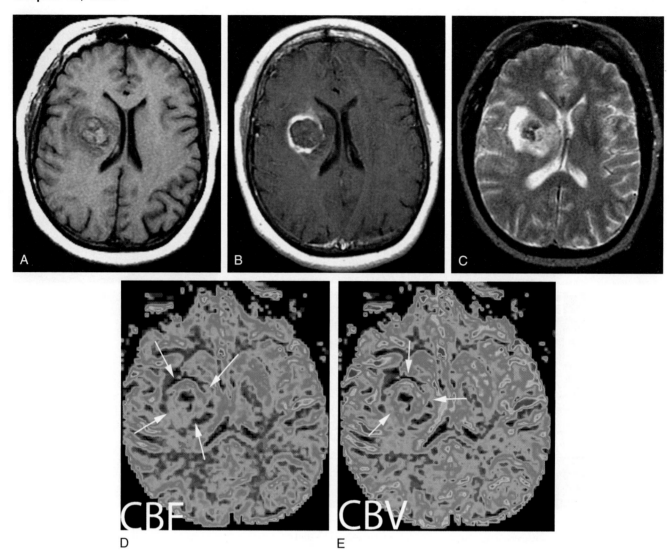

FIGURE 8A. Axial T1-weighted precontrast image. A heterogeneous mass with areas that are intrinsically bright on T1-weighted imaging is centered in the right basal ganglia.

FIGURE 8B. Axial T1-weighted postcontrast image. The mass demonstrates rim enhancement.

FIGURE 8C. Axial T2-weighted image. The mass is heterogeneous on T2 with areas of low and high T2-weighted signal.

FIGURES 8D AND 8E. Cerebral blood flow (CBF) (D) and cerebral blood volume (CBV) (E) perfusion images. There is increased CBF and increased CBV around the rim of the mass *(white arrows)*.

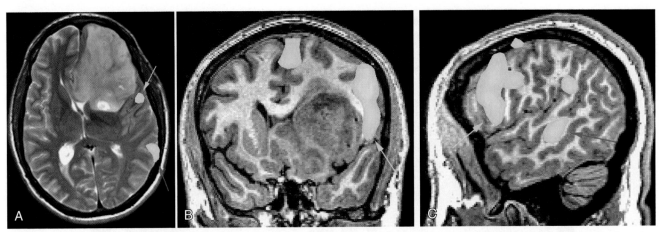

FIGURES 1A THROUGH 1C. Functional magnetic resonance imaging (fMRI) data obtained during language mapping. Color-coded statistical data from the fMRI has been co-registered to axial (A), coronal (B), and sagittal (C) T1- and T2-weighted images for anatomic localization. A large mass (biopsy-proven glioblastoma multiforme [GBM]) is identified in the left frontal lobe. The left inferior frontal gyral activation *(yellow arrows)* is consistent with the dominant expressive speech area. This lies within 1 cm of the posterolateral border of the left frontal mass. The left posterior superior temporal gyrus activation *(red arrows)* is consistent with the dominant receptive speech area and is separated from the mass by the sylvian fissure.

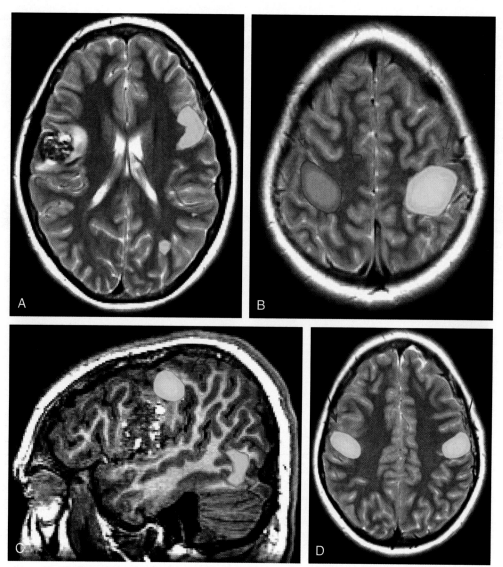

FIGURE 2A. Language mapping fMRI overlaid on axial T2-weighted image. The active area in the inferior left frontal lobe *(blue arrow)* represents Broca's expressive speech area. A cavernoma is centered in the inferior right frontal gyrus, on the contralateral side of the expressive speech area.

FIGURE 2B. Hand motor mapping fMRI overlaid on axial T2-weighted image. The active areas *(red arrows)* correspond to the hand motor and sensory cortex.

FIGURES 2C AND 2D. Mouth motor mapping fMRI overlaid on sagittal T1-weighted (C) and axial T2-weighted (D) images. The mouth motor strips *(maroon arrows)* are lateral and inferior to the hand motor strips. The mouth motor strip in the right frontal lobe is within 1 cm of the cavernoma.

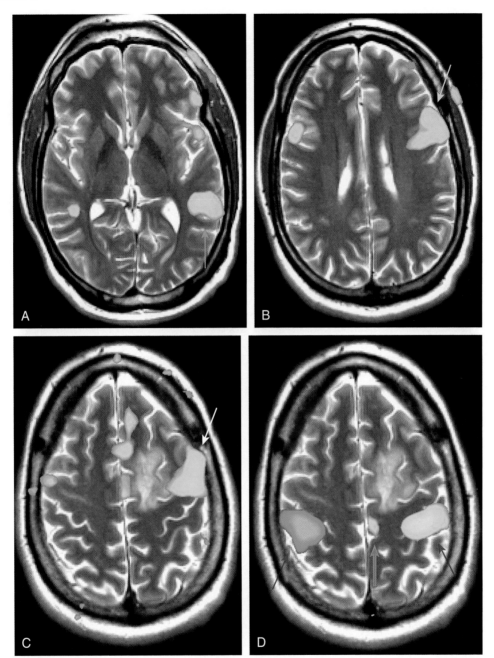

FIGURES 5A THROUGH 5C. fMRI data from a language mapping study overlaid on axial T2-weighted images. A T2 bright mass (biopsy-proven oligodendroglioma) is identified in the apex of the medial aspect of the left frontal lobe. The receptive speech area (*green arrow,* A) and expressive speech area (*yellow arrow,* B) are identified in the posterior aspect of the left superior temporal gyrus and inferior frontal gyrus, respectively. Additionally, activity is noted more superiorly in the left frontal lobe (*white arrow,* C) that is consistent with activity in the frontal eye fields. This activity is immediately adjacent to the mass in the left frontal lobe.

FIGURE 5D. fMRI data from a hand motor mapping study overlaid on axial T2-weighted image. The left hemisphere hand motor and sensory cortices *(blue arrows)* are within 1 cm of the posterior-lateral aspect of the mass. Additionally, a supplementary motor area *(red arrow)* is seen medial and posterior to the left frontal lobe mass.

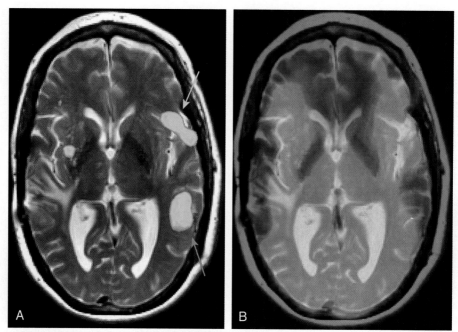

FIGURE 6A. fMRI language mapping data overlaid on axial T2-weighted image. A poorly defined T2 bright mass is partially visualized in the right temporal and parietal lobe. Dominant expressive *(yellow arrow)* and receptive *(green arrow)* speech areas are identified in the left hemisphere.

FIGURE 6B. Source fMRI echo-planar image overlying an anatomic axial T2-weighted image. On the source data, there is loss of signal from the cortex in the right frontal and parietal lobes adjacent to the patient's right pterional craniotomy site.

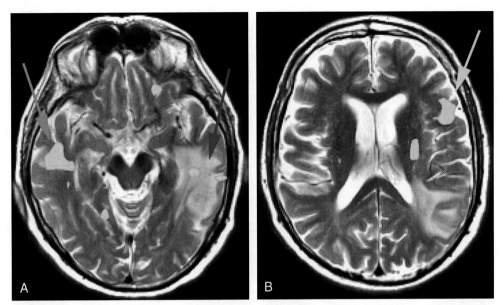

FIGURE 7A AND 7B. Color-coded language mapping fMRI data overlaid on axial T2-weighted images. A T2 bright mass (biopsy-proven GBM) is centered in the left temporal lobe. Activation in the inferior left inferior frontal gyrus (*yellow arrow,* B) is consistent with the expressive speech area. Activation within the right superior temporal gyrus (*green arrow,* A) is most consistent with the right-sided receptive speech area. Tiny foci of activation in the superior left temporal lobe (*blue arrow,* A) are seen in and adjacent to the T2 signal abnormality.

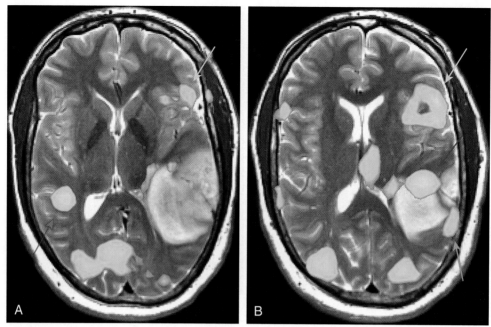

FIGURE 8A AND 8B. Color-coded fMRI data from a language mapping study overlaid on anatomic fast spin echo (FSE) T2-weighted sequence. A large T2 bright mass (biopsy-proven anaplastic astrocytoma) is centered in the left temporal lobe. Activation in the inferior left inferior frontal gyrus *(yellow arrows)* is consistent with a dominant expressive speech area. Left posterior superior temporal gyrus activation *(green and blue arrows, B)* is seen wrapping around the anterior, superior, and lateral margins of the tumor. This is consistent with dominant receptive speech areas being distorted by the mass. Activation in the right superior temporal gyrus *(red arrow, A)* is most consistent with an accessory receptive speech activation center.

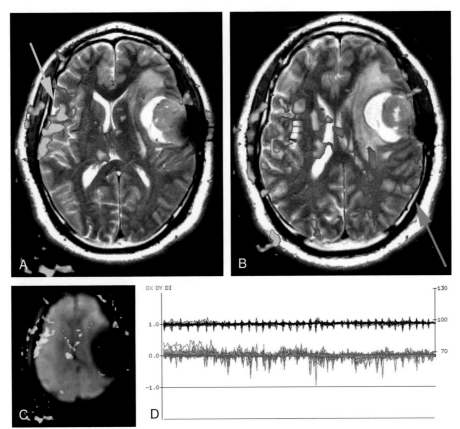

FIGURES 9A AND 9B. Color-coded language mapping fMRI data overlaid on anatomic axial T2-weighted images. Partially cystic and partially solid mass (biopsy-proven pleomorphic xanthoastrocytoma) is identified in the left frontal lobe. Activity is noted outside of the brain and field of view of the brain consistent with significant motion artifact. This artifact limits the ability to confidently characterize the expressive and receptive speech areas. Activity in the right inferior frontal lobe (*yellow arrow*, A) may represent an expressive speech area. Activity in the left superior temporal gyrus (*green arrow*, B) may represent a receptive speech area.

FIGURE 9C. Color-coded language mapping fMRI overlaid on axial echo-planar image. A large signal void is noted in the left frontal and temporal lobe from susceptibility artifact related to prior craniotomy. This susceptibility artifact could mask activation in the left frontal and temporal lobes.

FIGURE 9D. Graph demonstrating the motion of the head in three planes after motion correction. The *y*-axis represents how far the head has moved (measured in cm). The *green and red plots* measure motion in the *x* and *y* planes. The *black line* measures the signal intensity over time. Note the rhythmicity of the motion caused by this patient's hiccups.

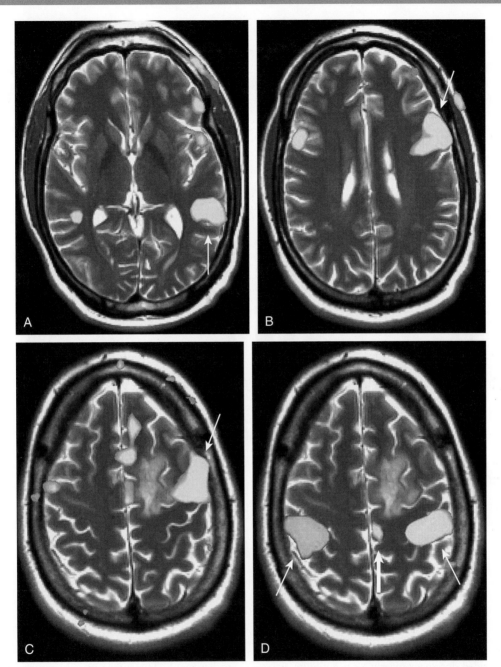

FIGURES 5A THROUGH 5C. fMRI data from a language mapping study overlaid on axial T2-weighted images. A T2 bright mass (biopsy-proven oligodendroglioma) is identified in the apex of the medial aspect of the left frontal lobe. The receptive speech area *(arrow,* A) and expressive speech area *(arrow,* B) are identified in the posterior aspect of the left superior temporal gyrus and inferior frontal gyrus, respectively. Additionally, activity is noted more superiorly in the left frontal lobe *(arrow,* C) that is consistent with activity in the frontal eye fields. This activity is immediately adjacent to the mass in the left frontal lobe.

FIGURE 5D. fMRI data from a hand motor mapping study overlaid on axial T2-weighted image. The left hemisphere hand motor and sensory cortices *(thin arrows)* are within 1 cm of the posterior-lateral aspect of the mass. Additionally, a supplementary motor area *(thick arrow)* is seen medial and posterior to the left frontal lobe mass. *(See Color Plate.)*

Diagnosis: The oligodendroglioma is immediately adjacent to the left frontal eye fields and within close proximity to the left hemisphere hand motor cortex and supplementary motor area.

Clinical Discussion: The patient underwent an awake craniotomy. Cortical stimulation revealed the location of the primary motor strip. No language center was identified in the operative field by cortical stimulation. The tumor was then surgically removed starting anteriorly away from the motor area. At follow-up, the patient did not have any motor or neurologic deficits and the seizures had resolved.

Discussion

This case also demonstrates the complexity of cortical mapping using fMRI. Interpreting fMRI requires a correlation between the expected location of a cortical function and the actual fMRI data. Idealized maps of cortical function should be known to the interpreting radiologist (see Fig. 1). In Case 5, we see the expressive speech area in the expected location of the inferior frontal gyrus. This activity is contiguous with the activity more superiorly and posteriorly in the left frontal lobe. However, this posterosuperior area is not the expected area of expressive speech function. Instead, this is the expected location of the frontal eye fields, areas of the brain that are also active when the patient is reading a sentence. Such areas can be considered "participatory" in the language task, however, not "eloquent" (i.e., essential) language cortex. Only by combining the information from the fMRI data with the idealized maps of cortical function can the radiologist correctly interpret what is represented by task-related locally increased levels of oxyhemoglobin.

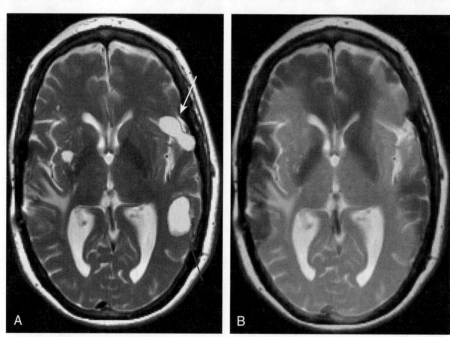

FIGURE 6A. fMRI language mapping data overlaid on axial T2-weighted image. A poorly defined T2 bright mass is partially visualized in the right temporal and parietal lobe. Dominant expressive *(white arrow)* and receptive *(gray arrow)* speech areas are identified in the left hemisphere.

FIGURE 6B. Source fMRI echo-planar image overlying an anatomic axial T2-weighted image (the echo-planar signal is the intermediate signal seen centrally, if this image is confusing, please see the color image in the insert). On the source data, there is loss of signal from the cortex in the right frontal and parietal lobes adjacent to the patient's right pterional craniotomy site. *(See Color Plate.)*

Diagnosis: Left-sided dominant speech; a susceptibility artifact from right pterional craniotomy limits evaluation of the right superior temporal gyrus.

Clinical Discussion: The clinical history in this patient is highly relevant. The patient is left handed. This increases the concern that the patient has right language dominance or that the patient is codominant. Additionally, the patient's original presenting concern was speech difficulty. At the time of the fMRI, the patient was already status post partial resection of the right parietal GBM and was returning for a repeat resection. The fMRI was ordered to help localize language function prior to a surgical resection.

After the fMRI, an awake craniotomy was performed with intraoperative cortical stimulation. The surgeons stimulated the area adjacent to the tumor in the right temporal lobe and could not find an area that caused the patient to be unable to say her name. The tumor was then surgically resected. The patient did not have any postoperative language deficits.

Physics Discussion

This case demonstrates how susceptibility artifact can be problematic in fMRI. fMRI sequences need to be particularly sensitive to the T2* effects of deoxyhemoglobin and oxyhemoglobin. One such susceptibility-sensitive sequence is gradient refocused EPI. This is useful in distinguishing between oxyhemoglobin and deoxyhemoglobin, but has a side effect of resulting in increased sensitivity to artifactual susceptibility effects.[11] This susceptibility is commonly present in the frontal lobes adjacent to the air-filled frontal sinuses and in the temporal lobes adjacent to the mastoid air cells and petrous ridge. Patients with intracranial hemorrhage or patients with metal from prior surgery will also have pronounced susceptibility effects.

In this case, the metal and blood products from the right pterional craniotomy result in susceptibility-induced loss of signal in the right temporal lobe. This is most evident when viewing the source echo-planar image. This loss of signal masks any underlying activity. As a result, the interpreting radiologist could not rule out the possibility that receptive speech was also located in the right temporal lobe, even though none was detected. When interpreting fMRI, the interpreting radiologist should be aware of any susceptibility effects that may distort the fMRI data, or instruct the technologists to apply appropriate magnetic field compensation strategies (such as z-shimming) to recover these signal losses in the source echo-planar images.[12]

CASE 7

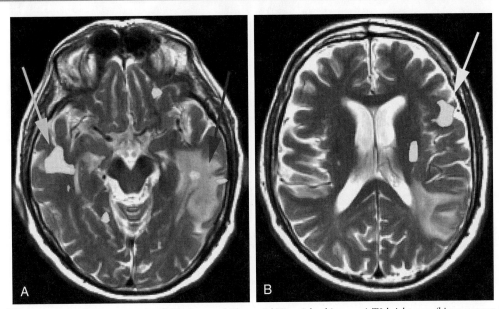

FIGURE 7A AND 7B. Color-coded language mapping fMRI data overlaid on axial T2-weighted images. A T2 bright mass (biopsy-proven GBM) is centered in the left temporal lobe. Activation in the inferior left inferior frontal gyrus (*arrow,* B) is consistent with the expressive speech area. Activation within the right superior temporal gyrus (*light gray arrow,* A) is most consistent with the right-sided receptive speech area. Tiny foci of activation in the superior left temporal lobe (*dark gray arrow,* A) are seen in and adjacent to the T2 signal abnormality (please also see color images in the insert to better depict this finding). (*See Color Plate.*)

Diagnosis: fMRI reveals left-dominant expressive speech and right-dominant receptive speech.

Clinical Discussion: The patient presented with word finding difficulty. An fMRI was ordered for preoperative management. An awake craniotomy was performed with intraoperative cortical stimulation, which demonstrated speech area in the superior aspect of the left middle temporal lobe gyrus. The GBM was then removed by working through the inferior temporal gyrus (and avoiding the speech area).

Physics Discussion

Intraoperative mapping at the time of surgery demonstrated that receptive speech was located in the superior aspect of the left middle temporal gyrus. In retrospect, there is faint activity in this location (see *dark gray arrow* in Fig. 7A) on the fMRI images. However, this level of activity was not called prospectively, and it is still unclear whether these tiny foci of activation on the fMRI correspond to the site of the receptive speech area defined by intraoperative cortical mapping.

In order to understand the source of this possible negative result, one first needs to recall our earlier discussion about the hemodynamic response. Functionally active cortical tissue normally recruits additional blood flow through autoregulatory arteriolar dilation. The increased blood flow results in a decrease in the level of deoxyhemoglobin and consequently an increase in signal on fMRI. Tumors can locally disrupt normal blood flow autoregulation. As a result, functionally active areas of the brain near a tumor may not be able to recruit additional blood flow and thus may not be bright on fMRI. Highly vascular tumors are particular adept at causing dysautoregulation. It is thought that these tumors are so aggressive at recruiting blood flow that they cause maximal vasodilation of the neighboring arterioles even when at rest. When the cortex next to the tumor does become active, the hemodynamic response fails because the arterioles are already maximally dilated. False-negative fMRI results are more commonly seen with higher grade tumors,[13] presumably because these tumors are more associated with dysautoregulation.[14] An alternative or possibly an additional reason why tumors decrease the sensitivity of fMRI is related to the mass effect of tumors. This mass effect may disrupt or displace venous return and, as a result, affect the hemodynamic response.[14]

Cerebrovascular disease and vascular malformations are additional causes for false-negative fMRI studies. These vascular diseases can also disrupt the brain's ability to autoregulate, limiting the hemodynamic response and decreasing or eliminating the BOLD effect during neuronal activation.[8] One strategy to assess for this source of a false-negative study in elderly patients with cerebrovascular disease or in patients with arteriovenous malformations is to use MRI perfusion imaging. If there is decreased cerebral perfusion to an area, then sensitivity of fMRI to cortical activity in that area will be decreased and the interpretation should reflect this limitation.[8]

275

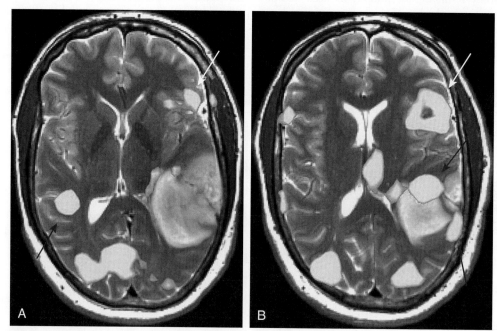

FIGURE 8A AND 8B. Color-coded fMRI data from a language mapping study overlaid on anatomic fast spin echo (FSE) T2-weighted sequence. A large T2 bright mass (biopsy-proven anaplastic astrocytoma) is centered in the left temporal lobe. Activation in the inferior left inferior frontal gyrus *(white arrows)* is consistent with a dominant expressive speech area. Left posterior superior temporal gyrus activation *(gray arrows,* B) is seen wrapping around the anterior, superior, and lateral margins of the tumor. This is consistent with dominant receptive speech areas being distorted by the mass. Activation in the right superior temporal gyrus *(black arrow,* A) is most consistent with an accessory receptive speech activation center. (*See Color Plate.*)

Diagnosis: The receptive speech area is seen wrapping around the anterior, superior, and lateral margin of the tumor.

Clinical Discussion: An awake craniotomy with intraoperative cortical stimulation was performed. Intraoperative cortical stimulation revealed a speech area superior and posterior to the mass (likely the area demarcated by the *lower gray arrow* in Fig. 8B). Surgical dissection was then performed with care to avoid this area. The tumor was resected to the level of the ventricle. As the surgeons worked close to the anterior aspect of the tumor (near the lateral ventricle), the patient did notice some speech errors (possibly the area demarcated by the *anterior gray arrow* in Fig. 8B). The dissection was then discontinued in this area.

Physics Discussion

Tumors can disrupt autoregulation and result in false negatives, but that is not always the case. This is more commonly seen with higher grade tumors, such as GBM.[13] In this example, even though the tumor is intimately involved with the dominant receptive speech area, the cortex has maintained its hemodynamic response and continues to be bright on functional MRI.

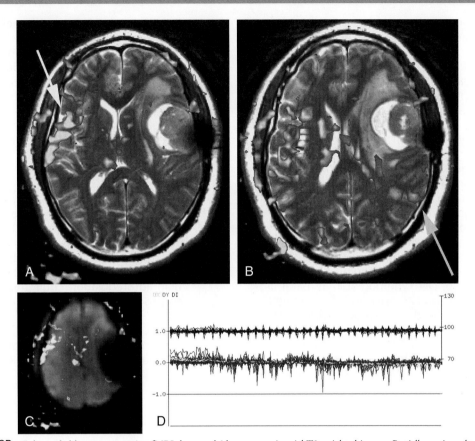

FIGURES 9A AND 9B. Color-coded language mapping fMRI data overlaid on anatomic axial T2-weighted images. Partially cystic and partially solid mass (biopsy-proven pleomorphic xanthoastrocytoma) is identified in the left frontal lobe. Activity is noted outside of the brain and field of view of the brain consistent with significant motion artifact. This artifact limits the ability to confidently characterize the expressive and receptive speech areas. Activity in the right inferior frontal lobe (*arrow,* A) may represent an expressive speech area. Activity in the left superior temporal gyrus (*arrow,* B) may represent a receptive speech area.

FIGURE 9C. Color-coded language mapping fMRI overlaid on axial echo-planar image. A large signal void is noted in the left frontal and temporal lobe from susceptibility artifact related to prior craniotomy. This susceptibility artifact could mask activation in the left frontal and temporal lobes.

FIGURE 9D. Graph demonstrating the motion of the head in three planes after motion correction. The *y*-axis represents how far the head has moved (measured in cm). The *light and dark gray plots* measure motion in the *x* and *y* planes. The *black line* measures the signal intensity over time. Note the rhythmicity of the motion caused by this patient's hiccups. (*See Color Plate.*)

Diagnosis: Motion artifact and susceptibility artifact severely limit the study. Possible right-dominant expressive speech and left-dominant receptive speech.

Clinical Discussion: The patient underwent an awake craniotomy and intraoperative cortical stimulation. Electrical stimulation revealed that the patient's expressive speech area was just anterior to the site of the tumor. The tumor was then resected with careful attention paid to not dissect into the speech area. The patient had no postsurgical speech problems.

Physics Discussion

This case demonstrates more limitations of functional MRI. Motion can often be a significant limitation to the study.

Motion correction algorithms are used to try to minimize these effects, but these algorithms have their own limitations. In this case, misregistered activity is seen outside of the head even after motion correction.

Additionally, this is another example of how susceptibility artifact can limit the study. The left frontal susceptibility artifact eliminated signal over the left frontal lobe, causing another false-negative case. Intraoperative cortical mapping at the time of surgery revealed the dominant expressive speech area to be just anterior to the mass in the left frontal lobe.

1. fMRI is a family of MRI techniques used to detect functionally active cortical areas of the brain.
2. Alternatives to fMRI:
   a. Wada test: Phenobarbital administered via an internal carotid artery to "numb" the brain perfused by that artery. Loss of function implies that the artery supplies the cortical area in question.
   b. Intraoperative cortical stimulation: Neurosurgeon uses electrical stimulation directly on the brain during an awake craniotomy. Loss of function implies that stimulated neurons are required for that function. Intraoperative cortical mapping is the gold standard.
3. How fMRI works:
   a. Hemodynamic response: Neuronal activation results in local arteriolar dilation and local decrease of the deoxyhemoglobin level.
   b. BOLD effect: Deoxyhemoglobin is paramagnetic and dark on T2* sequences. Consequently, reduction of the deoxyhemoglobin level (as a result of the hemodynamic response) results in increased signal on T2*-weighted images.
   c. Statistical analysis: The color images are statistical representations of the fMRI data. Brighter areas are more functionally active. The color images are overlaid on an anatomic sequence to improve anatomic localization because fMRI usually has low spatial resolution.
4. Popular clinical techniques to activate the cortex:
   a. Motor: Patient squeezes hand, or puckers mouth.
   b. Language mapping: Patient is asked to read or listen to assess language reception; patient speaks or think of words to assess language expression.
5. Limitations of fMRI:
   a. Motion.
   b. Susceptibility artifact: While T2*-weighted imaging is sensitive to the BOLD effect, it is also greatly impacted by susceptibility artifacts.
   c. Proximity to tumor: Adjacent tumors (especially high-grade tumors) can disrupt vascular autoregulation, null the hemodynamic response, and result in false-negative fMRI results.
   d. Cerebrovascular disease: Cerebrovascular disease can also disrupt vascular autoregulation and cause a false-negative fMRI.

References

1. Medina LS, Bernal B, Dunoyer C, et al: Seizure disorders: functional MR imaging for diagnostic evaluation and surgical treatment—prospective study. *Radiology* 236:247-253, 2005.
2. Petrella JR, Shah LM, Harris KM, et al: Preoperative functional MR imaging localization of language and motor areas: effect on therapeutic decision making in patients with potentially resectable brain tumors. *Radiology* 240:793-802, 2006.
3. Smits M, Visch-Brink E, Schraa-Tam CK, et al: Functional MR imaging of language processing: an overview of easy-to-implement paradigms for patient care and clinical research. *RadioGraphics* 26(Suppl 1):S145-S158, 2006.
4. Klöppel S, Büchel C: Alternatives to the Wada test: a critical view of functional magnetic resonance imaging in preoperative use. *Curr Opin Neurol* 18:418-423, 2005.
5. Ogawa S, Lee TM, Kay AR, Tank DW: Brain magnetic resonance imaging with contrast dependent on blood oxygenation. *Proc Natl Acad Sci USA* 87:9868-9872, 1990.
6. Huettel SA, Song AW, McCarthy G: *Functional Magnetic Resonance Imaging*, 2nd ed. Sunderland, MA: Sinauer Associates, Inc., 2009.
7. Malonek D, Grinvald A: Interactions between electrical activity and cortical microcirculation revealed by imaging spectroscopy: implications for functional brain mapping. *Science* 272:551-554, 1996.
8. Atlas SW: *Magnetic Resonance Imaging of the Brain and Spine*, 4th ed. Philadelphia: Lippincott Williams & Wilkins, 2009.
9. Wilkinson ID, Romanowski CAJ, Jellinek DA, et al: Motor functional MRI for pre-operative and intraoperative neurosurgical guidance. *Br J Radiol* 76:98-103, 2003.
10. Fandino J, Kollias SS, Wieser HG, et al: Intraoperative validation of functional magnetic resonance imaging and cortical reorganization patterns in patients with brain tumors involving the primary motor cortex. *J Neurosurg* 91:238-250, 1999.
11. Ojemann JG, Akbudak E, Snyder AZ, et al: Anatomic localization and quantitative analysis of gradient refocused echo-planar fMRI susceptibility artifacts. *Neuroimage* 6:156-167, 1997.
12. Song AW: Single-shot EPI with signal recovery from the susceptibility-induced losses. *Magn Reson Med* 46:407-411, 2001.
13. Bizzi A, Blasi V, Falini A, et al: Presurgical functional MR imaging of language and motor functions: validation with intraoperative electrocortical mapping. *Radiology* 248:579-589, 2008.
14. Holodny AI, Schulder M, Liu W-C, et al: The effect of brain tumors on BOLD functional MR imaging activation in the adjacent motor cortex: implications for image-guided neurosurgery. *AJNR Am J Neuroradiol* 21:1415-1422, 2000.

Note: Page numbers followed by f refer to figures; page numbers followed by t refer to tables; page numbers followed by b refer to boxes.

Time-of-flight (TOF) imaging *(Continued)*
  key points on, 184b
  limitations of, 177
  in middle cerebral artery infarction, 183, 183f
  in middle cerebral artery stenosis, 178, 178f
  in Moyamoya disease, 159f
  multiple overlapping thin-slab technique in, 178
  of right carotid artery, 184, 184f
  in stenosis, 178, 182
  in subclavian steal, 182f, 183
  three-dimensional, 178
  venous flow on, 179–180
  venous signal on, 181, 181f
  in venous sinus thrombosis, 179, 179f
  of vertebral artery, 182f, 183
Time to inversion (T1), 86
Tongue, fatty atrophy of, 10f, 11
Total parenteral nutrition, manganese deposition with, 16, 16f
Triquetrum contusion, 125, 125f
Truncation artifact. *See* Gibbs artifact

U
Ureteral calculi, 120, 120f
Ureteral jet, 137–138, 137f
Uterus, 34
  leiomyoma of, 37, 37f, 243, 243f
  septate, 34, 34f

V
Vector sum, 4
Veins. *See* Femoral vein; Iliac vein; Jugular vein; Portal vein

VENC value, 205
Venous sinus thrombosis, 179, 179f, 207, 207f
Vertebral artery, 182f, 183
  dissection of, 76, 76f
VIBE (volumetric interpolated breath-hold examination) sequence, 147f, 148, 224f
View sharing, 192
Voids. *See* Flow-related contrast, voids on

W
Wada test, 268–269
Water
  frequency-selective fat saturation suppression of, 89, 89f
  on T1-weighted MRI, 6
  on T2-weighted MRI, 22
Water-only sequence, 108, 108f–109f
Water saturation, 79, 79f
  in silicone implant rupture, 92, 92f
Watershed infarction, 219, 219f
White blood technique, 165–167, 165f
Wraparound artifact, 89f, 143, 143f

X
Xanthoastrocytoma, pleomorphic, 277, 277f

Z
Zinner's syndrome, 137–138